Ahmad HIJAZI

**KING WEST X-RAY &
ULTRASOUND**
1178 KING ST. W.
TORONTO, ONT.
M6K 1E6

Basic Doppler Echocardiography

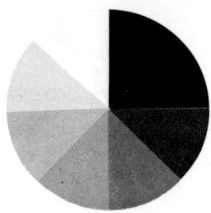

CLINICS IN DIAGNOSTIC ULTRASOUND
VOLUME 17

EDITORIAL BOARD

Kenneth J.W. Taylor, M.D., Ph.D., F.A.C.P., *Chairman*
Barry B. Goldberg, M.D.
John C. Hobbins, M.D.
Joseph A. Kisslo, M.D.
George R. Leopold, M.D.
Wesley L. Nyborg, Ph.D.
Arthur T. Rosenfield, M.D.
P.N.T. Wells, D.Sc.
Marvin C. Ziskin, M.D.

Volumes Already Published

Vol. 1 Diagnostic Ultrasound in Gastrointestinal Disease, Kenneth J.W. Taylor, Guest Editor

Vol. 2 Genitourinary Ultrasonography, Arthur T. Rosenfield, Guest Editor

Vol. 3 Diagnostic Ultrasound in Obstetrics, John C. Hobbins, Guest Editor

Vol. 4 Two-Dimensional Echocardiography, Joseph A. Kisslo, Guest Editor

Vol. 5 New Techniques and Instrumentation, P.N.T. Wells and Marvin C. Ziskin, Guest Editors

Vol. 6 Ultrasound in Cancer, Barry B. Goldberg, Guest Editor

Vol. 7 Ultrasound in Emergency Medicine, Kenneth J.W. Taylor and Gregory N. Viscomi, Guest Editors

Vol. 8 Diagnostic Ultrasound in Pediatrics, Jack O. Haller and Arnold Shkolnik, Guest Editors

Vol. 9 Case Studies in Ultrasound, Harris J. Finberg, Guest Editor

Vol. 10 Real-Time Ultrasonography, Fred Winsberg and Peter L. Cooperberg, Guest Editors

Vol. 11 Ultrasound in Inflammatory Disease, Anton E.A. Joseph and David O. Cosgrove, Guest Editors

Vol. 12 Ultrasound in Breast and Endocrine Disease, George R. Leopold, Guest Editor

Vol. 13 Vascular and Doppler Ultrasound, C. Carl Jaffe, Guest Editor

Vol. 14 Coordinated Diagnostic Imaging, Joseph F. Simeone, Guest Editor

Vol. 15 Gynecologic Ultrasound, William B. Steel and William J. Cochrane, Guest Editors

Vol. 16 Biological Effects of Ultrasound, Wesley L. Nyborg, Marvin C. Ziskin, Guest Editors

Forthcoming Volumes in the Series

Vol. 18 Genitourinary Ultrasound, Hedvig Hricak, Guest Editor

Vol. 19 Ultrasound in Perinatology, Nabil F. Maklad, Guest Editor

Vol. 20 Interventional Ultrasound, Eric vanSonnenberg, Guest Editor

Vol. 21 Controversies in Ultrasound, John P. McGahan, Guest Editor

Basic Doppler Echocardiography

Edited by

Joseph Kisslo, M.D.

Associate Professor of Medicine
Duke University Medical Center
Durham, North Carolina

David Adams, R.C.P.T., R.D.M.S.

Chief Echocardiography Technician
Duke University Medical Center
Durham, North Carolina

Daniel B. Mark, M.D., M.P.H.

Associate in Medicine (Cardiology)
Duke University Medical Center
Durham, North Carolina

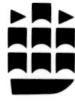

CHURCHILL LIVINGSTONE
NEW YORK, EDINBURGH, LONDON, MELBOURNE
1986

Acquisitions editor: Robert Hurley
Copy editor: Nancy R. Terry
Production designer: Charlie Lebeda
Production supervisor: Sharon Tuder
Compositor: Kingsport Press
Printer/Binder: The Murray Printing Co.

Accurate indications, adverse reactions, and dosage schedules for drugs are provided in this book, but it is possible that they may change. The reader is urged to review the package information data of the manufacturers of the medications mentioned.

© Churchill Livingstone Inc. 1986

All rights reserved. No part of this publication may be reproduced, stored in a retrieval system, or transmitted in any form or by any means, electronic, mechanical, photocopying, recording or otherwise, without prior permission of the publishers (Churchill Livingstone Inc., 1560 Broadway, New York, N.Y. 10036).

Distributed in the United Kingdom by Churchill Livingstone, Robert Stevenson House, 1–3 Baxter's Place, Leith Walk, Edinburgh EH1 3AF and by associated companies, branches and representatives throughout the world.

First published 1986

Printed in USA

ISBN 0-443-08431-9

7 6 5 4 3 2 1

Library of Congress Cataloging-in-Publication Data
Main entry under title:

Basic doppler echocardiography.

  (Clinics in diagnostic ultrasound ; v. 17)
  Includes bibliographies and index.
  1. Ultrasonic cardiography. 2. Doppler effect.
I. Kisslo, Joseph A. (Joseph Andrew), date.
II. Adams, David B. III. Mark, Daniel B. IV. Series.
[DNLM: 1. Echocardiography. W1 Cl831BC v. 17 /
WG 141.5.E2 B311]
RC683.5.U5B37 1986   616.1'207543   85-19506
ISBN 0-443-08431-9

Manufactured in the United States of America

Dedicated to our families
Kitty, Shelly, Connie, Andy, Tony,
Lee,
and Lee

Contributors

David Adams, R.C.P.T., R.D.M.S.
Chief Echocardiography Technician, Duke University Medical Center, Durham, North Carolina

Hugh D. Allen, M.D.
Professor of Pediatrics (Cardiology), Department of Cardiology, University of Arizona Health Sciences Center College of Medicine, Tucson, Arizona

Joshua A. Copel, M.D.
Fellow in Fetal-Maternal Medicine, Department of Obstetrics and Gynecology, Yale University School of Medicine, New Haven, Connecticut

Joseph Kisslo, M.D.
Associate Professor of Medicine, Duke University Medical Center, Durham, North Carolina

Charles S. Kleinman, M.D.
Associate Professor of Pediatrics, Departments of Diagnostic Imaging, and Obstetrics and Gynecology, Yale University School of Medicine, New Haven, Connecticut

Jack Krafchek, M.D.
Fellow in Cardiology, Duke University Medical Center, Durham, North Carolina

Daniel B. Mark, M.D., M.P.H.
Associate in Medicine (Cardiology), Duke University Medical Center, Durham, North Carolina

Gerald R. Marx, M.D.
Assistant Professor of Pediatrics (Cardiology), Department of Cardiology, University of Arizona Health Sciences Center College of Medicine, Tucson, Arizona

Jeffery H. Robertson, M.D.
Fellow in Cardiology, Duke University Medical Center, Durham, North Carolina

David J. Sahn, M.D.
Professor of Pediatrics, University of California, San Diego, School of Medicine; Chief, Division of Pediatric Cardiology, University of California, San Diego, Medical Center, San Diego, California

Peter X. Silvis, B.M.E.
Consumer Safety Officer, Office of Compliance, Center for Devices and Radiological Health, Food and Drug Administration, Rockville, Maryland

Stephen W. Smith, Ph.D.
Senior Scientist, Hydrodynamics and Acoustics Branch, Office of Science and Technology, Center for Devices and Radiological Health, Food and Drug Administration, Rockville, Maryland

Harold F. Stewart, Ph.D.
Chief, Hydrodynamics and Acoustics Branch, Office of Science and Technology, Center for Devices and Radiological Health, Food and Drug Administration, Rockville, Maryland

Steve M. Teague, M.D.
Assistant Professor of Medicine, Director, Adult Echocardiography, Department of Medicine, University of Oklahoma Health and Science Center, Oklahoma City, Oklahoma

Ellen M. Weinstein, M.D.
Fellow in Pediatric Cardiology, Department of Pediatrics, Yale University School of Medicine, New Haven, Connecticut

Contents

Preface — xiii

1. An Introduction to Doppler
   Joseph Kisslo, David Adams, and Daniel B. Mark — 1

2. The Doppler Principle and the Study of Cardiac Flows
   Daniel B. Mark, David Adams, and Joseph Kisslo — 7

3. Pulsed and Continuous Wave Doppler
   Joseph Kisslo, Daniel B. Mark, and David Adams — 25

4. Use of the Doppler Controls
   David Adams, Daniel B. Mark, and Joseph Kisslo — 47

5. The Doppler Examination
   David Adams, Daniel B. Mark, and Joseph Kisslo — 63

6. Doppler Evaluation of Valvular Regurgitation
   Daniel B. Mark, Jeffery H. Robertson, David Adams, and Joseph Kisslo — 91

7. Doppler Evaluation of Valvular Stenosis
   Joseph Kisslo, Jack Krafchek, David Adams, and Daniel B. Mark — 123

8. Measurement of Ventricular Function Using Doppler Ultrasound
   Steve M. Teague — 147

9. Doppler Echocardiography in Pediatric Cardiology
   Hugh D. Allen and Gerald R. Marx — 159

10. Pulsed Doppler Analysis of Human Fetal Blood Flow
    Charles S. Kleinman, Ellen M. Weinstein, and Joshua A. Copel — 173

11. Patient-Exposure Data for Doppler Ultrasound
    *Harold F. Stewart, Peter X. Silvis,
    and Stephen W. Smith*   187

12. Recommendations for Terminology and Display
    for Doppler Echocardiography
    *The Doppler Standards and Nomenclature
    Committee of the American Society of
    Echocardiography*   197

Index   209

Preface

We have prepared this volume in a simple and straightforward fashion in the hope of providing inexperienced users of Doppler echocardiography a means of getting started. The principles of Doppler and its clinical use are, indeed, complex, and beginners with this technique should not be lulled into overconfidence by our simplifications.

We thank those who stimulated our early interest in Doppler, Mr. Don Baker, Dr. Donald Kalmanson, and Dr. Simeon Rubenstein. We also thank those whose insights into the everyday clinical importance of this technique rekindled our interest: Dr. Bjorn Angelsen, Dr. Tony DeMaria, Dr. Liv Hatle, Dr. Walter Henry, Dr. Randy Martin, Dr. Alan Pearlman, Dr. Richard Popp, and Dr. David Sahn. We also thank Dr. Joseph C. Greenfield for providing us a means by which to study and prepare this volume.

Joseph Kisslo, M.D.
David Adams, R.C.P.T., R.D.M.S.
Daniel B. Mark, M.D.

1 An Introduction to Doppler

JOSEPH KISSLO
DAVID ADAMS
DANIEL B. MARK

The current interest in Doppler echocardiography has reached a remarkable level in just the past few years. Indeed, to many physicians, it may appear that Doppler instrumentation only recently became available and that this technique is a new innovation. Papers on Doppler echocardiography in the major cardiology journals are more abundant now than ever before. Manufacturers of ultrasound equipment estimate that over 85 percent of current sales of two-dimensional echocardiographic equipment will contain added Doppler capabilities.

From our conversations with beginning students of the cardiac Doppler technique, it appears that most consider Doppler to be difficult to perform, understand, and interpret. We have also noticed that the learning curve for Doppler echocardiography is much slower than that of two-dimensional echocardiography. Two-dimensional images portray anatomical configurations which are well known to physicians and sonographers. Doppler, on the other hand, provides flow information, and many of the phenomena associated with Doppler, such as aliasing and spectral displays, make this technique seem foreign and too technical.

With all the excitement about Doppler, it appears to us that there are few introductory explanations of the technique and its potential applications to the clinical care of patients. Thus, the purpose of this volume of *Clinics in Diagnostic Ultrasound* is to satisfy the needs of those individuals who are beginners with cardiac Doppler, those who are considering its acquisition, and even those who have only a casual interest in learning a little more about what Doppler is all about. The first several chapters in this volume will provide some background on the development of Doppler, the physical principles and instrumentation involved, and the performance of a Doppler examination with the currently available instrumentation. Later chapters will explore its uses in specific clinical situations and will examine its diagnostic utility in those situations.

DOPPLER ECHOCARDIOGRAPHY IN PRACTICE

In our echocardiography laboratory Doppler has been in use for several years. We have achieved what we believe to be acceptable quality and facility with the technique after some time and effort. Thus, we acknowledge to the beginner that the commitment to learn Doppler for everyday practice is great.

Full Doppler examinations now add an average of 30 minutes to the echocardiographic examination time for sonographer and patient. As subsequent chapters will reveal, Doppler tracings are not always of high quality and may be very difficult for a physician-interpreter to understand without the assistance of the person who performed the examination. Our laboratory is organized in a way that allows the sonographer who performed the Doppler examination to be present and interact with the physician during the interpretive session.

UNDERSTANDING DOPPLER

Understanding Doppler echocardiography begins with an understanding of certain basic principles about Doppler. The first principle is that the Doppler effect can be used to examine and record flow through the heart. The second principle is that a Doppler machine is a device specifically designed to measure the Doppler effect. These principles will be discussed in detail in Chapter 2.

The next step is to understand a bit of the history of Doppler echocardiography, for the technique is not new. The physical principles involved in its use have been understood for well over a century, and Doppler has been used in echocardiography for over 25 years. A brief review of the history of Doppler helps us to understand its current role in the noninvasive laboratory.

THE DOPPLER EFFECT DESCRIBED

The first scientific description of the physical principle commonly termed the "Doppler effect" is credited to Johann Christian Doppler, an Austrian mathematician and physicist who lived during the first half of the nineteenth century. In 1842, Doppler read a paper before the Royal Bohemian Society of Learning[1] in which he postulated that certain properties of wave phenomena (such as light or sound) depend on the relative motion of the observer and the wave source. Unfortunately, he followed an accurate description of the Doppler effect with the suggestion that the colored appearance of certain stars was caused by their motion relative to the earth, the blue ones moving toward earth and the red ones moving away. Thus, despite his correct description of the principle, he drew some erroneous conclusions, largely because of a misunderstanding about the composition of the electromagnetic wave spectrum, of which visible light is a part.

Accordingly, the Doppler effect drew great criticism at first. Experimental verification of the principle was difficult, since there was little instrumentation available at the time to accurately measure the frequency of any light or sound wave.

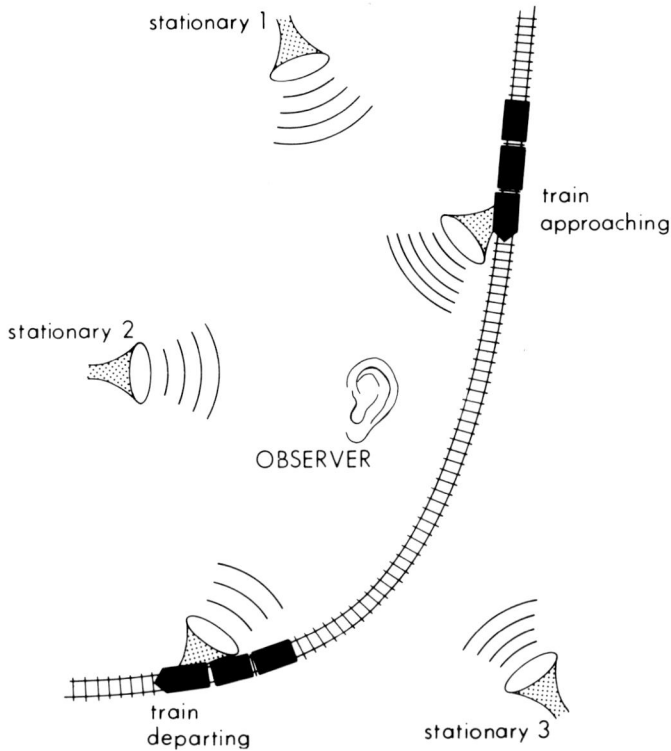

FIG. 1.1 A schematic recreation of the experiment of 1845 which proved the Doppler hypothesis. The observer with perfect musical pitch heard the sounds emanating from three stationary trumpets, each playing the same note. As the trumpeter on the approaching train played the note, it sounded higher pitched to the observer. From the train departing, the note sounded lower in pitch.

The ingenuity of one of Doppler's critics provided a means for the first known experimental test of the hypothesis in 1845 (Fig. 1.1). The "measurement instrument" used was an observer with the ability to describe the absolute pitch of musical sounds. This person compared the pitch of a trumpet sounded from several stationary positions with the pitch of a trumpet sounded from the top of a moving railroad car. He concluded that the sounds from the various stationary trumpets all had the same pitch, whereas the pitch of the moving trumpet increased as it approached and then decreased as it moved away from him, just as Doppler had predicted.

As often happens in the scientific community, the same hypothesis was independently put forward by H. Fizeau, a French physicist, and John Scott Russell, a British scientist, in 1848. In 1868, the British astronomer, William Huggins, presented the idea again. Huggins and subsequent workers demonstrated the correctness of Doppler's hypothesis in the realm of light and sound. In this century, the Doppler effect has become a major tool in astronomy.

Among other things, the "big bang" theory of the origin of the universe is based in part on observations using the Doppler effect.

THE DOPPLER EFFECT AND SOUND WAVES

There was little practical application of the Doppler acoustic effect until the second decade of this century. The sinking of the Titanic by an iceberg in 1912 sparked an interest in developing some method for detecting underwater objects. The advent of submarine warfare in World War I made the development of such instruments necessary, and practical sonar devices came into being.

Sonar developed as a technique which used reflected sound waves to detect objects underwater. Research on sonar between the two world wars provided important advances in transducer technology as well as improved understanding of the principles of ultrasound generation and reception. At the same time, intensive research was being carried out on the use of radio waves for detecting flying objects; the result was radar.

MEDICAL APPLICATIONS

Following World War II, the technological advances of sonar concerned with ultrasound generation and transducer design were joined with the methods of pulsed echo generation and signal processing from radar to produce the earliest ultrasound machines for medical use.

Pioneering work in the early 1950s culminated in the report of 1954 by Edler and Hertz[2] describing the first M-mode echocardiograph system for imaging cardiac structures. Interestingly, the first medical Doppler instrument was built in Japan by Satomura[3] in 1955 and described in a report published 2 years later. During the later 1950s and early 1960s, Doppler instruments were developed by Franklin, Rushmer, Baker, and their colleagues[4-6] that measured mean or average blood flow velocity.

Although the use of ultrasound for imaging the heart rapidly advanced through M-mode to two-dimensional echocardiography, the interest of the medical community in Doppler did not develop concurrently. During the 1960s, work by McLeod,[7] Baker et al.,[8] Peronneau et al.,[9] and Wells[10] resulted in pulsed Doppler systems for medical use that were able to examine the direction of blood flow and localize qualitative disturbances of flow in selected areas of the heart.

During the same period, Light,[11] Kalmanson et al.,[12] and others were in the process of developing continuous wave Doppler ultrasound for medical use. By 1980, the main accomplishments of pulsed and continuous wave Doppler echocardiography were in the investigation of patterns of blood flow in the heart and great vessels. Doppler could be used to differentiate abnormally fast from normal blood velocity. It provided a detector for the presence of valvular lesions, both stenosis and regurgitation, and for the presence of common congenital lesions such as atrial or ventricular septal defects.

What standard echocardiographic methods were for visualization of cardiac anatomy, Doppler was for the assessment of flow through the heart. Still, the general popularity of Doppler echocardiography could not keep pace with its imaging counterparts. Worldwide applications of M-mode and two-dimensional echocardiography boomed, whereas Doppler had its support among only a few determined individuals who saw its potential.

The limitations of Doppler echocardiography that prevented its more general use were many. First, the sensitivity of the early systems, especially in the realm of signal processing, was limited, and determination of absolute blood flow velocity was not easy. Second, system records of disturbed flow were poor, and Doppler examiners were generally limited to the audio output of the instrument for use in diagnostic studies. Third, Doppler studies were generally conducted in a blind fashion or with crude M-mode images, since interfaces of Doppler instruments with two-dimensional instruments had not yet been readily accomplished. Combined with the difficulty physicians had in understanding the nature of Doppler-detected flows, these factors made Doppler less appealing when compared with two-dimensional echocardiography.

DOPPLER TODAY

Today, however, there is a great deal of excitement concerning the clinical applications of Doppler. Much of this can be attributed to the efforts of Hatle and Angelsen[13] to make Doppler readily understandable to physicians and applicable to clinical care of patients. Doppler can now give reliable information about flow velocities through the heart. New developments in electronic components have provided the means to achieve excellent sensitivity in most instruments, making detection of normal and disturbed flows easier. Likewise, recent technological advances have made it feasible to generate spectral velocity recordings that serve as a permanent record of the Doppler study. In addition, interfaces with the two-dimensional echocardiographic system are providing means for physicians and sonographers to familiarize themselves with the relationships between anatomy and blood flow through the heart. Finally, based upon the work of early pioneers in the field, there is now a general agreement that Doppler echocardiography provides unique information regarding the patterns of normal and abnormal blood flow and estimates of pressure gradients and output that, heretofore, were not obtainable in a noninvasive way.

REFERENCES

1. White DN: Johann Christian Doppler and his effect: A brief history. Ultrasound Med Biol 8:583, 1982
2. Edler I, Hertz CH: Use of the ultrasonic reflectoscope for continuous recording of movements of heart wall. Kung Fysiograf Sallsd Lund Fordhandl 24:40, 1954
3. Nimura Y: History of pulse and echo Doppler ultrasound in Japan. In Spencer MP (ed): Cardiac Doppler Diagnosis. Martinus Nijhoff Publishers, Boston, 1983

4. Franklin DL, Schlegel W, Rushmer RF: Blood flow measured by Doppler frequency shift of back-scattered ultrasound. Science 134:564, 1961
5. Stegall HF, Rushmer RF, Baker DW: A transcutaneous ultrasonic blood-velocity meter. J Appl Physiol 21:707, 1966
6. Rushmer RF, Baker DW, Johnson WL, Strandness DE: Clinical applications of a transcutaneous ultrasonic flow detector. JAMA 199:104, 1967
7. McLeod FD: A directional Doppler flowmeter. In Jacobson B (ed): Digest of the 7th International Conference on Medical and Biological Engineering. Almqvist and Wiksell Publishers, Stockholm, 1967
8. Baker DW, Rubenstein SA, Lorch GS: Pulsed Doppler echocardiography: Principles and applications. Am J Med 63:69, 1977
9. Peronneau P, Xhaard M, Nowicki A, Pellet M, Delouche P, Hinglais J: Pulsed Doppler ultrasonic flowmeter and flow pattern analysis. In Roberts C (ed): Blood Flow Measurement. Sector Publishing Limited, London, 1972
10. Wells PNT: A range-gated ultrasonic Doppler system. Med. Biol Eng 7:641, 1969
11. Light H: Non-injurious ultrasonic technique for observing flow in the human aorta. Nature 224:1119, 1969
12. Kalmanson D, Veyrat C, Derai C, Chiche P: Diagnostic value of jugular venous flow velocity trace in right heart diseases. In Roberts C (ed): Blood Flow Measurement. Sector Publishing Limited, London, 1972
13. Hatle L, Angelsen B: Doppler Ultrasound in Cardiology. 2nd Ed. Lea and Febiger, Philadelphia, 1985

2 The Doppler Principle and the Study of Cardiac Flows

DANIEL B. MARK
DAVID ADAMS
JOSEPH KISSLO

Doppler instruments allow us to use the Doppler principle to study normal and abnormal blood flows through the heart. To perform or interpret cardiac Doppler examinations, it is necessary to understand the basics of blood flow and some basics of Doppler physics. Our purpose in this chapter is to present the elementary principles and avoid complex and detailed discussions. For the reader desiring greater detail, excellent reviews of the basic physics of Doppler are provided in the book by Hatle and Angelsen,[1] as well in previous issues of *Clinics in Diagnostic Ultrasound* by Beach and Phillips[2] and Woodcock and Skidmore.[3]

FLOW PATTERNS

Blood flow through the heart and great vessels has certain characteristics that can be measured using Doppler instruments. For the purpose of understanding flow patterns in the heart, it is important to recognize the difference between laminar (or normal) flow and turbulent (or disturbed) flow. Laminar flow is flow that occurs along smooth parallel lines in a vessel when all the red cells in an area are moving at approximately the same speed and in the same direction (Fig. 2.1). With the pulsations of the heart, the red cells generally accelerate and decelerate at approximately the same speed. Flow in most of the cardiovascular system, including the heart and great vessels, is normally laminar. Normal blood flow through the heart rarely exceeds the maximum speed of 1.5 m/sec.

In contrast, turbulent or disturbed flow is said to be present when there is some obstruction that results in a disruption of the normal laminar pattern. This causes the orderly movement of red blood cells to become disorganized and produces various whirls and eddies of differing velocities and directions.

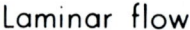
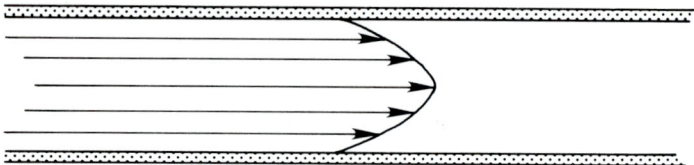

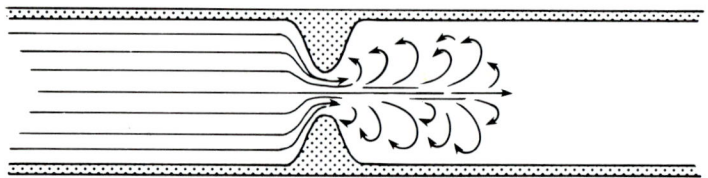

FIG. 2.1. Top section shows a vessel with normal laminar flow where all red blood cells are moving at approximately the same speed. The bottom section shows an example of turbulent flow where the normal laminar pattern has been disrupted and results in whirls and eddies of many different velocities. Such obstructions usually lead to some increase in velocity.

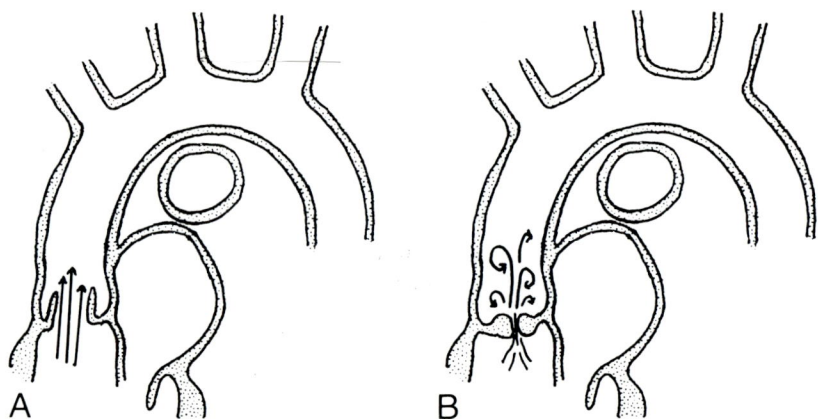

FIG. 2.2. Examples of (A) normal laminar flow through the aortic valve and (B) disturbed or turbulent flow resulting from aortic stenosis.

Obstruction to flow usually also results in some increase in velocity. Thus, turbulent flow is characterized by disordered directions of flow in combination with many different red cell velocities. If the obstruction is significant, some of the red blood cells may be moving at higher velocities than normal and may reach speeds of 5 or 6 m/sec. Turbulent flow is usually an abnormal finding and is considered indicative of some underlying cardiovascular pathology.

As an example, let us consider blood flow in the ascending aorta during systole. If the aorta and aortic valve are normal, then this flow is laminar. However, the presence of a valvular stenosis will induce a turbulent flow pattern. Figure 2.2 shows that a narrowed aortic valve orifice interrupts the parallel lines of normal laminar flow and creates turbulent flow. As will be discussed in more detail later, the stenosis also causes blood crossing the valve to be accelerated to an abnormally high velocity. The resulting jet of blood creates a short segment within the proximal aorta with complex flow characteristics.

Recognizing these various characteristics of normal (laminar) flow and disturbed (turbulent) flow allows us to understand which physical properties of flow can be measured by a Doppler echocardiographic system. Such systems use the Doppler effect to measure the direction, velocity, and degree of turbulence, thereby enabling us to differentiate normal from abnormal flow patterns and, in some cases, to quantitate these characteristics.

THE DOPPLER EFFECT

Doppler ultrasound systems work quite differently from standard ultrasound imaging devices. In standard echocardiographic imaging a given pulse of ultrasound is transmitted into the body and then reflected back from the various

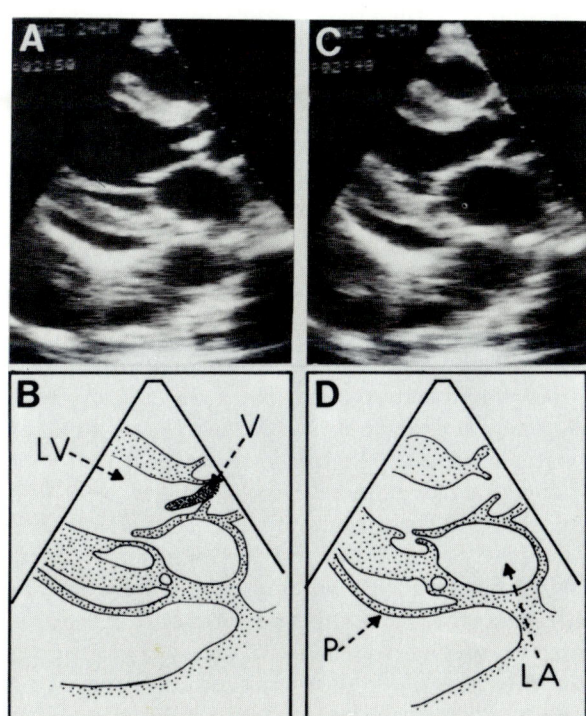

FIG. 2.3. Stop-frame two-dimensional echocardiograms in (A) diastole and (C) systole with accompanying schematic drawings (B and D, respectively) from patient with aortic valve endocarditis. Such images are made with standard reflected pulsed ultrasound. The best images are made when the interrogating beam is perpendicular to the target. Abbreviations: LV = left ventricle, V = vegetation, LA = left atrium, P = pericardium.

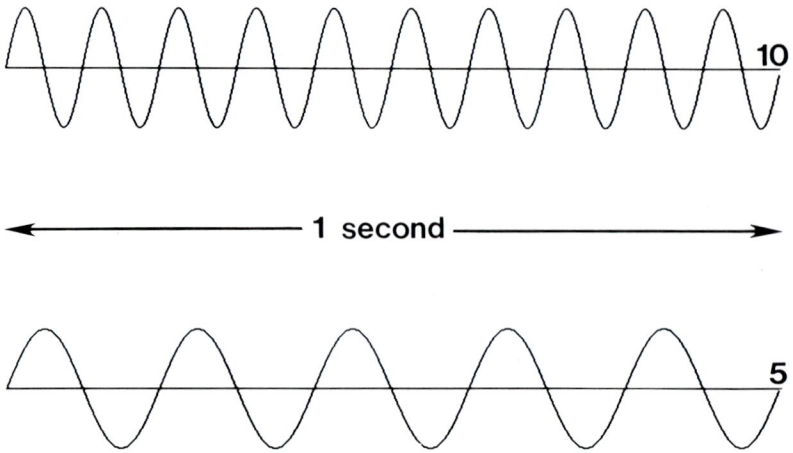

FIG. 2.4. Example of the frequency of any wave form. The top example shows 10 waves per second or 10 Hz, and the bottom shows 5 waves per second or 5 Hz. The top wave form has a higher frequency than the bottom.

tissues. Since the speed of sound in tissue is known (approximately 1,540 m/sec), a standard ultrasound imaging system can measure the time required for the transmitted pulse to travel to a target (time X) and then back (time 2X), and use this information to create an image of the target. In complex two-dimensional imaging systems this alternating process is repeated in a variety of directions thousands of time each second (Fig. 2.3). The best ultrasound images are made when the target is perpendicular to the sound waves. A standard M-mode or two-dimensional echocardiographic system does not measure the frequency of the transmitted or returned signal.

Doppler echocardiography, on the other hand, depends on measurement of the *relative change* in the returned ultrasound frequency when compared with the transmitted frequency. This principle was described in its simplified form in Chapter 1 (Fig. 1.1).

The example of the first experimental test of the Doppler principle highlighted two important features of the Doppler effect. First, the note sounded by all the trumpets, stationary or moving, was identical. Second, there was an apparent change in pitch noted by the stationary observer which was caused by the motion of the sound source.

The pitch or note of a sound is a subjective feature that is appreciated by the ear. The corresponding objective characteristic that can be measured and quantified is frequency. Frequency is a fundamental characteristic of any wave phenomenon, including sound and light, and refers to the number of waves that pass a given point in 1 second (Fig. 2.4). It is usually described in units of cycles per second or hertz (Hz). Thus, the top of the illustration shows an example of a wave form of 10 Hz whereas the bottom is 5 Hz.

The relationship between pitch and frequency is simple: The pitch of any given sound is proportional to its frequency. As sound wave frequency goes up, pitch gets higher; as frequency goes down, pitch declines.

What makes the altered frequency of the Doppler effect more than just an interesting curiosity is the fact that it actually provides a method which is used by many familiar devices that measure the direction and speed of moving objects.

The radar unit used by police to monitor the speed of cars on a highway is one such device that uses the Doppler effect in a quantitative manner. Almost every motorist is aware that police radar is set up in a position where it can be directed along the line of traffic flow. When activated, it sends a beam of radar waves of a known, uniform frequency at the oncoming cars. Each time the beam encounters an oncoming car, waves of higher frequency are reflected back to the police unit. The frequency of these returning waves is measured and compared with the transmitted frequency. The magnitude of this change in frequency, or Doppler frequency shift, is proportional to the speed or velocity of the car that produced it. By using the Doppler equation (discussed below), an estimate of the speed or velocity of the car can be calculated.

If the radar beam strikes a stationary car, then the reflected wave will have a frequency identical to the transmitted waves, and no Doppler shift is recorded. However, if a vehicle is moving toward the radar, the returned frequency will be higher than the transmitted frequency, and a positive Doppler shift will be noted. On the other hand, if the vehicle is moving away from the radar source, the returned frequency will be less than that transmitted, and the Doppler shift will be negative.

Although the car in this example is not the source of the sound the way the trumpets were in the first example, it is, nevertheless, the "effective" source. This is true because its action on the transmitted radar waves results in a change, or shift, of the reflected frequency that characterizes the Doppler effect.

There are important similarities between the example of the police radar and how Doppler systems work in the body. In both cases, transmitted waves of some type encounter moving objects and are reflected back with altered frequencies. And, in both cases, the magnitude of the induced frequency change or Doppler shift allows the velocity of the moving objects to be calculated.

One important difference between the radar unit and the Doppler ultrasound machine is that radar is used to measure the speed of single objects (cars),

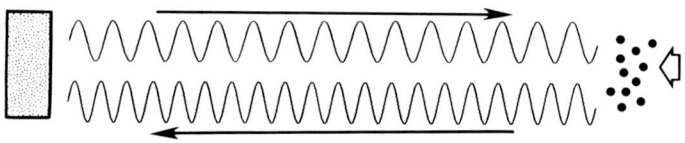

FIG. 2.5. Example of the Doppler effect resulting from red blood cells traveling toward the transducer at the left. A burst of ultrasound is sent into the tissues at a given frequency and is reflected off the red cells moving toward the transducer at a higher frequency. This is a positive Doppler shift.

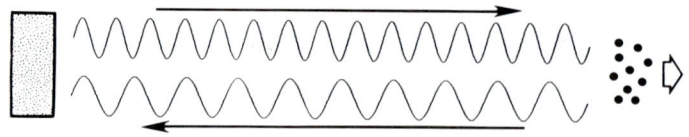

FIG. 2.6. Example of the Doppler effect resulting from red blood cells traveling away from the transducer at the left. A burst of ultrasound is sent into the tissues at a given frequency and is reflected off the red cells moving away, and the reflect wave is returned at a lower frequency. This is a negative Doppler shift.

whereas the Doppler ultrasound system measures the speed of millions of objects (red blood cells) at a time. Thus, the Doppler device can be regarded as a complex speedometer designed to detect red cell motion (i.e., blood flow) and measure its velocity.

Figure 2.5 shows a transducer on the left that is emitting a given frequency of ultrasound toward the right and into the tissues. The transmitted sound waves encounter a group of red cells moving toward the transducer and are reflected back at a higher frequency than what was sent, producing a positive Doppler shift. Figure 2.6 shows the opposite effect when a given frequency sent into the tissues encounters red cells moving away. The result is the return of a frequency lower than what was transmitted, and the Doppler shift is negative.

THE DIRECTION OF FLOW

A good example of the ability of Doppler to determine the direction of flow is noted in Fig. 2.7 in which a Doppler transducer is held in the suprasternal notch, first being angled toward the ascending aorta, and then toward the right where it encounters the descending aorta. When angled into the ascending aorta, flow is toward the transducer, and the Doppler shift is positive (Fig. 2.8) or upward from the baseline of the display. When angled into the descending aorta, flow is away from the transducer and the Doppler shift is negative (Fig. 2.9) or downward from the baseline. If the beam intercepts stationary targets, the returned frequency is the same as that transmitted, and no shift occurs.

Doppler ultrasound systems do measure the frequency change between emitted and returned frequency caused by moving objects. The relationship between the Doppler frequency shift produced by moving objects, such a red cell, and the velocity or speed of those moving objects is expressed formally in the Doppler equation shown in Fig. 2.10. From our discussion thus far, it is apparent that Doppler instruments know the transmitted frequency (f_0) and can be programmed for the velocity of sound in blood (c). Similarly, the frequency of the returning ultrasound (f_2) can be measured. If the transducer is positioned as parallel to blood flow as possible, then the angle between the beam and velocity is zero degrees and cos θ becomes 1.

Clinically, we are most interested in measuring velocity since it is altered

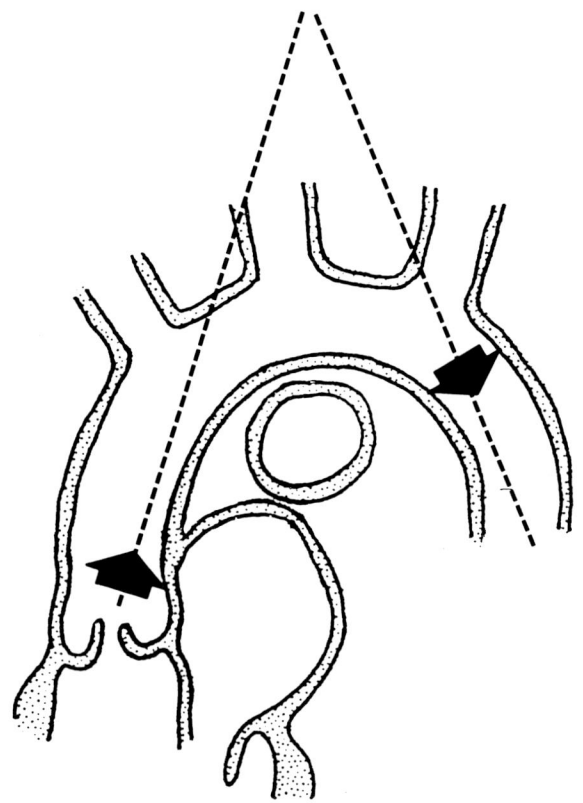

FIG. 2.7. If a Doppler transducer is held in the suprasternal notch and angled toward the ascending aorta, it will encounter flow toward it (left arrow). If then angled toward the descending aorta, the beam will encounter flow away from the transducer (right arrow).

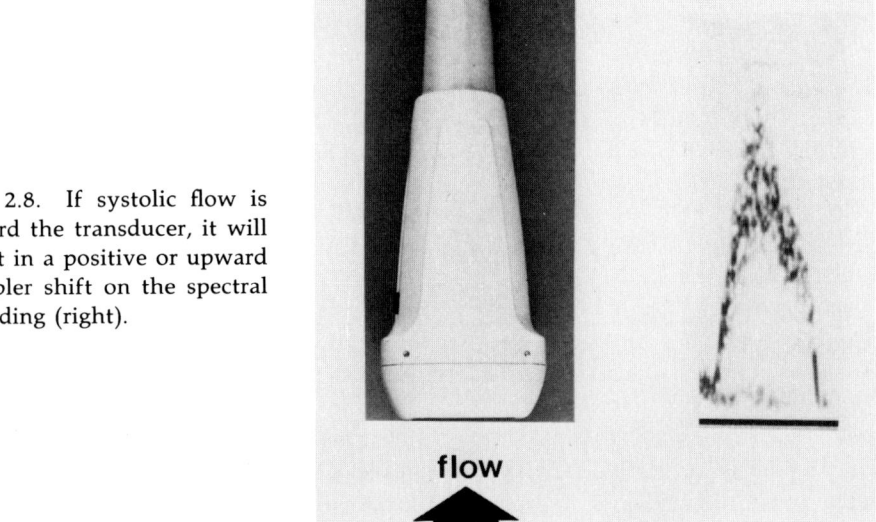

FIG. 2.8. If systolic flow is toward the transducer, it will result in a positive or upward Doppler shift on the spectral recording (right).

14 BASIC DOPPLER ECHOCARDIOGRAPHY

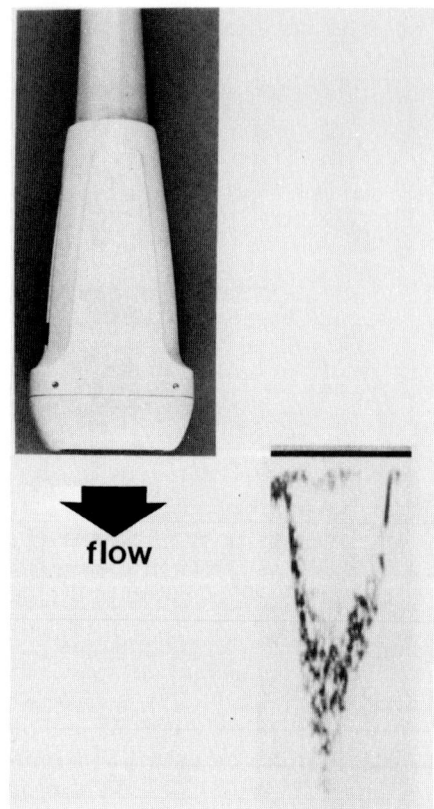

FIG. 2.9. If systolic flow is away from the transducer, it will result in a negative or downward Doppler shift on the spectral recording (right).

$$f_2 = \frac{2f_o}{c} v \cos\theta$$

where : f_2 = returned frequency
f_o = transmitted frequency
v = maximal velocity
$\cos\theta$ = angle between beam and velocity
c = velocity of sound in blood

FIG. 2.10. The Doppler equation.

$$V = \frac{c}{2f_o \cos\theta} f_2$$

FIG. 2.11. The Doppler equation rearranged for velocity.

in disease states. All components of the Doppler equation, except velocity, are readily measured by the Doppler instrument.

Since the primary variable desired for clinical work is velocity (V), the Doppler equation can be rearranged to that shown in Fig. 2.11. What these complex formulas tell us is that the Doppler principle can be used to tell us the direction and velocity of flow. What is important to recognize is:

$$\text{Frequency shift} \rightarrow \text{Doppler Equation} \rightarrow \text{Velocity data}$$

A Doppler machine, therefore, is a velocity detector (speedometer) that tells the direction and speed of blood flow.

THE DOPPLER DISPLAY

The most important Doppler output is the audio, and some background on this has already been gained in our discussions of the Doppler effect. It is the most common type of output and is available on all cardiac Doppler systems.

As we will see in later chapters, listening to the audio output is very helpful during the conduct of a Doppler examination. The changing velocities (frequencies) detected by the Doppler instrument are converted into audible sounds and, after some filtering and other processing, are emitted from speakers placed within the machine.

High-pitched sounds are obviously the result of large Doppler shifts and indicate the presence of high velocities, whereas low-pitched sounds are the result of lesser Doppler shifts. Flow direction information (relative to the transducer) is provided by a stereophonic audio output in which all flow toward the transducer comes out of one speaker, and all flow away comes out of the other speaker.

The audio output also allows the operator to easily differentiate laminar from turbulent flow. Laminar flow produces a smooth, pleasant tone because of the narrow, uniform shape of the Doppler spectrum. Turbulent flow, because of the presence of many different velocities, commonly results in a high-pitched and whistling or harsh and raspy sound.

Audio output is one of the oldest and simplest forms of Doppler display. Nevertheless, it remains an indispensable guide to the machine operator for achieving proper orientation of the ultrasound beam, even when the Doppler is being used in conjunction with an ultrasound imaging technique. The reason is that the trained ear can more readily appreciate minor changes in spectral composition than can the eye, given the same information displayed graphically. In occasional patients, it may be possible to pick up the flow characteristics of interest using the audio output alone and not be able to get an adequate separation of signal from noise on a hard-copy graphic display. The major limitations of audio Doppler outputs are the requirements for subjective interpretation and, in some cases, the lack of a permanent objective record. It is difficult to publish the audio output of a Doppler system in this book.

The audio output from a Doppler machine may superficially resemble the sounds produced by an amplified stethoscope or a phonocardiogram. It is, therefore, worth emphasizing that the Doppler is neither of these. The sounds detected with a stethoscope are transmitted vibrations or pressure waves from the heart and great vessels that are believed to be the result of rapid accelerations and decelerations of blood. The Doppler audio output, in contrast, is an audible display of the Doppler frequency-shift spectrum produced by red cells moving in the path of the ultrasound beam. It is a sound produced by the Doppler that does *not* occur in nature and, therefore, it does not originate in the heart.

There have been many formats for the hard-copy graphic display of Doppler information, including those used throughout this book and seen in Figs. 2.8 and 2.9. Over the years, several approaches to create a hard-copy record of the Doppler examination have been attempted and include zero-crossing detectors and sound spectrographs. All of these hard-copy methods had considerable drawbacks, and the advent of digital technology and relatively inexpensive microcomputer chips has made their use obsolete.

The new generation of Doppler echocardiography equipment contains sophisticated sound frequency or velocity spectrum analyzers. The advances made possible by this equipment have helped promote physician interest in Doppler because practical recording systems are now available. Most commercially available Doppler systems display velocity spectral outputs, and most of the hard-copy recordings in this book are of velocity spectra.

As can be seen in Figs. 2.8 and 2.9, the Doppler velocity information is displayed vertically (up or down), depending on the Doppler shift. Time is on the horizontal axis. The internal workings of such systems are complex,

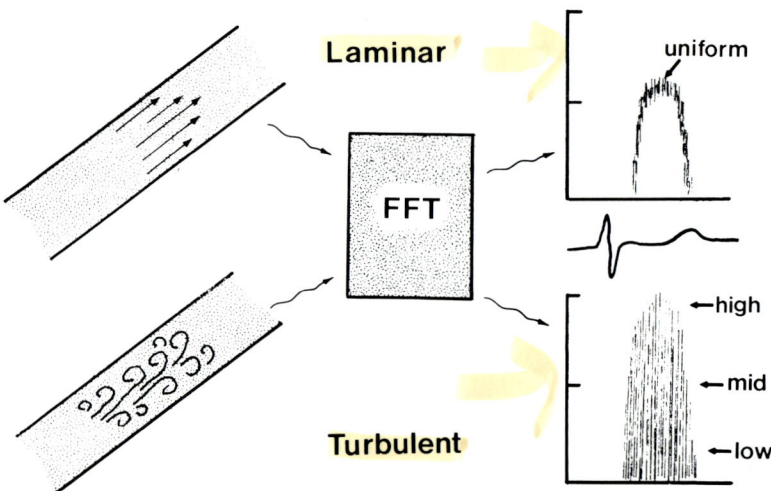

FIG. 2.12. Fast Fourier Transform (FFT) is a complex method of decifering the various velocities encountered by the returning signal. In the case of laminar flow there are generally uniform velocities as the blood accelerates and decelerates during systole. Turbulent flow, however, results in a great many different velocities and broadens the velocity spectrum into high, mid, and lower velocities. There also is usually some increase in velocity with turbulence resulting from obstruction.

DOPPLER PRINCIPLE AND CARDIAC FLOWS   17

but the results are rather simple. Flow toward the transducer is recorded by the Doppler system as a positive or upward deflection. Likewise, flow away from the transducer is recorded as a negative or downward deflection.

When flow is laminar and all the red cells are accelerating and decelerating at approximately the same velocities, a very nice envelope of these similar velocities is recorded over time (Fig. 2.12). When flow is turbulent, however, there are many different velocities detected at any one time (a wide spectrum of velocities). Such turbulence, produced by an obstruction to flow, results in the spectral broadening (display of velocities that are low, mid, and high) and increase in peak velocity seen in disease states.

This display of the spectrum of the various velocities encountered by the Doppler beam (Fig. 2.13) is accomplished by very sophisticated microcomputers that are able to decifer the returning complex Doppler signal and process it into its various velocity components. There are two basic methods for this to be accomplished. The most popular is Fast Fourier Transform (FFT), and the other is called Chirp-Z transform.

A better understanding of the somewhat complex creation of a spectral velocity recording aids one in performing and interpreting Doppler studies. Figure 2.14 demonstrates that the spectral recording is really made up of a series of "bins" (vertical axis) that are recorded over time (horizontal axis). At any given point in time, there is a differential speed of movement of red cells with more red blood cells moving at the velocity of the most intense bin

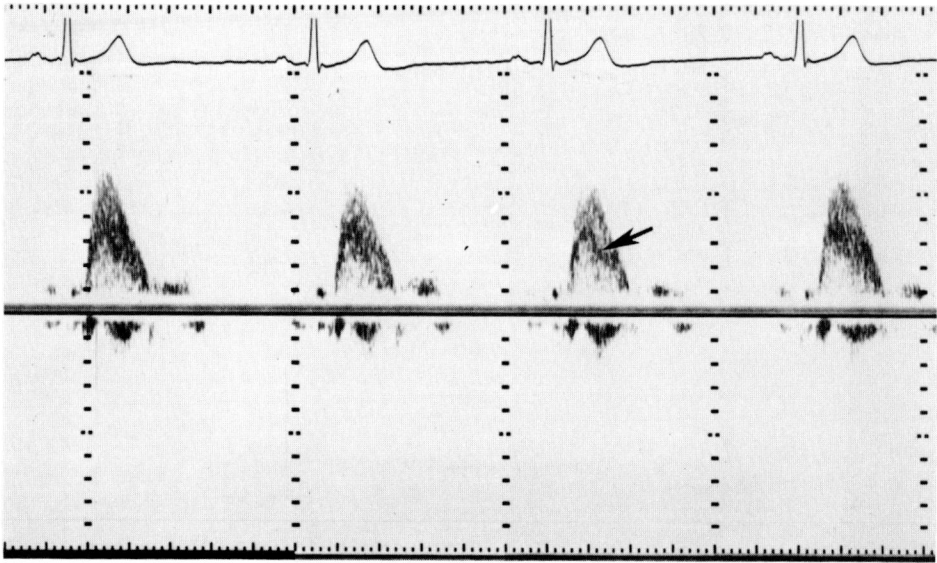

FIG. 2.13. A spectral analysis of the ascending aorta taken from the suprasternal notch. Flow is toward the transducer in systole. Note the darker areas (arrow) in comparison with the lighter shades of gray. The darker areas indicate that more red blood cells of this velocity were detected in comparison with the lighter areas.

18 BASIC DOPPLER ECHOCARDIOGRAPHY

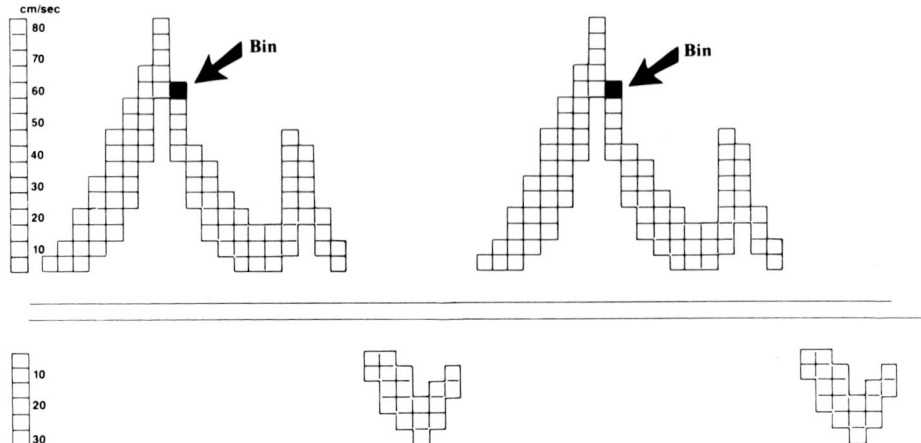

FIG. 2.14. A simplified representation of bins in the spectral velocity recording. Time is on the horizontal axis. (Reproduced by permission of Hewlett-Packard, Inc.)

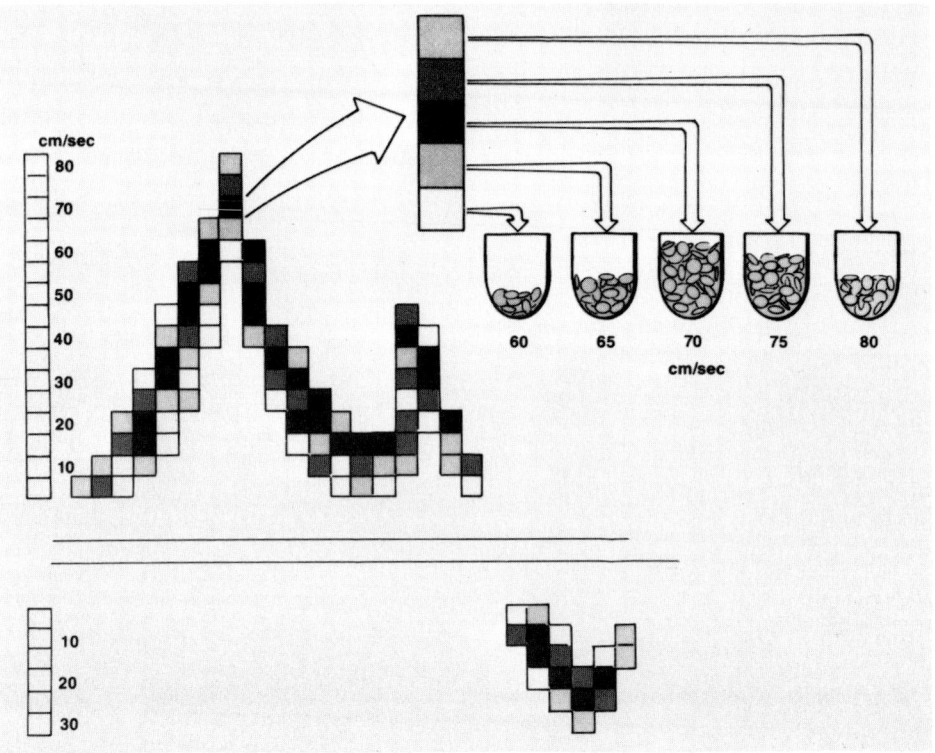

FIG. 2.15. The more blood cells detected at any given velocity, the greater the intensity in the bin. Thus, the spectral recording reflects information as to the relative number of cells at any velocity. (Reproduced by permission of Hewlett-Packard, Inc.)

DOPPLER PRINCIPLE AND CARDIAC FLOWS 19

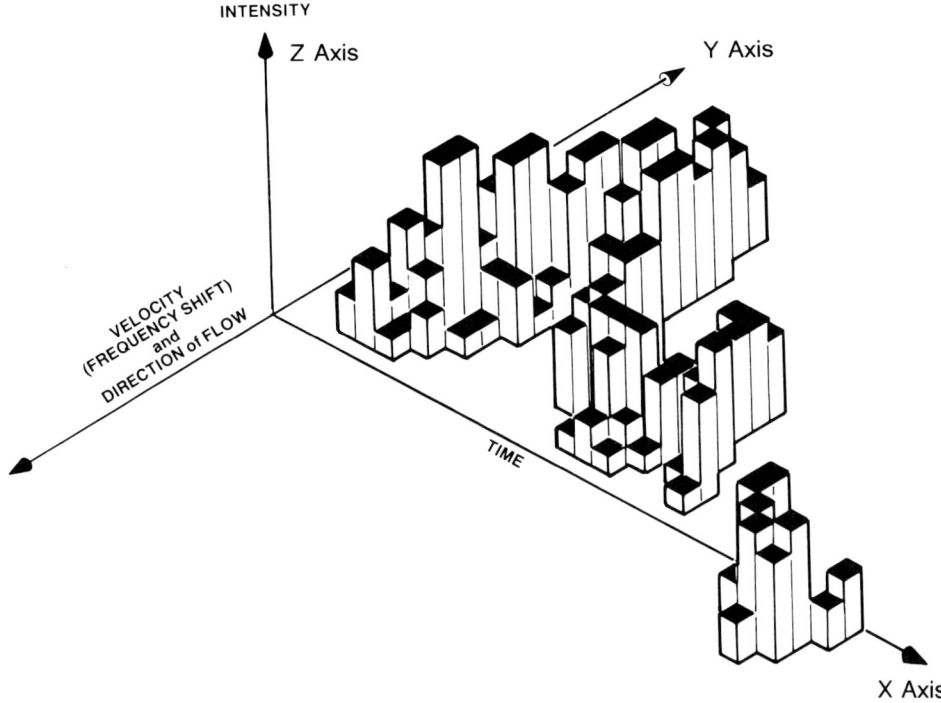

FIG. 2.16. The spectrum has time on the X axis, velocity on the Y axis, and amplitude (or numbers of red cells) on the Z axis. (Reproduced by permission of Hewlett-Packard, Inc.)

than are moving at the other velocities, which are represented by the less intense bins (Fig. 2.15).

Thus, the velocity spectral analysis is really a complex plot of the various velocities over time (Fig. 2.16). Time is on the X axis and velocity is on the Y axis. As time progresses, various velocities are detected moving forward and backward with the phases of the cardiac cycle. The amplitude, or number of red cells at any given velocity, is on the Z axis and is represented by differential intensities, gray scale, on the display. As will be discussed later, the operator does have some control of the gray scale display, and various possible settings are provided on most machines. Improper gray scale adjustments can obscure or eliminate useful information (see also Chapter 4).

Since this full spectral display is so highly processed, there are a variety of other outputs which can be displayed, and they are electronically derived from the spectral data (Fig. 2.17). These include mean velocity and maximum velocity. A line drawn as an envelope around the spectrum at the peak Doppler shift at any point during the cardiac cycle is the peak velocity profile. Mean Doppler shift can be estimated from a line drawn through the darkest part of the spectrum. Structures such as heart valves reflect a great deal more ultrasound than red cells. This intensity of reflected sound is referred to as the

20   BASIC DOPPLER ECHOCARDIOGRAPHY

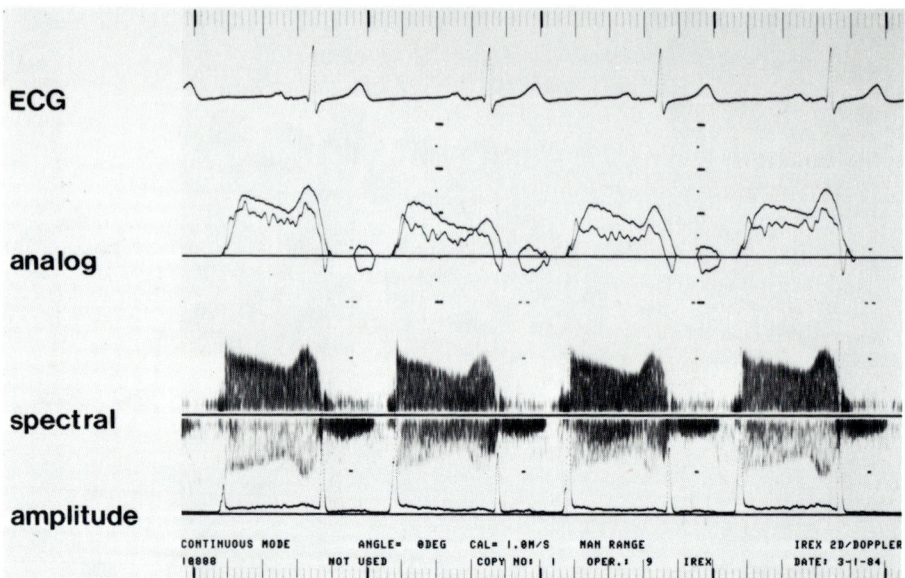

FIG. 2.17. An example of the various Doppler displays from a patient with mitral stenosis with the transducer held at the apex. Flow in diastole is toward the transducer. The ECG is at the top. The analog outputs are of maximum and mean velocities. The spectral recording shows spectral broadening toward the transducer in diastole. Because the diastolic flow signal is so strong, there is some "mirroring" into the opposite channel.

amplitude, which is useful for timing the opening and closing of heart valves. For standard clinical purposes the full spectrum is generally used.

Current velocity spectral analyzers have provided the means for graphic representation of the Doppler shift data in a more reliable way than ever before. As we shall see in later chapters, however, dependence on and operator interaction with the audio outputs are still necessary. It is not infrequent that abnormalities can be "heard" but not readily recorded.

THE EFFECT OF ANGLE

The Doppler equation also tells us that the angle the Doppler beam makes with the lines of flow being evaluated is very important. This angle, theta (written as θ), is of crucial importance in the calculation of velocities from Doppler shift data (Fig. 2.18).

When the ultrasound beam is directed parallel to blood flow, angle θ is 0° (cosine $\theta = 1$), and measured velocity on the recording will be true velocity. In contrast, with the ultrasound beam directed perpendicular to flow, angle θ = 90° (cosine 90 = 0), and measured velocity will be 0. Therefore, the smaller the angle θ, the closer angle cosine θ is to 1, and the more reliable is the recorded Doppler velocity. A wider-angle θ will result in a greater reduction in measured velocity compared with true velocity.

FIG. 2.18. Schematic diagram showing the importance of being parallel to flow. The solid arrows represent the direction of a systolic jet of 2 m/sec. If the interrogating beam is only 10° from parallel, the maximum velocity that can be recorded is 1.97 m/sec. Moving 60° from parallel only allows a peak velocity of 1.0 m/sec to be recorded.

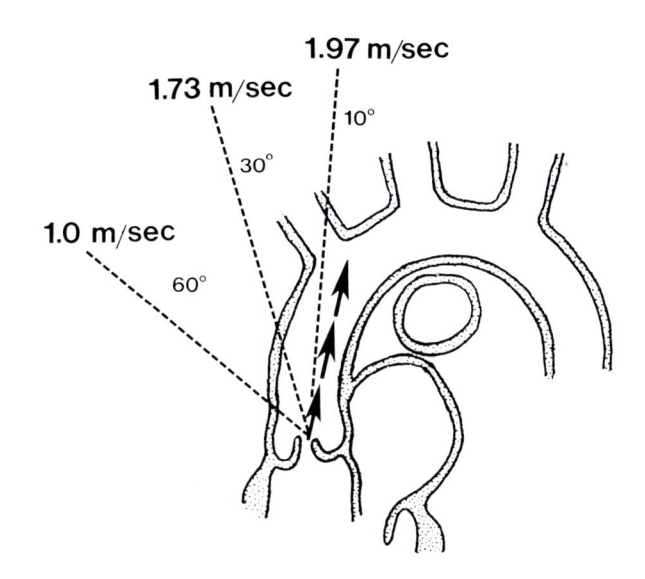

Thus, the more parallel to flow the Doppler ultrasound beam is directed, the more faithfully the measured velocity will reflect true velocity. For practical purposes, angles of greater than 25° between the ultrasound beam and the blood flow being studied will generally yield clinically unacceptable quantitative estimates of velocity.

An operator using Doppler and desiring the best quantitative estimates of

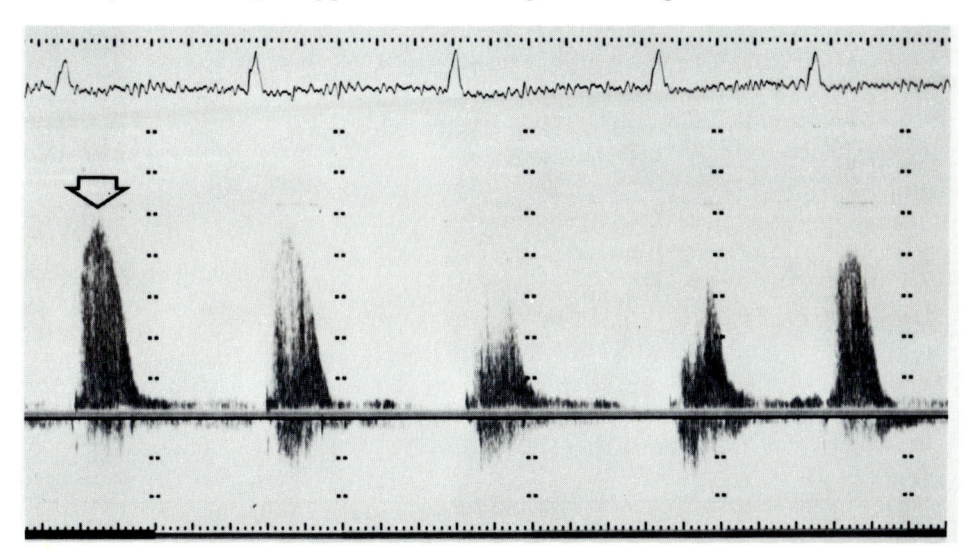

FIG. 2.19. The effect of varying angulation in relationship to a systolic jet in a patient with aortic stenosis. The recording was taken from the suprasternal notch, and flow is toward the transducer in systole. Note that the peak jet is nearly 5 m/sec (open arrow). In subsequent beats the beam profile is angled away from parallel, and the full profile is lost.

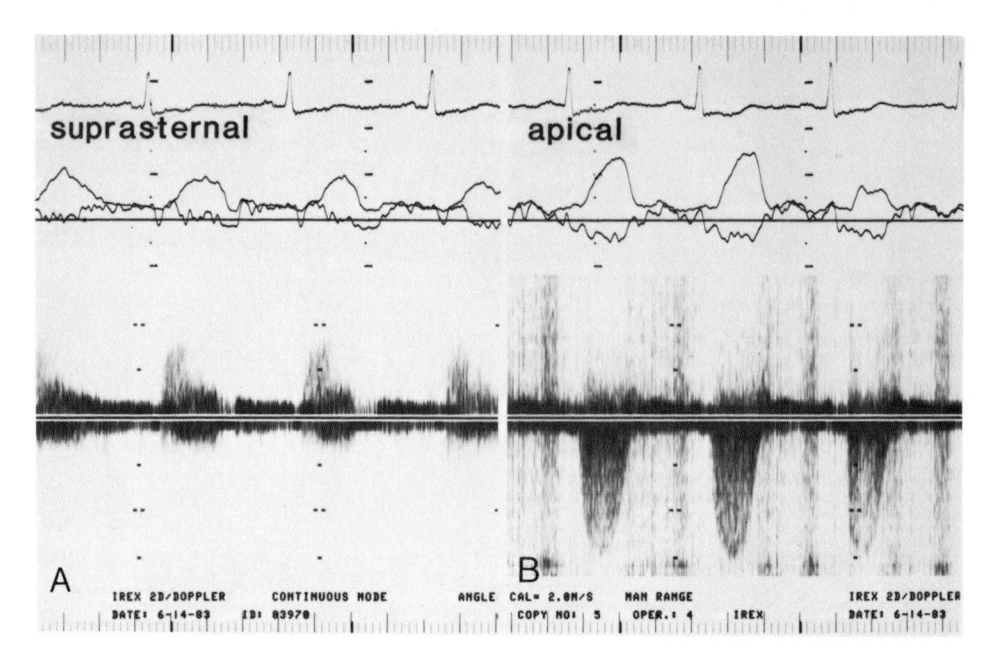

FIG. 2.20. (A) Suprasternal (with flow toward the transducer) and (B) apical (with flow away from the transducer) recordings from a patient with aortic stenosis. Note the differences in profiles between the two recording sites. The best profile was taken from the apical position.

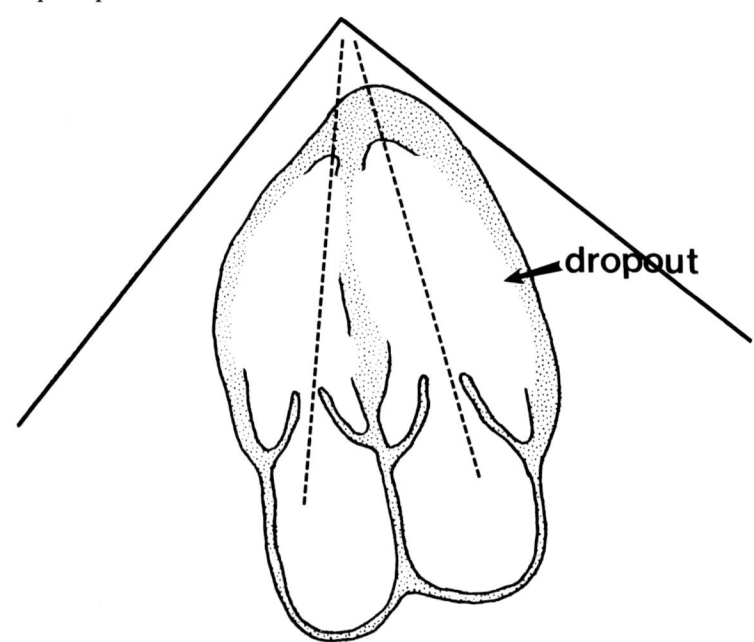

FIG. 2.21. Doppler recordings are best taken when the interrogating beam is parallel to flow. As this schematic diagram depicts, there is often "target dropout" in the two-dimensional recording as the imaging beam is parallel to the targets. Good Doppler recording sites are rarely good imaging sites.

flow must, therefore, always attempt to be parallel to flow, and this concept is of fundamental importance in the conduct of a clinical examination. Figure 2.18 shows the effect of varying angle on the measurement of peak velocity of an aortic stenotic jet. Figure 2.19 shows the actual effect of changing angle on a systolic aortic stenotic jet toward a transducer in the suprasternal notch. The first beat (open arrow) shows the only fully formed profile.

The great importance of this concept in the conduct of a clinical examination for aortic stenosis is demonstrated in Fig. 2.20. Such abnormal jets are often eccentric, and their directions cannot always be predicted. This requires a Doppler examiner to interrogate the jet from a variety of angles. Note that the full jet is not seen from the suprasternal area in this patient but is detected from the apical approach.

This need to be parallel to flow leads the Doppler examiner to depend on some windows for examination that may sacrifice the quality of the two-dimensional image. For example, Fig. 2.21 shows the direction of the ultrasound beam through either the mitral or tricuspid orifices from the apical position, an excellent Doppler window but one which may allow significant echocardiographic "dropout" since the imaging beams are parallel to the endocardium.

REFERENCES

1. Hatle L, Angelsen B: Doppler Ultrasound in Cardiology. 2nd Ed. Lea and Febiger, Philadelphia, 1985
2. Beach KW, Phillips DJ: Doppler instrumentation for the evaluation of arterial and venous disease. Clin Diagnostic Ultrasound 13:11, 1984
3. Woodcock JP, Skidmore R: Principles and applications of Doppler ultrasound. Clin Diagnostic Ultrasound 5:166, 1980

3 Pulsed and Continuous Wave Doppler

JOSEPH KISSLO
DANIEL B. MARK
DAVID ADAMS

Justification for the use of Doppler echocardiography stems from the realization that certain forms of cardiac disease, such as valvular heart disease, produce changes in the direction and/or velocity of blood flow. Just as imaging echocardiography can be used to detect abnormalities of cardiac anatomical structures, Doppler echocardiography can be used to assess these abnormalities of flow.

Since both approaches use ultrasound, it is logical to assume that both Doppler and imaging functions can be combined into one ultrasound instrument. Ideally, this compound system would provide high-quality images with a high frame rate and wide field of view. These images would also assist the operator in precisely positioning the Doppler beam within various cardiac chambers. The optimal system would allow both of these functions to be carried out simultaneously while preserving the capability to accurately measure the full range of normal and abnormal blood flow velocities, from 0 to approximately 6 m/sec. (Velocities are usually expressed in meters or centimeters per second.)

Unfortunately, this fully simultaneous capability is not currently possible with existing technology. Doppler and imaging systems actually make competing demands on an ultrasound device. The limiting factor in combining the two is the relatively slow (and constant) speed of ultrasound in tissue. In the imaging mode, a two-dimensional echocardiographic machine rapidly and repeatedly transmits and then receives bursts or pulses of ultrasound while mechanically or electronically (as with phased array) sweeping the beam back and forth. If one desires a wide field of view (nominally between 60 and 90°) and high frame rates (30 or more full frames per second), there is little time left over for the system to perform Doppler functions properly.

Similarly, when using a selective Doppler mode to assess an area of turbulence deep into the heart (e.g., 8 to 10 cm from the transducer face), the transit time of the ultrasound to and from the area of interest is such that there is little time left over to create a two-dimensional image. This problem is compounded by the fact that abnormal velocities associated with valvular heart disease frequently exceed 1.5 m/sec, and faithful recording of these elevated velocities requires very high-pulse repetition rates (and thus a lot of time spent in the Doppler mode).

Other factors make this ideal mixture of capabilities difficult. The optimal echocardiographic image is obtained by orienting the transducer perpendicular to the surfaces of interest. As we have previously noted, optimal Doppler information is obtained in a position parallel to flow. Commonly, the ideal transducer position for imaging is not suitable for obtaining Doppler information. The converse is also true.

There are now many different commercial cardiac Doppler instruments with various mixtures of capabilities available, and the market may appear confusing to the uninitiated. Certain terms have been used recently to describe the new dual-capability ultrasound machines. When Doppler is physically combined into the same housing as the imaging system this Doppler is called an "add-on." An add-on Doppler that can be used with some combined, but limited, imaging capabilities is generally referred to as a "duplex" Doppler. A Doppler system without simultaneous two-dimensional imaging capabilities is generally referred to as a "stand-alone" Doppler. When a Doppler system is added-on to an existing imaging device but no provision is made for some form of combined imaging, it is functionally the same as a stand-alone device.

PULSED AND CONTINUOUS WAVE DOPPLER

There are two main types of Doppler echocardiographic systems in common use today, continuous wave and pulsed wave. They differ in transducer design and operating features, signal-processing procedures, and in the types of information provided. Each has important advantages and disadvantages and, in our opinion, the current practice of Doppler echocardiography requires some capability for both forms.

Continuous wave (CW) Doppler is the older and electronically more simple of the two kinds. As the name implies, CW Doppler involves continuous generation of ultrasound waves coupled with continuous ultrasound reception. This dual function is accomplished by a two-crystal transducer with one crystal devoted to each function (Figs. 3.1 and 3.2).

The main advantage of CW Doppler is its ability to measure high blood velocities accurately. Indeed, CW Doppler can accurately record the highest velocities in any valvular and congenital heart disease. Since velocities exceeding 1.5 m/sec are frequently seen in such disorders, accurate high-velocity measurement is of particular importance for allowing the recognition of the full abnormal flow profile. It is also of considerable importance for the quantitative evaluation of abnormal flows, as will be seen later.

The main disadvantage of CW Doppler is its lack of selectivity or depth discrimination. Since CW Doppler is constantly transmitting and receiving from two different transducer heads (crystals), there is no provision for imaging or

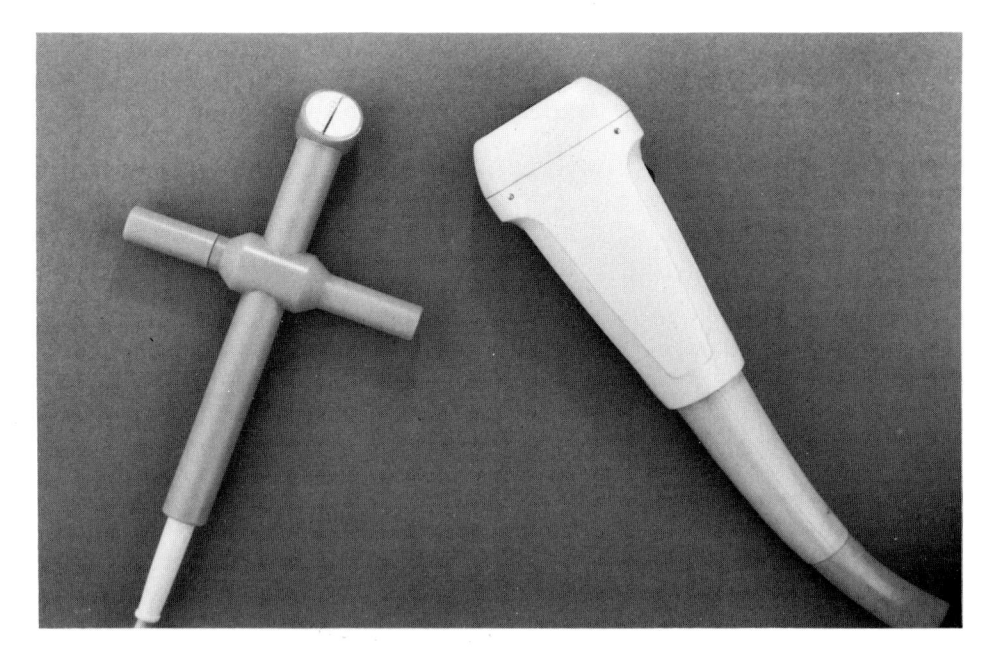

FIG. 3.1. The transducers used for Doppler examination of the heart. On the left is the continuous-wave transducer. Note the split face for independent transmit and receive. On the right is a typical phased-array transducer which contains pulsed-mode capabilities.

range gating to allow selective placing of a given Doppler sample volume in space. The output from a CW examination contains Doppler shift data from every red cell reflecting ultrasound back to the transducer along the course of the ultrasound beam.

Thus, true CW Doppler is functionally a stand-alone technique whether or not the capability is housed within a two-dimensional imaging system.

FIG. 3.2. Modes of transmission and reception. In CW there is constant transmission and reception, whereas in PW the system must alternate between transmit-and-receive functions using the same transducer.

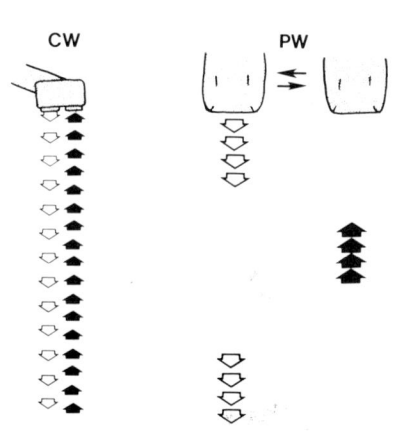

28 BASIC DOPPLER ECHOCARDIOGRAPHY

The absence of anatomical information during a CW examination may lead to interpretive difficulties, particularly if more than one heart chamber or blood vessel lies in the path of the ultrasound beam.

It is possible, however, to program a phased-array system to perform both two-dimensional and CW Doppler functions nearly simultaneously, and some of these systems are available on today's market. The quasi-simultaneous Doppler two-dimensional technique uses a time-sharing arrangement in which the transducer rapidly switches back and forth from one type of examination to the other. Because this switching is done at very high speeds, the operator gets the impression that both studies are being done continuously and in real-time. During the imaging period, no Doppler data are being collected, so an estimate is generated, usually from the preceding data. During the Doppler collection period, previously stored image data are displayed. This arrangement usually degrades the quality of both the two-dimensional and Doppler data.

Pulsed wave (PW) Doppler machines use a single-crystal transducer which alternates transmission and reception of ultrasound similar to the way an M-mode transducer does (Figs. 3.1 and 3.2). One main advantage of PW Doppler is its ability to provide Doppler shift data selectively from a small segment along the ultrasound beam, referred to as the sample volume (Fig. 3.3). This location of the sample volume is operator controlled. An ultrasound pulse is transmitted into the tissues, travels for a given time (time X) until it is reflected back by a moving red cell, and then returns to the transducer over the same time interval (at a new frequency as predicted by the Doppler equation). The total transit time to and from the area sampled is 2X. Since the speed of ultrasound in the tissues is constant, there is a simple relationship between roundtrip travel time and the location of the sample volume relative to the transducer face (i.e., distance to sample volume equals ultrasound speed divided by round-trip travel time). This process is alternately repeated through many transmit–receive cycles.

This range gating is basically a timing mechanism that only samples the returning Doppler shift data from a given region. It is calibrated so that as the operator chooses a particular location for the sample volume, the range

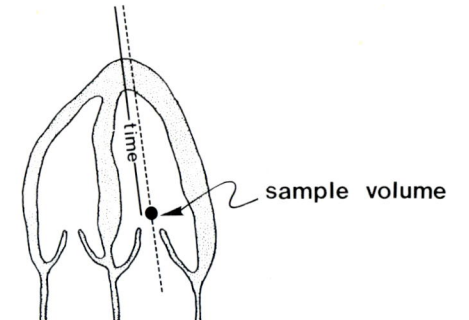

FIG. 3.3. Pulsed wave is able to obtain a Doppler signal at a given range in the heart called the sample volume.

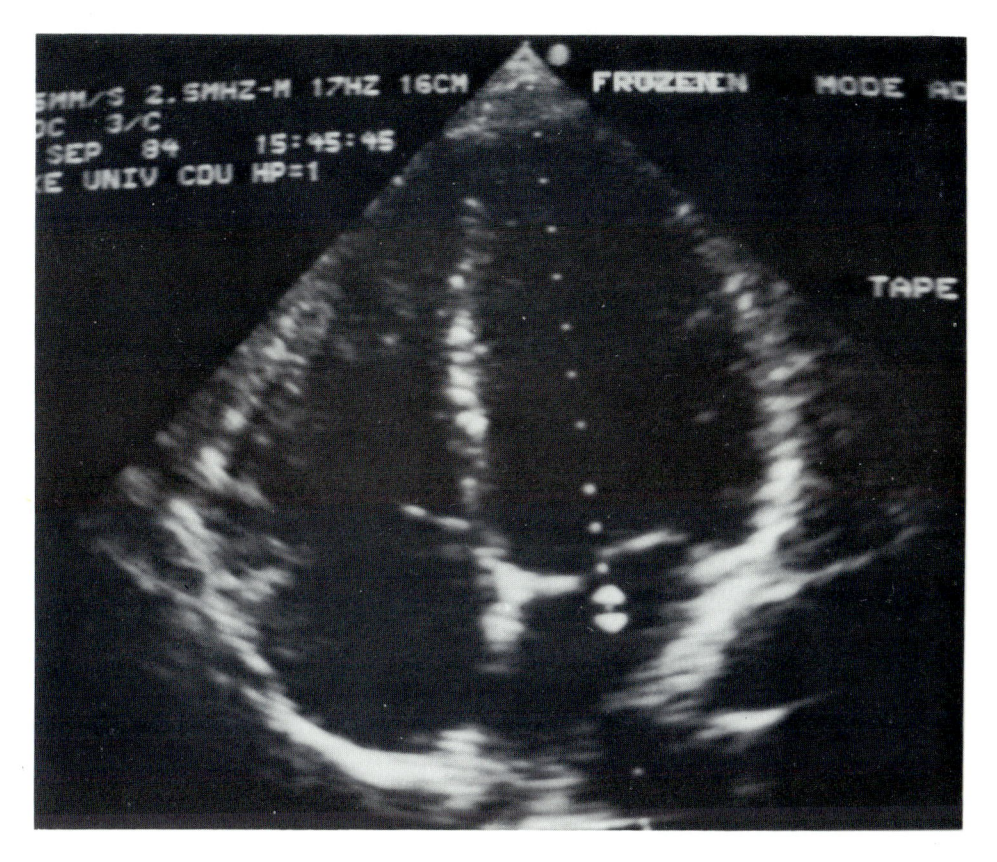

FIG. 3.4. Pulsed wave echocardiography allows some interaction between imaging and Doppler modes. Here the PW cursor and sample volume site are shown on the two-dimensional image.

gate circuit will permit only Doppler shift data from inside that area to be displayed as output. All other returning ultrasound information is essentially "ignored."

Another main advantage of pulsed Doppler is the fact that some imaging may be carried on alternatively with the Doppler, and thus the sample volume may be shown on the actual two-dimensional display for guidance (Fig. 3.4). PW Doppler capability is possible in combination with imaging from a mechanical or phased-array imaging system. It is also generally steerable through the two-dimensional field of view, although not all systems have this capability.

In reality, since the speed of sound in body tissues is constant, it is not possible to simultaneously carry on both imaging and Doppler functions at full capability in the same ultrasound system. In mechanical systems, the cursor and sample volume are positioned during real-time imaging, and the two-dimensional image is then frozen when the Doppler is activated. With most phased-array imaging systems the Doppler is variably programmed to allow

30   BASIC DOPPLER ECHOCARDIOGRAPHY

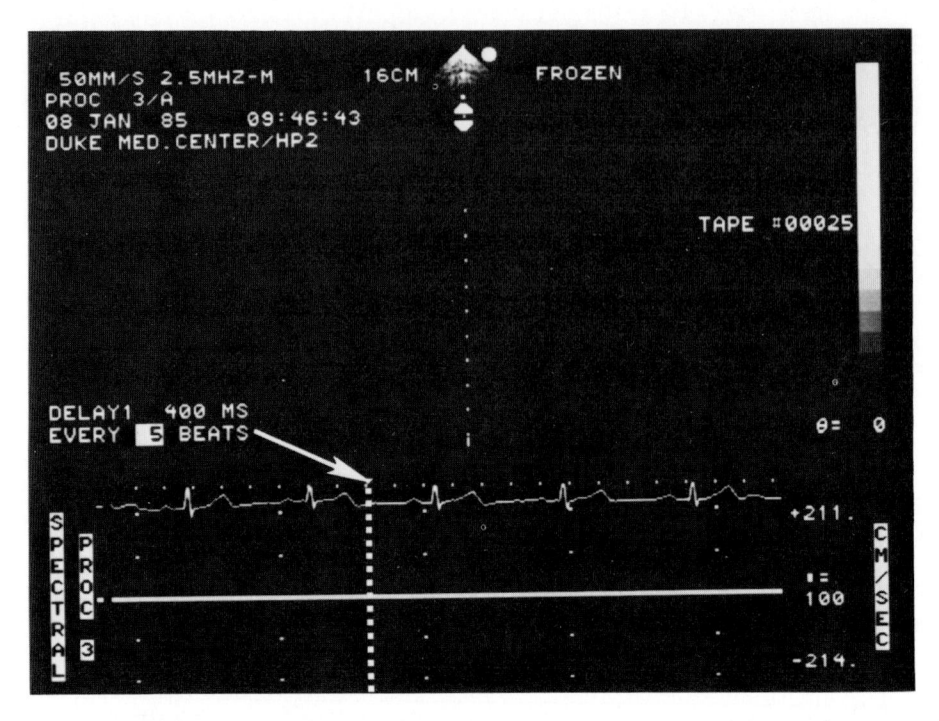

FIG. 3.5. When the pulsed wave Doppler operates, it causes the two-dimensional image to be updated intermittently. In this case the system is set for updating the image 400 msec after the QRS every five beats. This update will usually appear as a blank on the spectral display (dashed line).

periodic update of a single-frame two-dimensional image every several beats (Fig. 3.5). In other phased arrays, two-dimensional frame rate and line density are significantly decreased to allow enough time for the pulsed Doppler to sample effectively. This latter arrangement gives the appearance of near simultaneity.

Thus, true simultaneous Doppler and imaging are not possible. The beginner should keep in mind that the maximum Doppler capabilities are available when in full Doppler mode, and maximum imaging capabilities are available when in full imaging mode.

The sample volume is really a three-dimensional, teardrop-shaped portion of the ultrasound beam (Fig. 3.6). Its volume varies with different Doppler machines, different size and frequency transducers, and different depths into the tissue. Its width is determined by the width of the ultrasound beam at the selected depth. Its length is determined by the length of each transmitted ultrasound pulse. Therefore, the farther into the heart the sample volume is moved, the larger it effectively becomes. This happens because the ultrasound beam diverges as it gets farther away from the transducer.

The main disadvantage of PW Doppler is its inability to accurately measure high blood flow velocities, such as may be encountered in certain types of

FIG. 3.6. The sample volume of pulsed wave Doppler is actually a three-dimensional volume that changes in size as its location relative to the transducer is changed. When placed in the far field, it becomes very large.

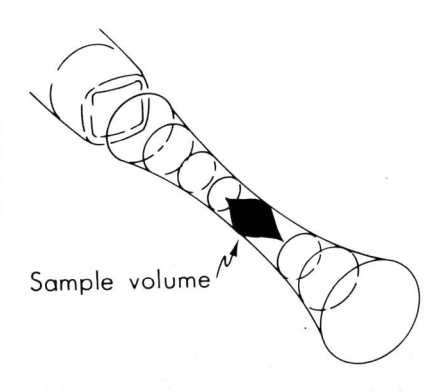

FIG. 3.7. Schematic rendering of the full spectral display of a high-velocity profile fully recorded by CW. The PW display is aliased, or cut off, and the top is placed at the bottom.

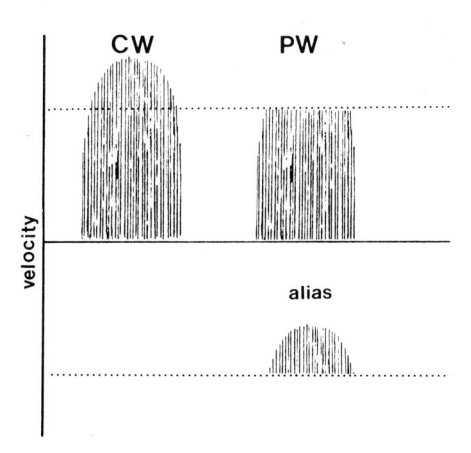

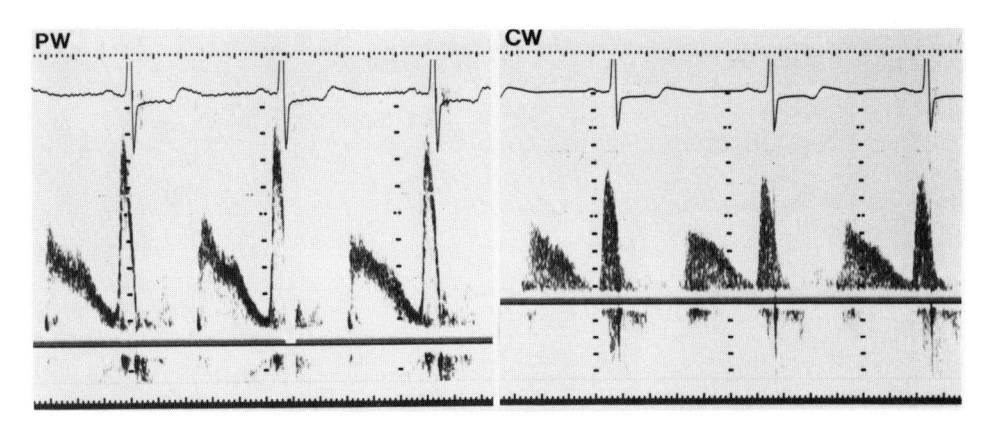

FIG. 3.8. Spectral displays of diastolic flow through the mitral orifice. The transducer is located at the apex, and diastolic flow is toward the transducer (positive). Note the laminar appearance of the PW display. The CW does not usually display the same laminar flow pattern since it receives flow information from all portions of the ultrasound beam.

32 BASIC DOPPLER ECHOCARDIOGRAPHY

TABLE 3.1 Comparison of Pulsed and Continuous Wave Techniques

	Range Resolution	Limitation on Maximum Velocity
Pulsed wave	Yes	Yes
Continuous wave	No	No

valvular and congenital heart disease. This limitation is technically known as "aliasing" and results in an inability of pulsed Doppler to faithfully record velocities above 1.5 to 2 m/sec, when the sample volume is located at standard ranges in the heart (Fig. 3.7). Aliasing is represented on the spectral trace as a cutoff of a given velocity with placement of the cut section in the opposite channel or reverse flow direction. Because aliasing is so common in disease states, it will be considered in detail in the next section.

The spectral outputs from PW and CW appear differently (Fig. 3.8). When there is no turbulence, PW will generally show a laminar (narrow band) spectral output. CW, on the other hand, rarely displays such a nice narrow band of flow velocities because all the various velocities encountered by the ultrasound beams are detected by CW.

It can be said roughly that when an operator wants to know where a specific area of abnormal flow is located that pulsed wave Doppler is indicated. When accurate measurement of elevated flow velocity is required, then continuous wave Doppler should be used. The various differences between pulsed and continuous wave Doppler are summarized in Table 3.1.

ALIASING

The aliasing phenomenon occurs when the abnormal velocity being studied exceeds the ability of the pulsed wave system to record it properly. Figure 3.9 shows a PW Doppler spectral tracing from an individual with aortic insufficiency with the transducer positioned at the apex. In this situation, abnormal diastolic flow is detected toward the transducer and recorded in a positive, or upward, direction. The system first detects a pulsed (and aliased) spectral profile. After the third beat, the system is switched into CW and the full profile is recognized. The aliased portion in the first three beats is cut off the top of the velocity spectrum and placed in the reverse channel, or below the baseline (arrow).

Figure 3.10 shows a similar phenomenon from another Doppler system where the full-spectral recording of aortic insufficiency is easily recorded in diastole by CW. Note that the baseline has been moved to the bottom of the recording paper. The right-hand panel demonstrates aliasing, and again the top of the diastolic velocity profile is cut off.

The phenomenon of aliasing is best explained using a simple example (Fig. 3.11). A mark is placed on a turning wheel, and the wheel rotates in a clockwise

PULSED AND CONTINUOUS WAVE DOPPLER   33

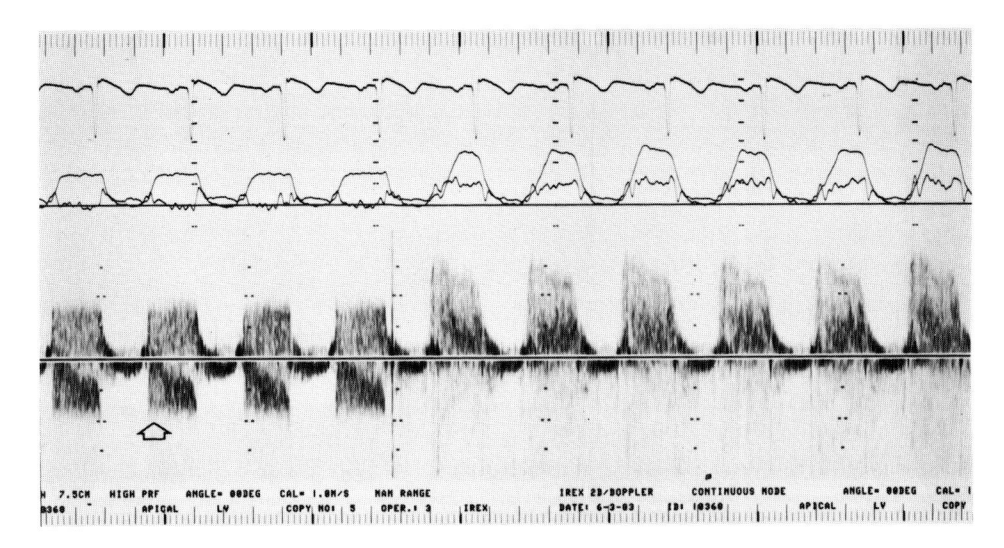

FIG. 3.9. Aliased spectral display of aortic insufficiency (arrow) in pulsed wave mode. After three beats the system is switched into continuous wave and the full profile is seen. The tracing was obtained from the ventricular apex, and the abnormal diastolic flow is toward the transducer. Note that in this system there is no automatic change in the velocity range calibration. Mean and maximum velocity analog tracings are shown above the full spectral display. The maximum velocity tracing corresponds to an envelope drawn aroung the full spectral display. The mean velocity tracing represents an average of all the velocities present. Note that both are significantly depressed when aliasing is present.

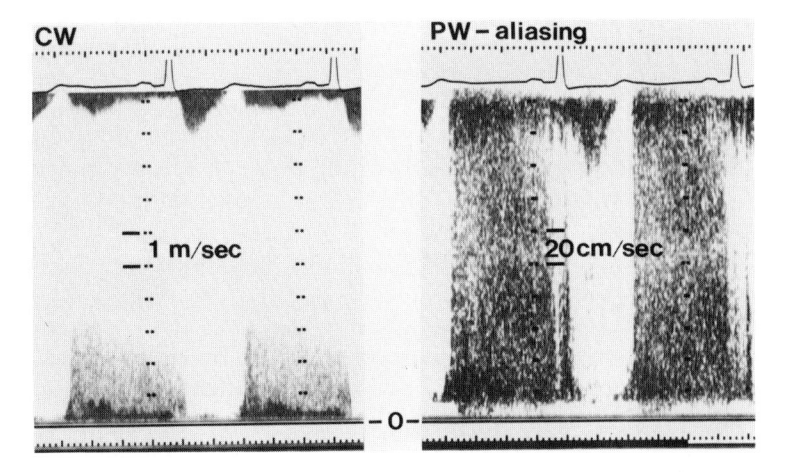

FIG. 3.10. The full abnormal flow velocity is displayed in CW mode. When switched into PW mode, aliasing occurs and the top of the profile appears cut off. The baseline, or zero shift, is at the bottom of the figure. Notice in this system there is an automatic shift in the calibration.

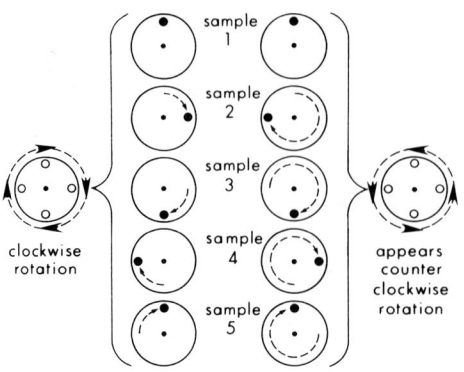

FIG. 3.11. Schematic representation of differing sampling rates of a mark on a turning wheel. The sequence in the left column is adequate to record the clockwise rotation, whereas the sequence in the right column is inadequate and shows the wheel rotating in an apparent counterclockwise fashion, resulting in aliasing. For details, see text.

fashion at a speed of one turn every 4 seconds. If the sample rate (or pulse repetition frequency) is one sample per second, the mark is recorded at each progressive 90° position. The final recording would then show the proper clockwise direction of motion of the wheel (left column).

If the sample rate (or pulse repetition frequency) is slowed to only one sample every 3 seconds, a strange phenomenon occurs (right column). Note that the mark is moving 180° between sampling times and that while actually turning clockwise the recording makes the wheel appear to be apparently be moving in the opposite, or counterclockwise, direction. This is also the reason why propellers and wagon wheels appear to go backward on movie film since the film frame rate is too slow to accurately keep up with these rapidly moving structures.

Nyquist Limit

The Nyquist limit defines when aliasing will occur using pulsed wave Doppler (Fig. 3.12). The Nyquist limit specifies that measurements of frequency shifts (and, thus, velocity) are accurate only if the pulse repetition frequency (PRF) is at least twice the maximum velocity (or Doppler shift frequency) encountered in the sample volume.

It is obviously desirable to use as high a pulse repetition frequency as possible for recording abnormally elevated velocity jets. The problem is that the maximum PRF is limited by the distance into the heart the sample volume is placed.

The closer the sample volume is located to the transducer, the higher the maximum PRF that can be used. Conversely, the farther the sample volume

$$\text{Nyquist limit} = \frac{\text{number pulses/sec}}{2}$$

FIG. 3.12. When the Nyquist limit is exceeded, aliasing occurs. The Nyquist limit depends on the depth into the tissues the sample volume is placed, as well as transducer frequency.

PULSED AND CONTINUOUS WAVE DOPPLER 35

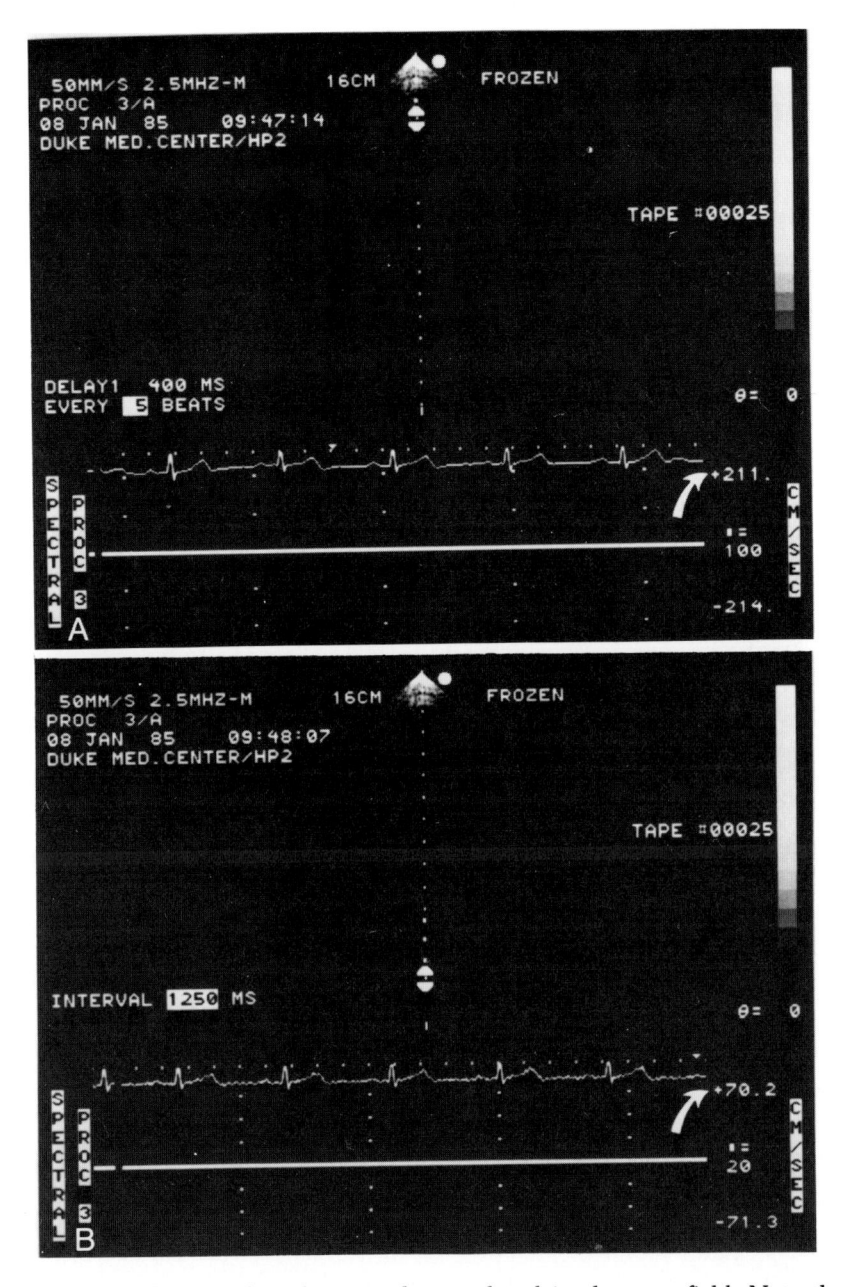

FIG. 3.13. (A) The sample volume is shown placed in the near field. Note that the velocity spectral display is able to accurately record velocities of approximately 211 cm/sec in either direction before aliasing would occur (curved arrow). (B) The sample volume is placed deeper into the two-dimensional display, and the Nyquist limit is accordingly reduced. In this case, the spectral velocity display is limited to only 70 cm/sec before aliasing would occur.

36 BASIC DOPPLER ECHOCARDIOGRAPHY

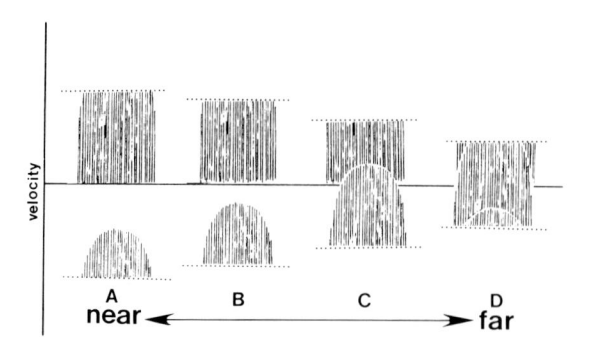

FIG. 3.14. Schematic drawing of the effect of a reduction in the Nyquist limit in pulsed wave echo when a high-velocity jet is encountered in the near field (A) or progressively deeper into the tissues (B, C, and D). Note the progressive and marked aliasing of the spectral signal the farther the jet is encountered away from the transducer.

is placed into the heart, the lower the maximum PRF becomes. This is true because the distance (and therefore pulse travel time) to and from the sample volume is much shorter in the near field and, therefore, pulse roundtrip transit time is much less when compared with greater distances. Figure 3.13 shows an example of the spectral velocity display with the sample volume located in the near field. The maximum velocity which can be recorded without aliasing is 2.11 m/sec in either direction (Fig. 3.13A, arrow). When the sample volume is positioned farther into the field, the maximum possible velocity in either direction is reduced to 0.702 m/sec (Fig. 3.13B, arrow).

Note that with the Doppler system used in the previous example, the scale of the spectral display automatically changes. In some systems, the scale is fixed and the size of the spectral tracing will alter. Figure 3.14 demonstrates mild aliasing when a high-velocity jet is in the near field (A). Progressively more severe aliasing with distortion of the full profile occurs if this same jet is encountered at progressively increasing distances from the transducer face (B, C, and D). At point D the aliased profile is so distorted as to be unrecognizable.

In a practical sense, the Nyquist limit is a descriptive term which specifies the maximum velocity that can be recorded without aliasing. This limit is controlled by two factors, depth into the tissue and transducer frequency.

When dealing with valvular heart disease, most abnormal jets exceed 1.5 to 2.0 m/sec and, therefore, beginning Doppler users should not expect to easily record the full flow profile of these abnormal jets using pulsed wave echocardiography. In fact, most beginners should simply attempt to recognize the presence of aliasing. As experience is acquired, it will become easier to identify an aliased signal.

The recognition of aliasing on the audio output is difficult without reference to the concomitant spectral display. If aliasing is severe, then the audio spectrum may sound broader than it really is, leading to an erroneous impression of turbulent flow. Also, aliasing will lead to flow erroneously assigned into the opposite channel so that it appears that there is flow both toward and away from the transducer.

The output from a mean velocity estimator when significant aliasing is present will show a large reduction in magnitude and often negative components with

FIG. 3.15. The relationship between the maximum possible velocities able to be recorded at any given range for a variety of transducer frequencies. Higher velocities can be recorded with lower-frequency transducers. This is a graphic representation of the Nyquist limit. On the Y axis, velocity has been substituted for Doppler shift frequency using the Doppler equation. (Courtesy Hewlett-Packard, Inc.)

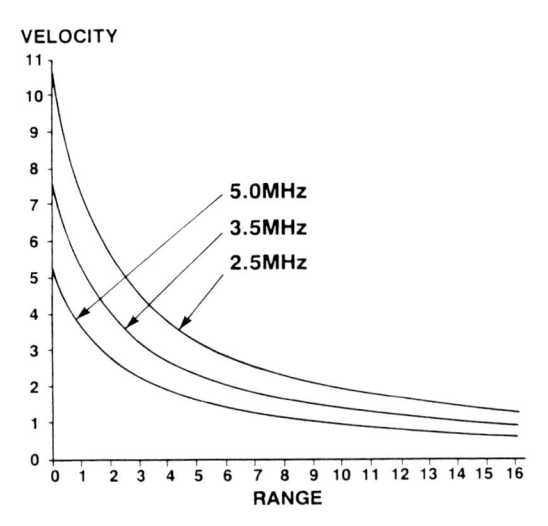

the mean falling below the zero line (Fig. 3.9). A maximum velocity estimator will also generate erroneously low estimates of peak velocity (Fig. 3.9).

Control of Aliasing

It is also important to realize that the maximum recordable velocities in any jet relate to the frequency of the PW transducer used (Fig. 3.15). Using a lower-frequency transducer increases the ability of a PW system to record high velocities. The main drawback of lowering the transducer frequency is a reduction in the signal-to-noise ratio of the resulting Doppler data (and thus the quality of the output). For this reason, most standard pulsed Doppler systems operate at approximately 2.5 MHz. Table 3.2 shows the differing velocities (or Nyquist limits) associated with different frequency transducers and varying depths. Based on these data, it is clear that if aliasing is encountered with a 5-MHz transducer at a given depth, use of a lower-frequency transducer may allow the operator to record the entire profile without distortion.

The second, and most practical, method to overcome aliasing is to take advan-

TABLE 3.2 Maximum Doppler Velocities (cm/sec)

	Transducer Frequency		
Depth (cm)	2.5 MHz	3.5 MHz	5 MHz
4	382	273	191
8	231	165	116
12	166	119	83
16	129	92	65

Note: Values are for HP 77020 Doppler Imaging System using zero baseline shift.
Source: Data supplied courtesy Hewlett-Packard, Inc.

38 BASIC DOPPLER ECHOCARDIOGRAPHY

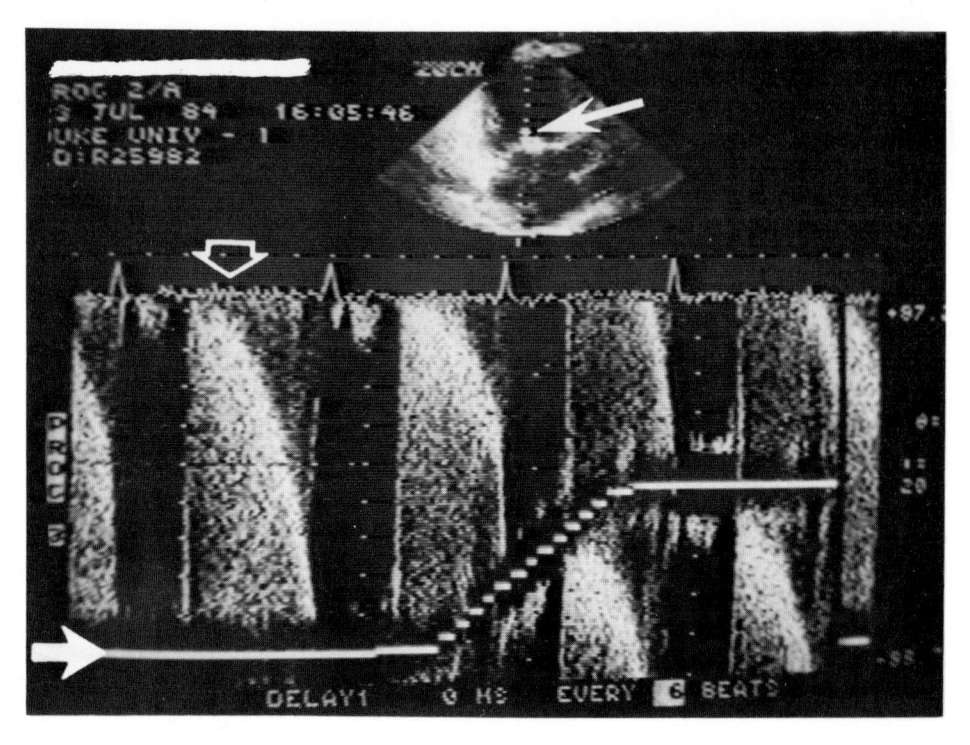

FIG. 3.16. With the transducer at the apex and the sample volume (top arrow) located just below the aortic root, the abnormal diastolic flow of aortic insufficiency is recorded as flow toward the transducer. Note the baseline (solid arrow, bottom) is located at the bottom of the trace, and almost all of the abnormal profile is recorded (open arrow). When the baseline is shifted upward to the center, severe aliasing occurs. Moving the baseline up or down will help somewhat in overcoming aliasing by using the opposite channel.

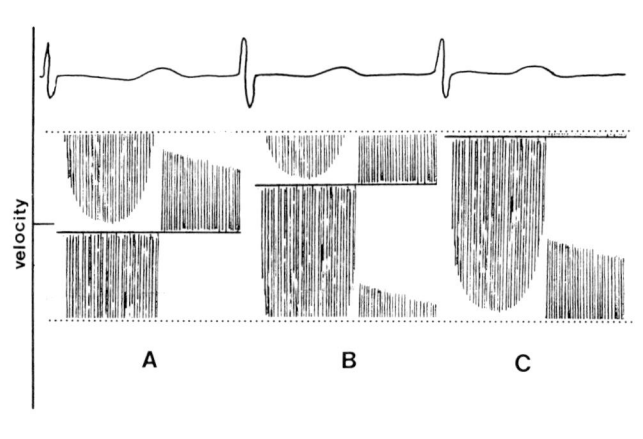

FIG. 3.17. Schematic diagram showing the effect of baseline movement on an aliased PW velocity spectral recording of bidirectional jets toward and away from the transducer. Flow away from the transducer is aliased in A. Progressive movement of the baseline upward first causes both signals to be aliased in B, whereas movement of the baseline all the way to the top (C) shows the full profile of both.

tage of the range of velocity available in the opposite channel by moving the baseline. Figure 3.16 shows almost the entire profile of an aortic insufficiency jet when the baseline is at the bottom of the display. In the left portion of this figure, the entire display represents flow toward the transducer. As the baseline is moved upward to the center of the display, the top of the spectral profile is aliased to the opposite channel.

Additional use of the baseline movement is shown in the schematic diagram in Fig. 3.17. Here the baseline is progressively raised to expose the full profiles of both flow jets. Aliasing occurs in this instance, but the display is made more identifiable by the operator. This baseline control may be called "zero shift" or "zero off-set" on some systems. Note that use of the baseline shift control as demonstrated in Figs. 3.16 and 3.17 doubles the Nyquist limit at any given depth.

High PRF Doppler

It seems reasonable that if the problem of aliasing is caused by an insufficiently high PRF, the way to reduce the problem is to find some method of increasing

FIG. 3.18. Conventional PW Doppler transmits a pulse and then waits for it to be received from a jet 8 cm into the tissues. The spectral signal from the high-speed jet is severely aliased (bottom left). High PRF PW Doppler uses higher sampling (or pulsing) rates and has the ability to record higher velocities without aliasing (lower right). The price of high PRF Doppler is that velocity data are also recorded from other depths (2, 4, and 6 cm) and are displayed together in the final Doppler output.

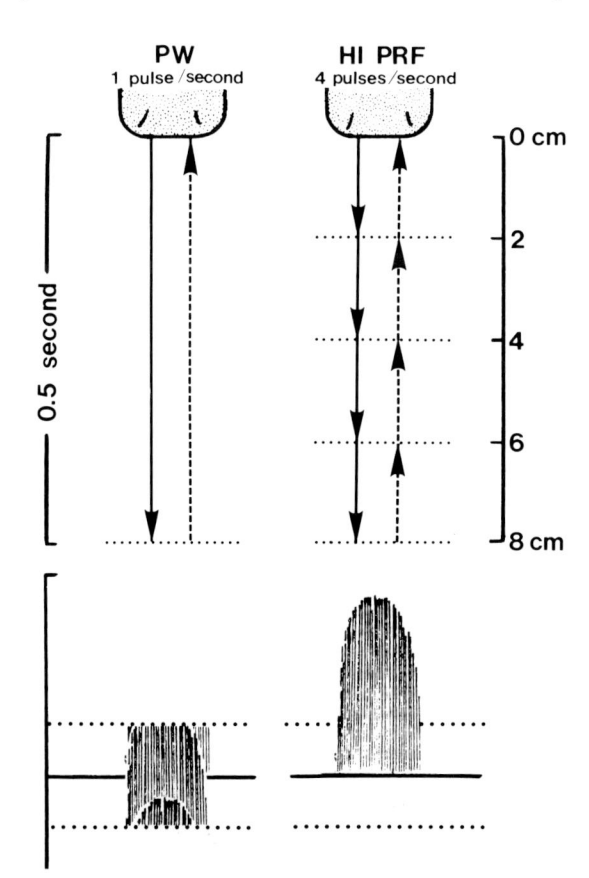

the PRF. Recently, some pulsed Doppler systems have been introduced which allow the operator to select a PRF above the Nyquist limit and thereby reduce aliasing. High PRF Doppler can use multiples of the PRF corresponding to the Nyquist limit at a given depth.

The basic principle of the so-called high PRF Doppler is illustrated in Fig. 3.18. In this example a given high velocity is located 8 cm into the body. If the pulse transit time to the jet and then back to the transducer is 1 second then the PRF is one pulse per second. Because the velocity being sampled exceeds the Nyquist limit (as discussed previously), aliasing is seen in the spectral display. High PRF systems emit multiple pulses without waiting for the original one to be received. In this example four pulses are emitted and received per second. This results in a fourfold increase in PRF and a spectral display that is not aliased.

The problem with this approach is that some of the range selectivity used in precisely locating the sample volume is relinquished. As this pulsing sequence is carried on repeatedly, some data are returned to the transducer from 8 cm simultaneously as data from 6, 4, and 2 cm. If other significant Doppler data were located at any one of these ranges, the operator would not be able to tell where the high-velocity jet of interest was located, as data from all these volumes are added together in the final output. This results in what is called "range ambiguity." The higher the PRF generated, the worse the ability to discriminate in range becomes.

This method of increasing the PRF for the aquisition of high-velocity data has been described as programming the machine to "think" that the high-velocity jet is much closer to the transducer than it really is. In reality, the machine knows exactly what it is doing, and the beginning operator is the one that is fooled.

With proper operator recognition of the range ambiguity created, high PRF Doppler can be a valuable addition to the Doppler laboratory. Early reports for the use of this approach for successfully extending the velocity measurement capability of pulse wave Doppler have been quite favorable. The ability to use some visual guidance and acquire higher velocities is obviously attractive.

When using the high PRF mode, it is best to first locate the high-velocity jet or turbulence using standard single-gate PW Doppler, and to ensure the absence of other areas of turbulence along the path of the ultrasound beam. The high PRF mode can then be used to record the unaliased Doppler signal.

COLOR FLOW MAPPING

Recent advances in technology allow the use of multiple complex-gating routines to display flow information as an overlay on the two-dimensional display. Although high PRF Doppler also uses multiple gates, it should not be confused with these "multigated" PW Doppler devices which use many more range gates (hundreds) to provide simultaneous information about flow in multiple adjacent areas of the heart or blood vessels. This latter type of multigated Doppler is not concerned with overcoming aliasing but with presenting a profile of flow or velocity characteristics along the course of the ultrasound beam while maintaining depth discrimination. Some of these systems are able to overlay the two-dimensional image with flow information coded in color instead of standard gray scale. This has the effect of "seeing" the flow through the heart on the two-dimensional image. Such systems are only now becoming available, and experience with them is still limited.

THE BERNOULLI EQUATION

There is clear justification for concern over accurate recording of very high-velocity jets within the heart. As will be discussed in more detail later, the presence of an obstruction to flow, such as aortic stenosis, will result in a significant increase in velocity across the aortic valve in systole. In practice, these jets attain speeds of up to 5 or 6 m/sec.

The Bernoulli equation is a complex formula that relates the pressure drop (or gradient) across an obstruction to many factors, as is seen in Fig. 3.19. For practical use in Doppler echocardiography this formula has been simplified to:

$$p_1 - p_2 = 4v^2$$

As we shall see in later chapters, Doppler recordings of velocity may, in certain situations, be used to estimate pressure gradients within the heart. When used for this purpose, it is important to keep in mind that the angle the Doppler beam is incident to any given jet may not be known since these examinations are frequently done blindly by CW. In these cases the operator always tries to orient a beam as parallel to flow as possible so that the full velocity recording is obtained (this assumes $\cos \theta = 1$).

Note that the full Bernoulli equation requires velocity data from below (V_1) and above (V_2) any given obstruction. Since V_1 is usually much smaller than V_2 (Fig. 3.20), it can usually be ignored in the calculation of a pressure gradient.

In the example cited, the peak velocity is approximately 3.5 m/sec, and this would correspond to an aortic gradient of 48 mmHg by the simplified Bernoulli equation. Obviously, faithful recording of abnormal velocities has great importance, not only for clear identification and recognition of abnormal profiles but also for quantitative purposes.

FIG. 3.19. The Bernoulli equation is a complex formula that may be reduced to its simplest expression.

$$p_1 - p_2 = 1/2\, \rho(v_2^2 - v_1^2) + \rho \int_1^2 \frac{d\vec{v}}{dt} d\vec{s} + R(\vec{v})$$

convective acceleration | flow acceleration | viscous friction

$$p_1 - p_2 \approx 4v^2$$

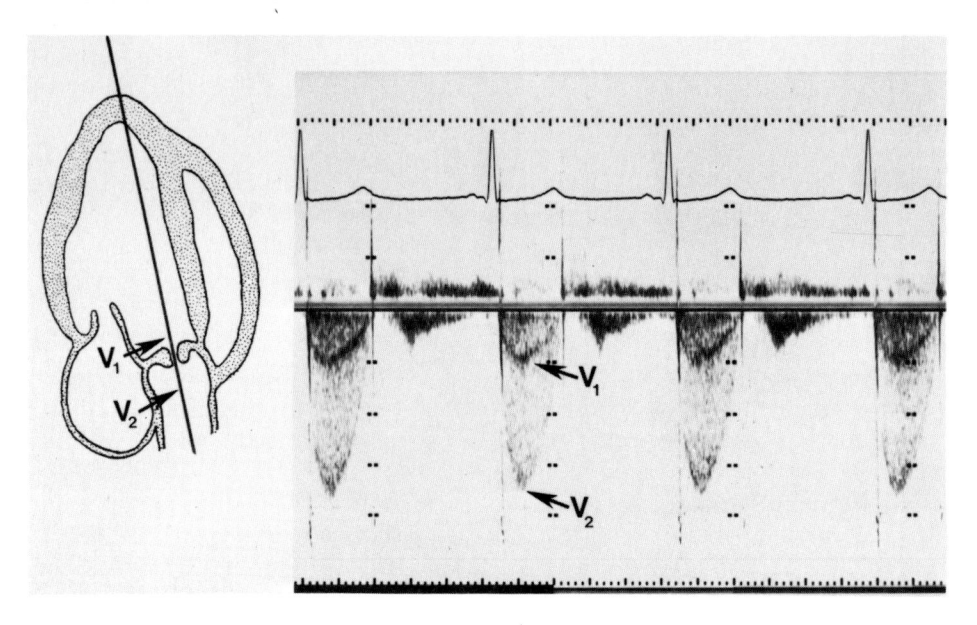

FIG. 3.20. An example of a CW spectral recording of aortic stenosis. There is a given velocity (V_1) on the ventricular side of the valve that is accelerated (V_2) as blood is ejected through the stenotic orifice. The full Bernoulli equation (Fig. 3.19) requires both velocities to be measured. Since V_1 is usually much smaller than V_2 and is rarely recorded, it is ignored in the simplified Bernoulli equation.

SYSTEM DISPLAY CAPABILITIES

All of the factors considered in this chapter may be brought together in a discussion of the various display functions of a combined Doppler imaging system. A regular two-dimensional echocardiographic examination may be conducted in real-time and operating at full frame-rate capabilities (Fig. 3.21). When the pulsed Doppler is switched on, the cursor and sample volume indicator appear along with a video picture of the spectral display, and the system goes into an automatic gating mode that, in this case, updates the two-dimensional image single frame every four beats (Fig. 3.22). Notice the location of the sample volume in the apical four-chamber view just below the aortic root. The spectral display in this image shows aortic insufficiency in diastole that is obviously aliased (arrow). The scale factors at the right of the spectral display indicate that the maximum velocity able to be detected before aliasing occurs is only around 83 cm/sec.

A hard-copy printout of the PW spectral recording is usually available on most machines from of a graphic recorder (Fig. 3.23). Again, note the aliasing of the high-velocity aortic insufficiency. The blanks in the spectral tracing indicate the time where the image was updated.

If a continuous-wave examination is then performed, the video screen on the system just shows the CW-mode spectral display since no imaging is possi-

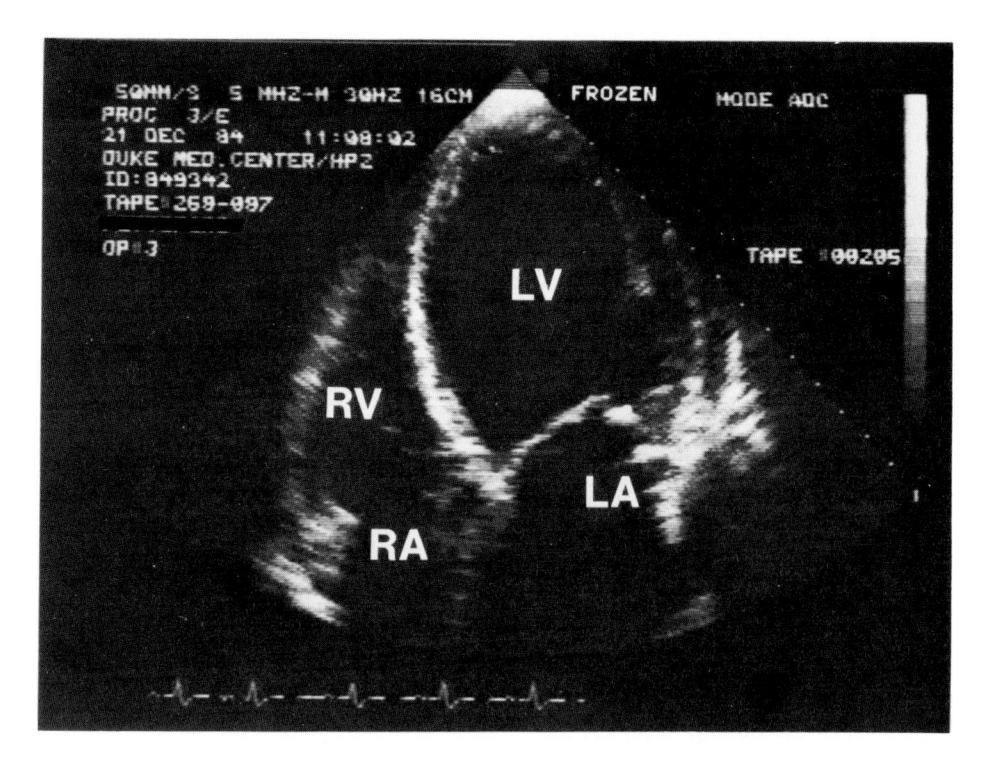

FIG. 3.21. Apical four-chamber view of a patient with aortic insufficiency. When in the full two-dimensional imaging mode, there is no time for Doppler.

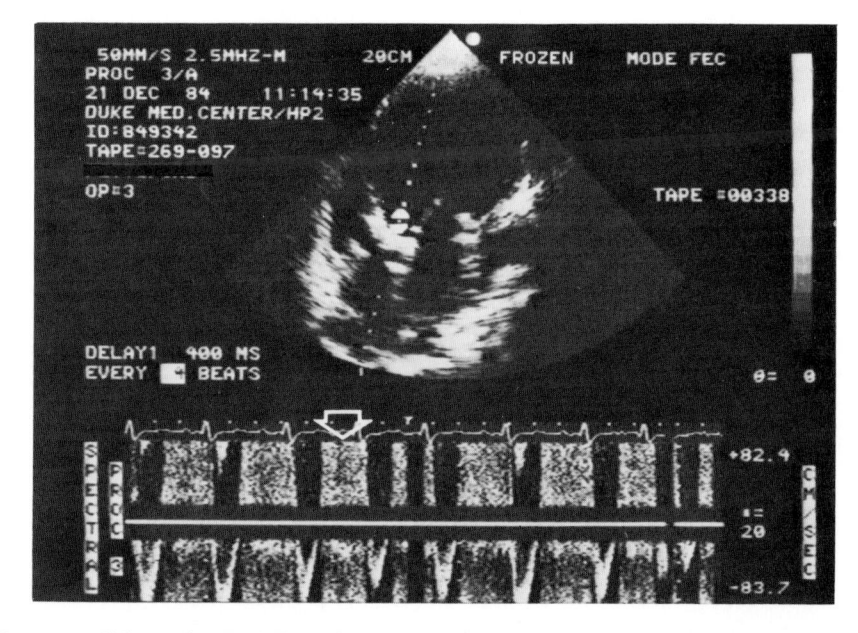

FIG. 3.22. When the PW Doppler is turned on and the sample volume positioned just below the aortic valve, the two-dimensional image is automatically gated to provide enough time for Doppler sampling. Aortic insufficiency is encountered and severe aliasing is noted (arrow).

44 BASIC DOPPLER ECHOCARDIOGRAPHY

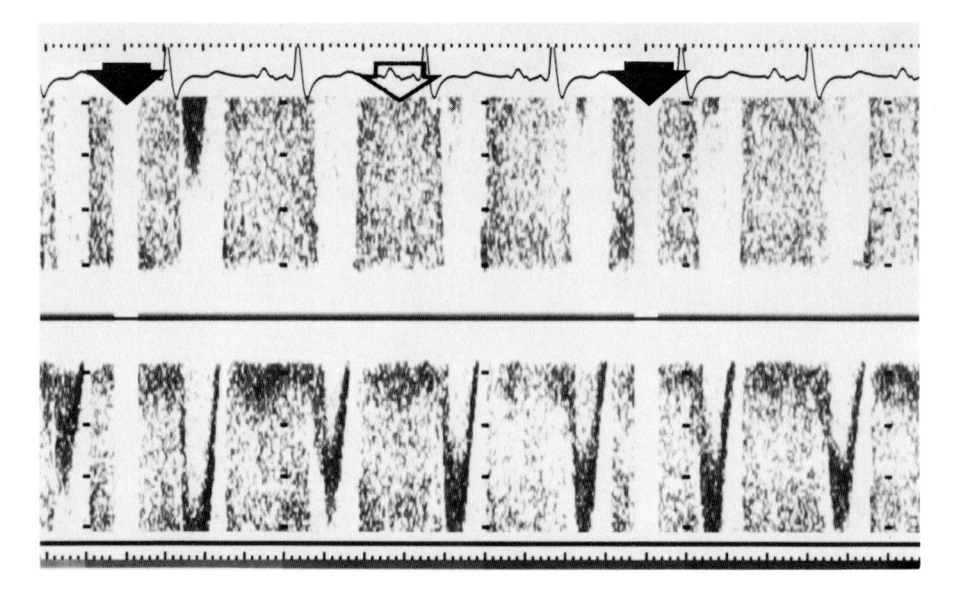

FIG. 3.23. Hard-copy paper recording of the aliased (open arrow) aortic insufficiency spectral recording. Note the blanks in the spectral tracing where the two-dimensional image was updated (closed arrows).

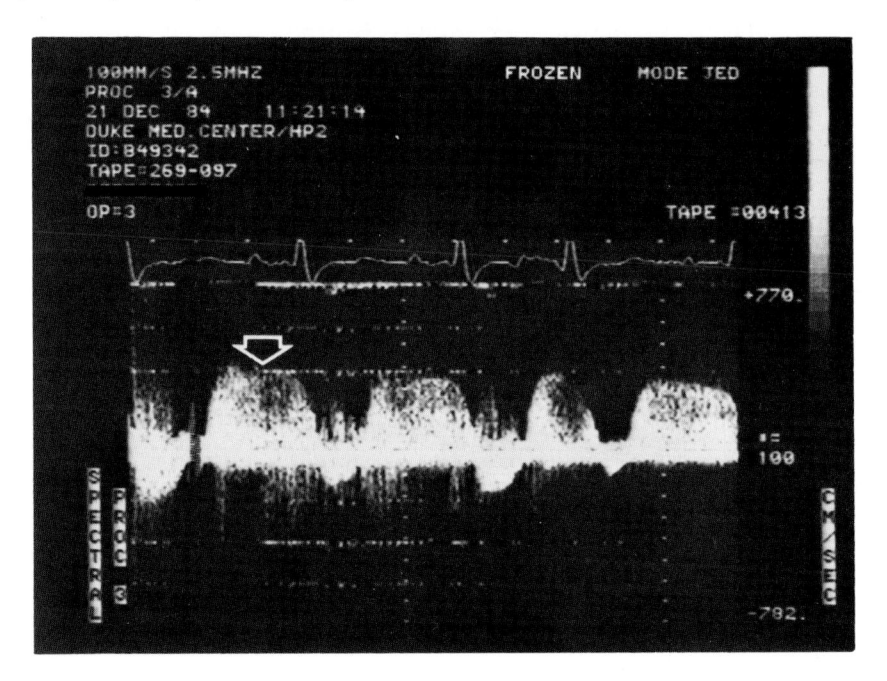

FIG. 3.24. Full-spectrum recording of the aortic insufficiency jet (open arrow) as it appears on the system video screen with the CW transducer positioned at the apical window. Note the range in the spectrum is markedly increased from that seen in PW in Fig. 3.22. No two-dimensional image is possible when operating in full CW mode.

PULSED AND CONTINUOUS WAVE DOPPLER   45

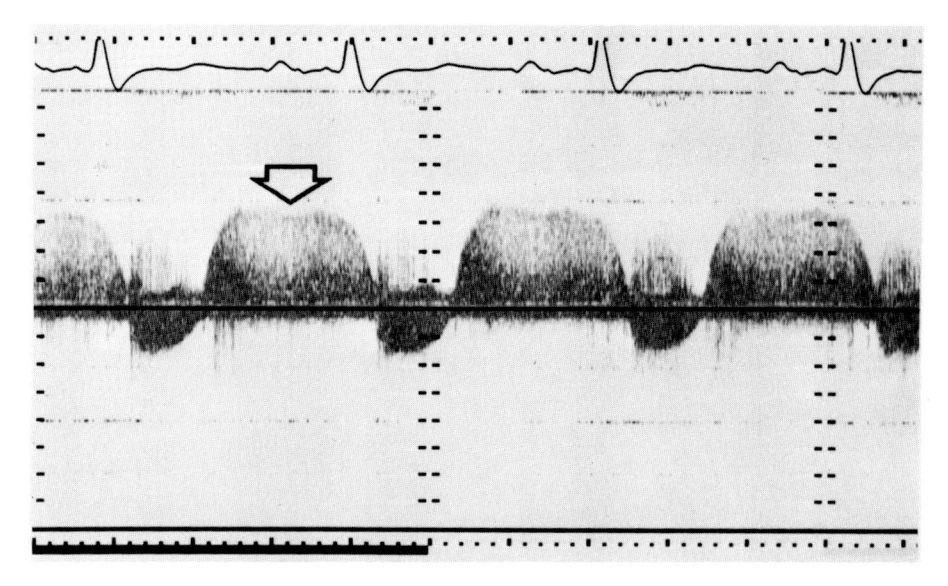

FIG. 3.25. Hard-copy paper recording of the CW spectral trace of aortic insufficiency (arrow). Scale marks are 1 m/sec.

ble in this mode. With the transducer at the apex of the left ventricle, the full profile of the aortic insufficiency is seen as a positive velocity shift on the spectral display (Fig. 3.24). Notice that in this mode it is possible to detect velocities of over 750 cm/sec in either direction. As before, hard copy of the spectral tracing is possible by means of the graphic recorder (Fig. 3.25).

From this series of figures, the uses of PW and CW Doppler become more evident. When using pulsed Doppler, aliasing of abnormal jets is generally accepted in order to gain depth and location discrimination. When a full-velocity spectrum is desired, continuous wave must be used to record the high velocities usually encountered in abnormal jets. The use of CW requires the sacrifice of depth and location information.

FIG. 3.26. Examples of the schematic illustration used throughout much of this text. CW is represented as a solid line, and PW is represented as a dashed line. The PW sample volume is a solid dot (arrow).

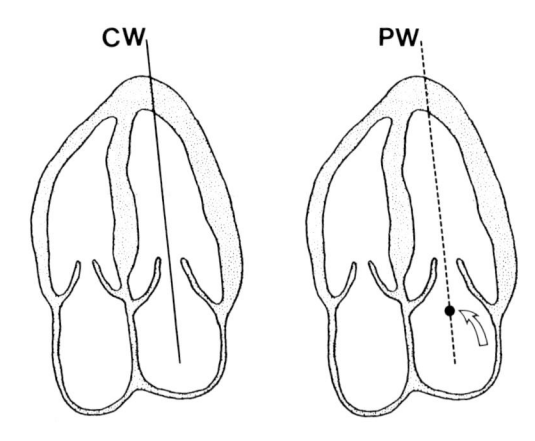

In many of the following chapters of this volume we have attempted to provide graphic orientation of the heart using familiar two-dimensional image views. The standard style of these illustrations is indicated in Fig. 3.26. The path of the CW beam is indicated by a solid line, and the path of the PW beam is indicated by a dashed line with a solid dot showing the position of the sample volume.

4 Use of the Doppler Controls

DAVID ADAMS
DANIEL B. MARK
JOSEPH KISSLO

This chapter deals with the controls of the Doppler machine and will discuss how the adjustment of these controls can increase or decrease the quality of the Doppler recordings. It is our experience that beginning users of Doppler echocardiographic systems are frequently intimidated by the many controls on a Doppler machine. The main point of this chapter is that there are relatively few controls of true importance.

We have attempted to depict all the important controls for a continuous wave and pulsed wave Doppler examination of the heart in (Fig. 4.1). The schematic drawing of the control panel is generic, and Doppler users should be able to find these controls on their system by the same or a similar name.

In this basic model, the eight controls can be divided into three categories. First is the group of controls that influence the quality of the Doppler recording (Doppler gain, gray scale, and wall filter). This group is of importance in both continuous wave and pulsed wave examinations. Second are the controls that change the appearance of the graphic display (scale factor and baseline position). These are also of importance for both continuous wave and pulsed wave examinations. The third group are of use *only* for pulsed wave examinations since they relate to the sample volume (cursor, sample depth, and angle).

OBTAINING THE DOPPLER SIGNAL

It is important for the Doppler novice to keep clearly in mind the differences between continuous wave and pulsed wave Doppler when learning how to use a system (see Chapter 3). Continuous wave examinations are usually conducted with a "stand-alone" transducer (Fig. 4.2) and without benefit of a two-dimensional image to guide the operator, but they have the advantage of allowing the operator to accurately record the high velocities seen in valvular heart disease.

48 BASIC DOPPLER ECHOCARDIOGRAPHY

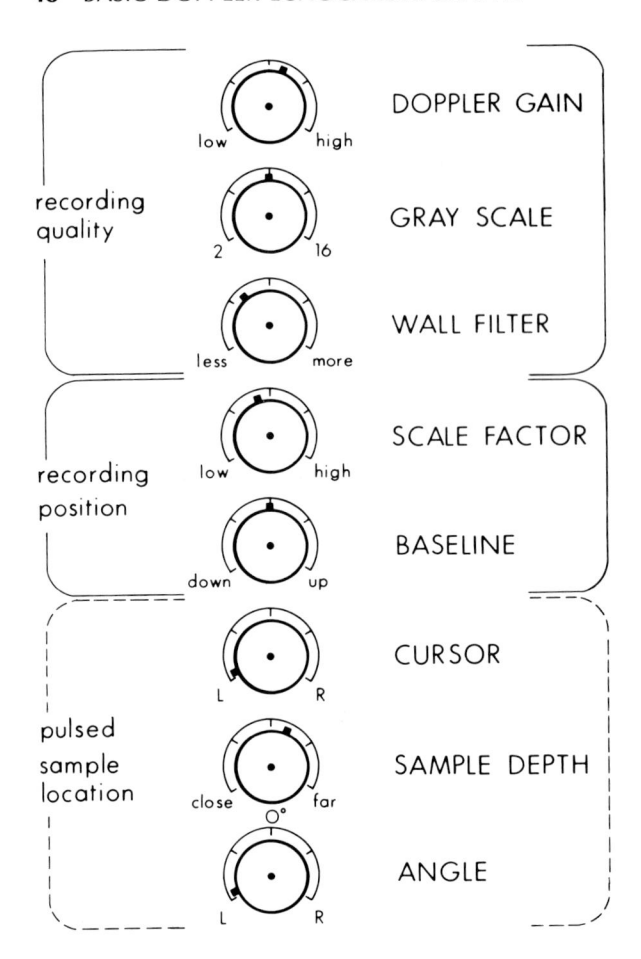

FIG. 4.1. Mock Doppler control panel showing the most common CW and PW Doppler controls. Almost every Doppler system with pulsed and continuous wave capabilities will contain these controls.

Pulsed wave examinations are usually conducted with the same transducer that is used for two-dimensional imaging (Fig. 4.3), and have the advantage of allowing the operator to see where the sample volume is positioned in relation to the actual heart image. The disadvantage of this operating mode is that the high-pulse repetition rates necessary for faithful recording of the full profile of abnormal velocities cannot be achieved without aliasing.

Not all Doppler systems have both continuous wave and pulsed wave capabilities, but we think that Doppler echocardiography is most useful when both capabilities are present. Although not pictured on our generic panel, Doppler instruments capable of both modes will have some control that allows the operator to switch between continuous and pulsed modes.

The following explanations of the Doppler controls apply to both operating modes, and beginners will generally find it helpful to familiarize themselves with the controls by performing initial self-examinations. For the beginning continuous wave self-examination, the system should be switched into this operating mode and the transducer positioned in the suprasternal notch. Slight

USE OF THE DOPPLER CONTROLS   49

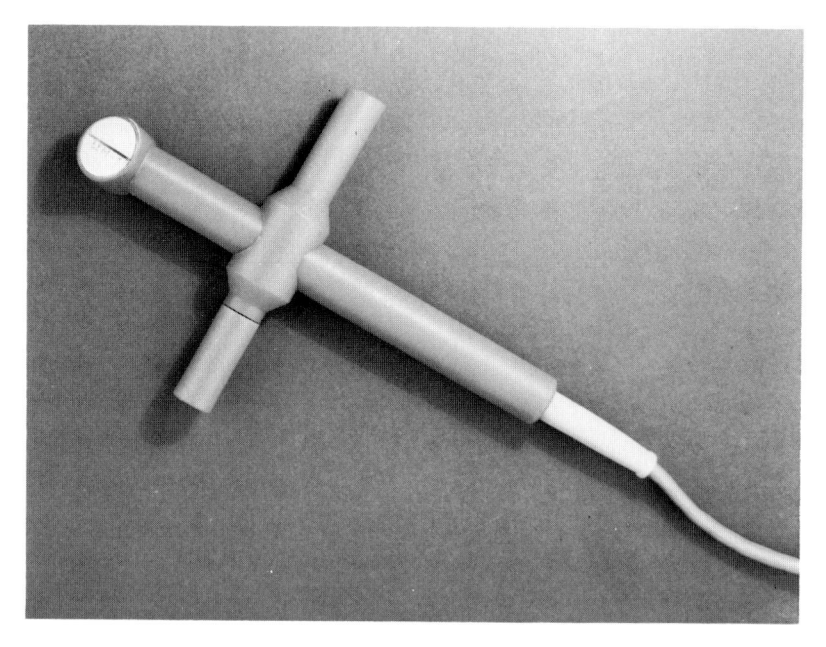

FIG. 4.2. The CW transducer. Note its small size and the two elements for simultaneous transmission and reception of Doppler signals.

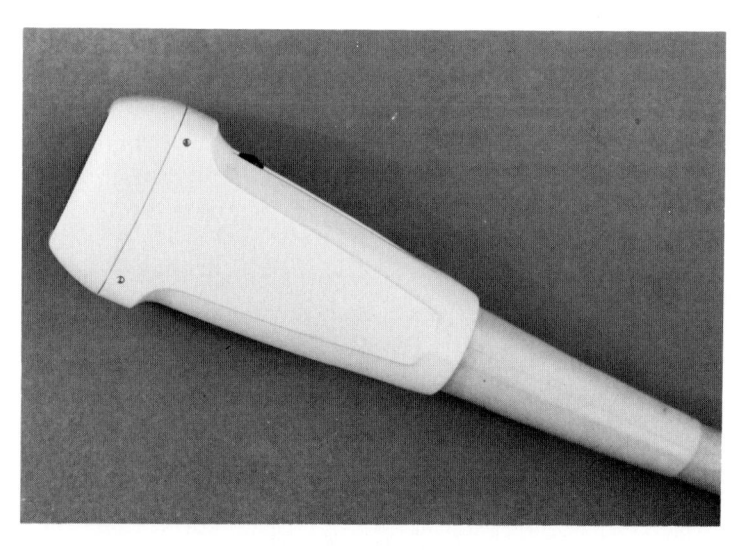

FIG. 4.3. A standard two-dimensional echocardiographic transducer. Many phased-array and mechanical systems have some ability for pulsed Doppler examinations.

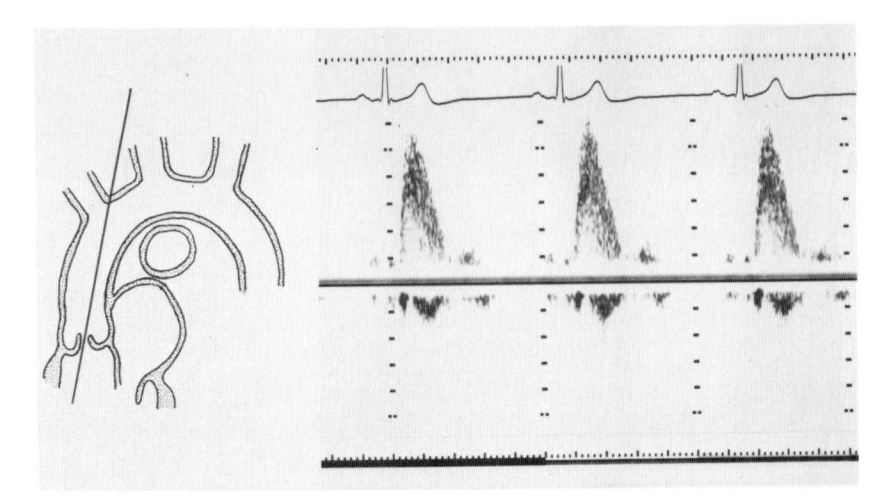

FIG. 4.4. CW spectral velocity trace from the suprasternal notch encountering the systolic flow toward the transducer.

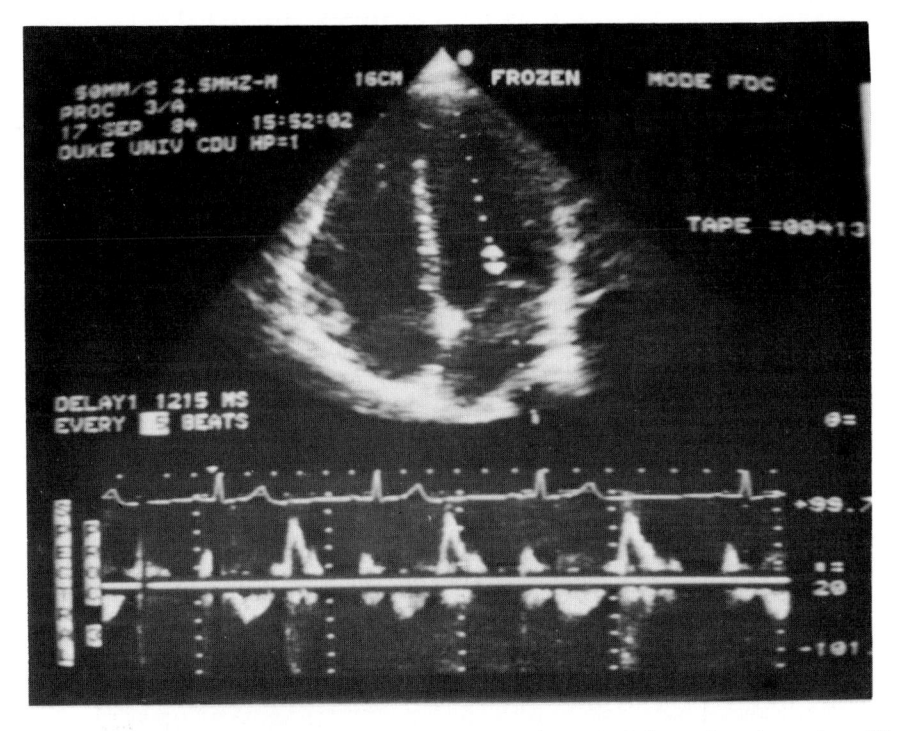

FIG. 4.5. Two-dimensional stop-frame image in the apical four-chamber view. The pulsed sample volume is located just on the ventricular side of the mitral valve. The spectral recording shows normal diastolic flow toward the transducer.

angulation anteriorly and toward the right hip will usually produce some evidence of aortic systolic flow toward the transducer (Fig. 4.4).

For the initial pulsed wave examination, the system should be switched into pulsed mode and the transducer positioned at the apical window with the sample volume positioned in front of the mitral valve (Fig. 4.5). In either mode, the gain control should first be adjusted to produce some Doppler flow signal.

DOPPLER GAIN

Beginners should start with the overall Doppler gain control (Fig. 4.1). Rotating between higher and lower settings will alter the strength of the Doppler signals from the audible output and will be perceived by the operator as a change in the volume of the audio output. Fig. 4.6 shows the range in appearance of the velocity spectral recording for excessively high-, correct-, and low-gain settings.

As with any ultrasound system, it is prudent to use the lowest-gain or power setting that allows the recording of adequate signals. More detailed examination of the recording in Fig. 4.6 shows a normal aortic spectral trace obtained from the suprasternal window. Systolic flow velocity toward the transducer is depicted as an upward profile and is laminar in appearance. The first two profiles show a gain setting that is too high. This results in excessive background noise that makes identification of the clear outline of systolic flow difficult and produces an overflow in the opposite channel represented below the baseline (this is called "mirroring" or "crosstalk"). The third profile (arrow) is set at an optimal-gain setting and displays a clear systolic envelope of flow with a minimum of background noise; the fourth profile demonstrates an incomplete spectrum due to an improperly low-gain setting.

The practical use of correct-gain setting is again shown in Fig. 4.7. In this continuous wave examination from the ventricular apex, tricuspid insufficiency is encountered as a systolic movement of the velocity spectrum away from the transducer. In the complexes without adequate gain, the full-velocity profile is not well seen (open arrows). It is not until the gain is increased to an adequate level that true spectral broadening and the true peak velocity are noted. A beginning operator should first detect some flow signal and then run through all of the possible gain settings to become familiar with the effect of too much or too little gain.

GRAY SCALE

The gray scale control provides a means of altering the various ranges of gray (from white to black) on the spectral display. Altering the position of this control has no effect on the audio output of the Doppler system. Different Doppler instruments have from two to more than eight different ranges of gray scale display.

Figure 4.8 demonstrates the use of this control at eight different gray scale

(Text continues on p. 54.)

52   BASIC DOPPLER ECHOCARDIOGRAPHY

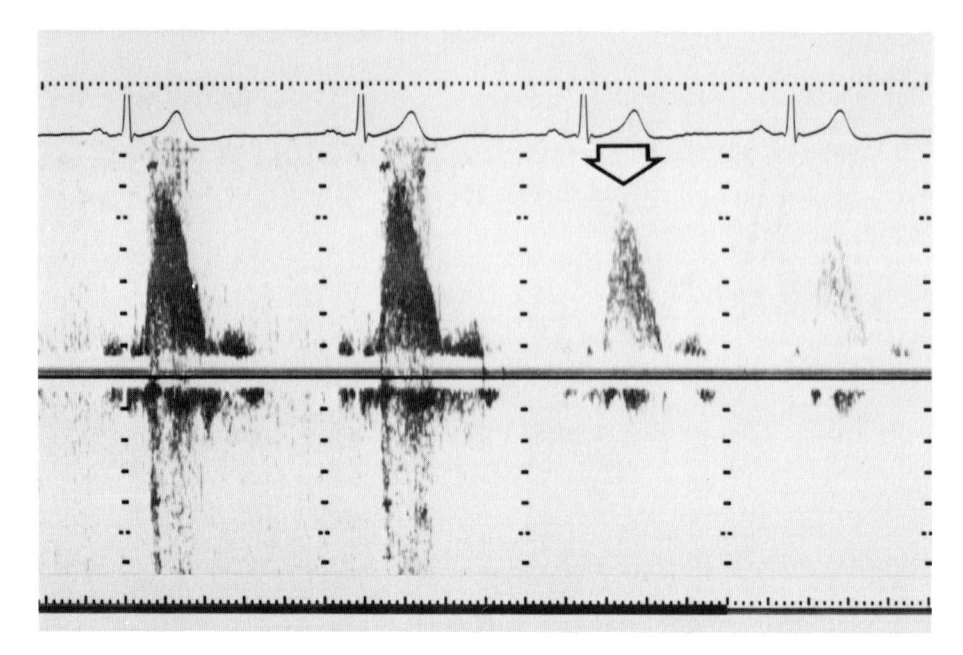

FIG. 4.6. Normal aortic spectral trace from the suprasternal window; arrow points to spectral trace with proper gain settings. Tracings on the left have too much gain whereas the trace on the right has too little.

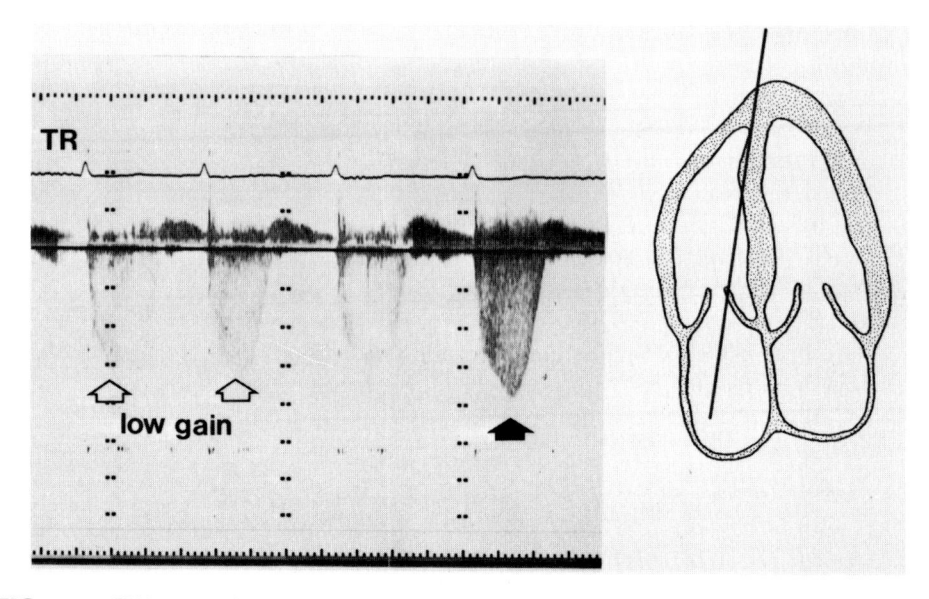

FIG. 4.7. CW spectral velocity trace of tricuspid insufficiency from a transducer located in the apical window. Note the low gain (open arrows) that fails to display the full-spectral profile. Proper gain is at the right (closed arrow), and spectral broadening is observed.

USE OF THE DOPPLER CONTROLS   53

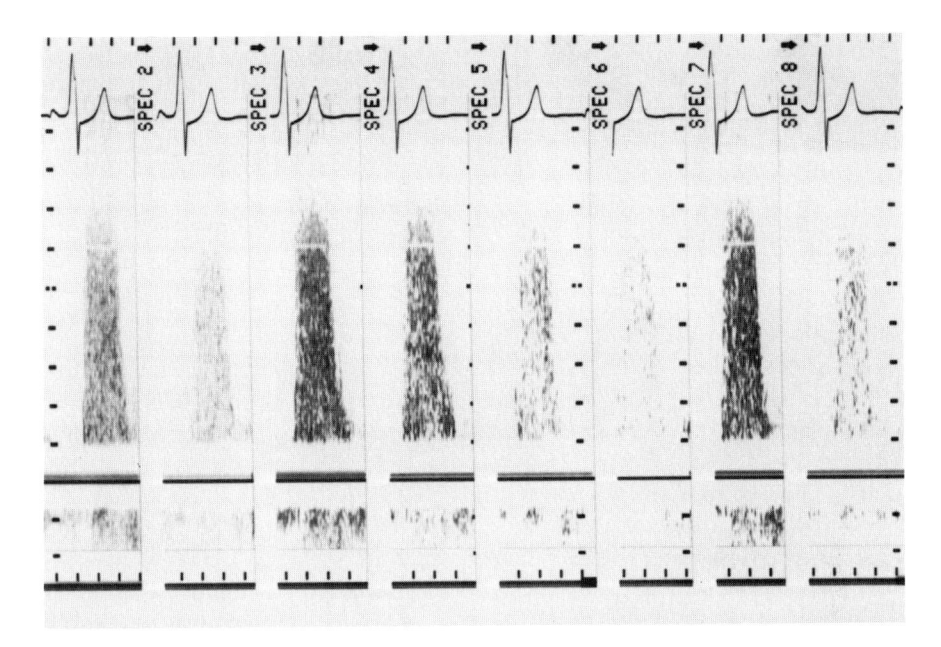

FIG. 4.8. A CW spectral velocity recording of eight different gray scale settings. The eight beats are continuous as the gray scale setting was changed.

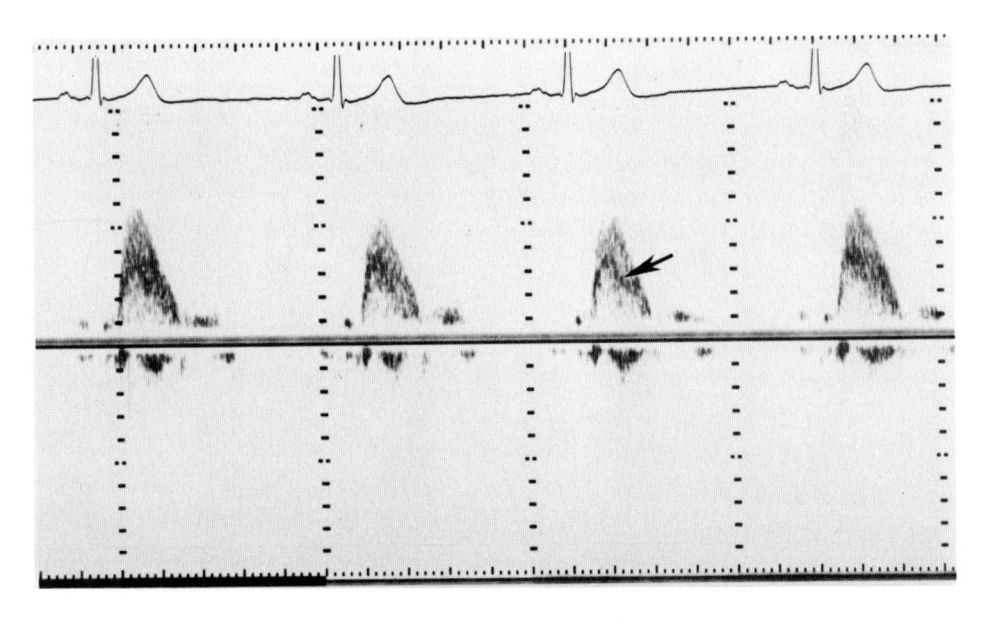

FIG. 4.9. PW spectral recording of systolic flow in the ascending aorta. The transducer was in the suprasternal window. Note the gray scale in the spectral display.

54 BASIC DOPPLER ECHOCARDIOGRAPHY

settings. This recording was produced from the suprasternal notch and shows eight consecutive beats, each with a different gray scale setting. Beginners should practice moving through all available gray scale settings of their Doppler instrument during the learning phase, as the effect of this control is frequently difficult to understand.

Ideally, it is desirable to have as many shades of gray as possible in the display. Careful inspection of Fig. 4.8 reveals that the full range of spectral velocities is not present in the first, second, fifth, sixth, and eighth profiles. Adequate gray scale is seen in the third, fourth, and seventh profiles.

Since the concentration of velocities within the spectral trace are displayed in varying intensities of gray (Fig. 4.9), complete operator understanding of this control is necessary. Lighter shades of gray indicate that there are few red cells moving at that velocity in comparison with darker shades of gray or black. These indicate that many more red cells are moving at the given velocity. Thus, when laminar flow is detected and all the red cells are accelerating, peaking, and decelerating at the same velocity, a very clean spectral tracing is produced with a central band of very dark gray (arrow).

When turbulence is encountered, there are many red cells moving at many different velocities, and the resulting spectral velocity recording is altered. In this case there is a wide range of differing shades of gray all over the spectral trace (Fig. 4.7, black arrow). This is usually referred to as spectral broadening.

The problem with leaving the gray scale control at the maximum setting is that a light level of gray is assigned to low-amplitude background noise in the spectral trace (Fig. 4.10). Thus, there must be a balanced adjustment between the gain control and the gray scale control so that the cleanest spectral trace with the most shades of gray is displayed.

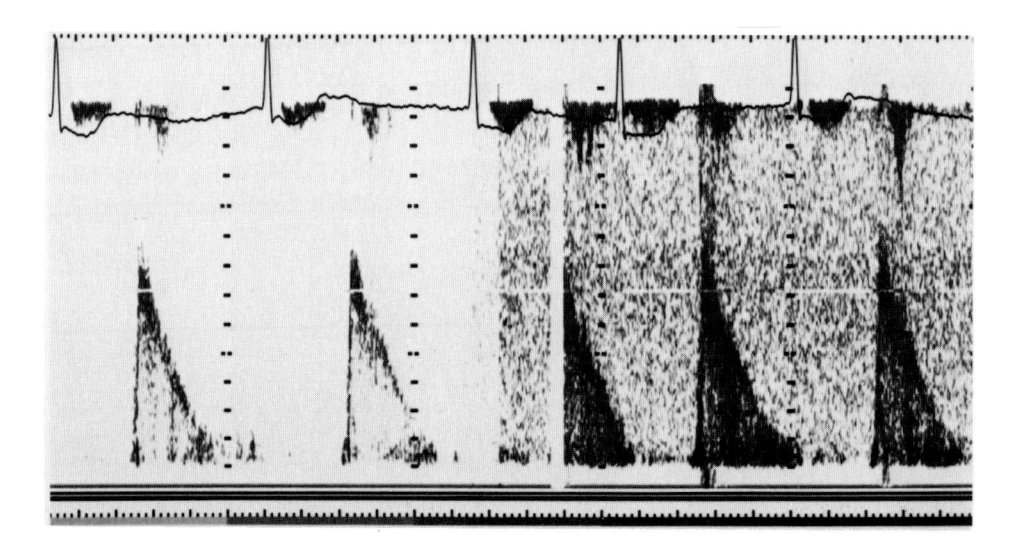

FIG. 4.10. PW spectral recording of early mitral diastolic flow from the apical window. Improper gray scale setting on the right-hand side brings up background noise.

WALL FILTER

The low frequency (velocity) of heart wall motion is easily detected by all Doppler instruments and commonly interferes with clear recording of blood flow profiles. Movement of the heart walls produces easily heard, low-pitched "clunking" sounds in the audio output. These may be so loud as to obscure the higher-frequency flow signals desired.

Thus, all Doppler systems have a variable wall filter control that sets the threshold below which low-frequency signals are removed from the display. Fig. 4.11 shows improper wall filter settings in a patient with aortic stenosis. The arrows point to where there is no filtering of the lower frequencies. Since we are mainly interested in these high-frequency flow signals, it is best to set the wall filter so that most, if not all, the lower-frequency signals are attenuated. For most Doppler echocardiographic studies, it is necessary to use some wall filter control.

A beginning Doppler operator should practice with this control to see its variable effect on the graphic display and on the audio output. The wall filter control has a very marked and obvious effect on the audible signal.

SCALE FACTOR

The scale factor control varies the range of velocity that can be displayed on the spectral recording. Altering this control has no effect on the audio output.

Figure 4.12 shows how increasing the scale factor (A versus B) increases the display range. The velocity of the spectral trace has remained at between 3 and 4 m/sec, even though the display size was decreased as well as the velocity calibration markers. The beginner should note that the actual velocity of the spectral trace does not change despite the differing appearances.

This control should be set so that the highest-velocity spectral trace can be displayed without fear of cutting off a part of the peak velocity. For continuous wave Doppler, the operator is usually allowed to move through a full range of scale factors. When operating in pulsed mode, however, many instruments will automatically limit the range of scale factors possible, depending on the depth of the sample volume and the pulse repetition rate. Scale velocity markers are usually expressed in meters per second or centimeters per second.

BASELINE CONTROL

The baseline control will vary the position of the velocity baseline (zero velocity) within the Doppler trace. Although altering this control has no effect on the audio output, it is very important for the graphic spectral display.

It is very important to recognize the position of the baseline when recording or inspecting a Doppler velocity spectral output. The proper use of this control is crucial in pulsed Doppler echocardiography since the higher velocities recorded in disease states usually result in aliasing. The graphic appearance of this aliasing may be remarkably different, depending on the location of the

56 BASIC DOPPLER ECHOCARDIOGRAPHY

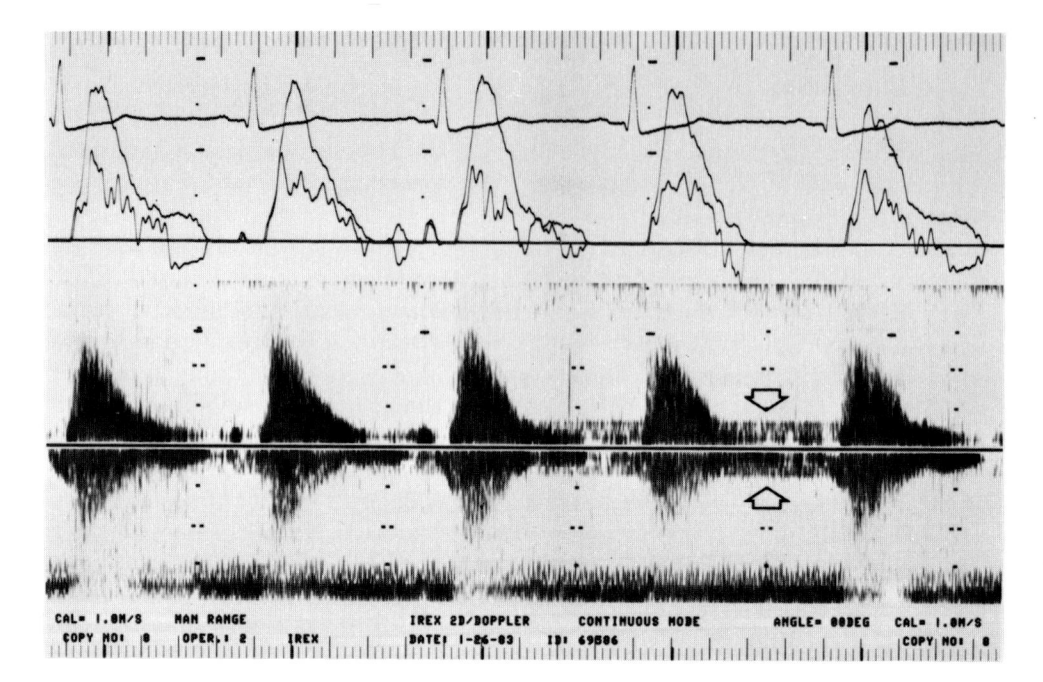

FIG. 4.11. CW spectral velocity recording of the ascending aorta from the suprasternal notch. Arrows point to where the wall filter control is turned off and shows too much low-frequency noise.

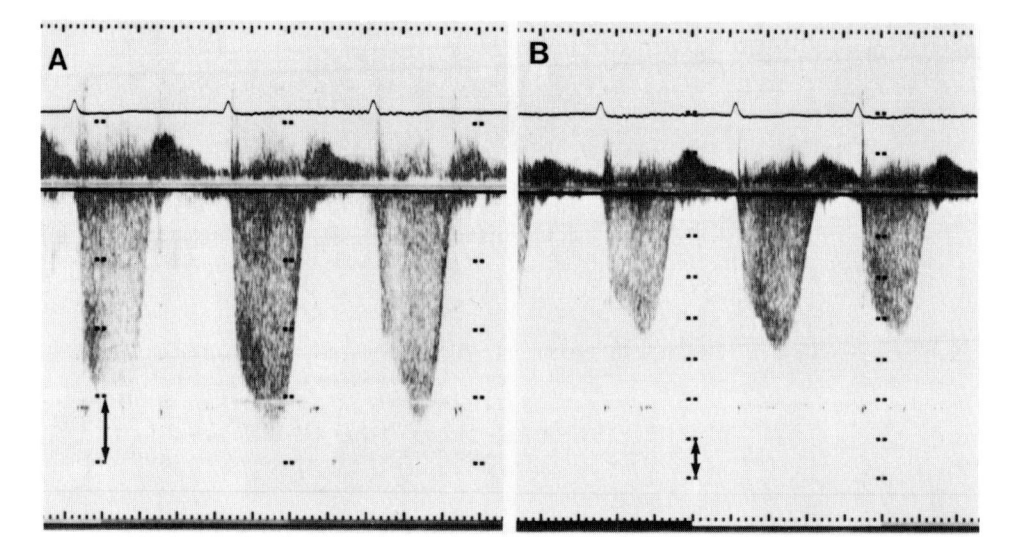

FIG. 4.12. CW spectral velocity recordings of mitral regurgitation from the apical window. The abnormal diastolic jet is away from the transducer. The scale factor is changed between A and B (note arrows).

USE OF THE DOPPLER CONTROLS   57

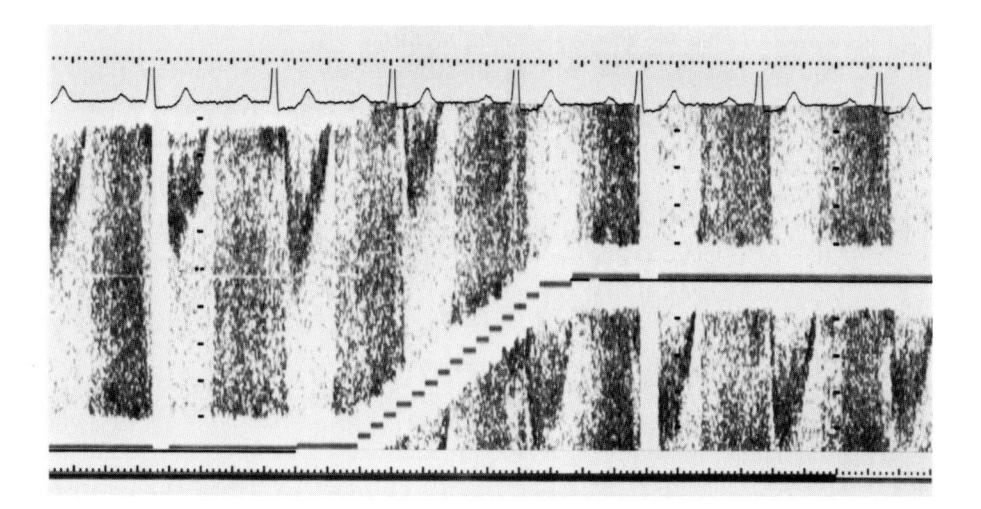

FIG. 4.13. Demonstration of movement of the Doppler baseline in a pulsed Doppler spectral velocity recording of aortic insufficiency obtained from the apical window. The few beats at the left display more of the aliased profile with the baseline at the bottom than is evident when the baseline is moved to the center. Aliasing becomes severe at the right.

baseline (Fig. 4.13). If an aliased signal is detected, it is usually helpful to position the baseline in one of its extreme positions (top or bottom) in order to display as much of the abnormal velocity as possible. This takes advantage of the range of velocity available in the opposite channel.

At first look to a beginner, almost all pulsed Doppler recordings of disease

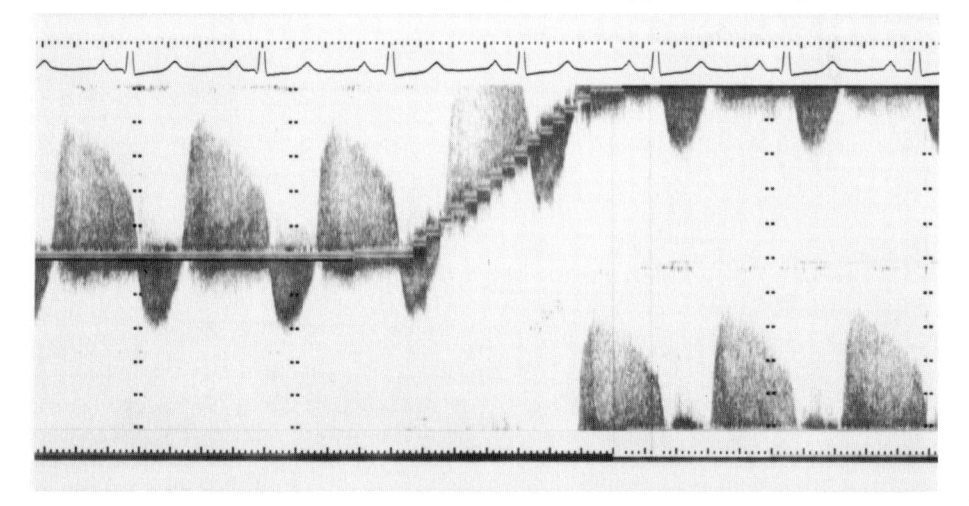

FIG. 4.14. Continuous wave recordings of spectral tracings are best when the baseline is near the center of the display. Movement of the baseline upward in this recording of mixed aortic valve disease shows incorrect positioning that has the same effect as aliasing in pulsed mode.

states look alike because of the resulting aliasing, and the entire spectral trace looks filled with signals from top to bottom. In studying such tracings, one should first find the baseline and then the EKG to help identify both the direction and timing of the aliased signal.

This control is of less importance for continuous wave echocardiography and is best left in some midrecording position so as to allow for display of the full forward and backward flow profiles both above and below the baseline. Figure 4.14 shows the effect of proper and improper positioning of the baseline in the continuous wave mode.

PULSED CURSOR POSITION

The Doppler cursor placement is controlled by the cursor switch or paddle (on some machines a joystick). It is important to remember that the cursor control is operational only in pulsed mode and has no effect in continuous wave.

This cursor allows movement of the Doppler beam to the left or right within the two-dimensional scan (Fig. 4.15). In common use the movement of this control allows for positioning the pulsed sample volume from one heart chamber to another. Occasionally, this control is used for positioning the Doppler beam as parallel to flow as possible. As will be seen later, the most important use of cursor positioning is in the mapping technique for semiquantitating regurgitant lesions.

Depending upon the location of the cursor and the flow intercepted, it has a variable effect on audio and spectral output.

PULSED SAMPLE DEPTH

In pulsed Doppler, the sample depth control selects the depth at which the sample volume gate is placed along the cursor line (Fig. 4.16). As with all cursor and sample volume controls, sample depth has no effect in the continuous wave mode.

This has very important use in positioning the sample volume properly for the detection of normal or abnormal flows, particularly in the mapping of various lesions. It should be remembered that deeper positioning of the sample volume into the heart results in an automatic decrease in pulse repetition rate and a decrease in the Nyquist limit (Fig. 4.17). In this schematic example of a spectral display, a jet of given velocity is encountered in the near field (A), and the signal is obviously aliased. If this same jet were encountered somewhere deeper into the tissues such as B or C, more severe aliasing would occur. The same jet encountered deep into the field would produce very serious aliasing and a signal of unrecognizable profile. Therefore, for a given velocity the display will be different, depending upon how deep the sample volume must be located. As a rule, the farther into the tissues a sample volume is placed, aliasing will occur at progressively lower velocities.

Some systems also allow variable control of the size of the pulsed Doppler

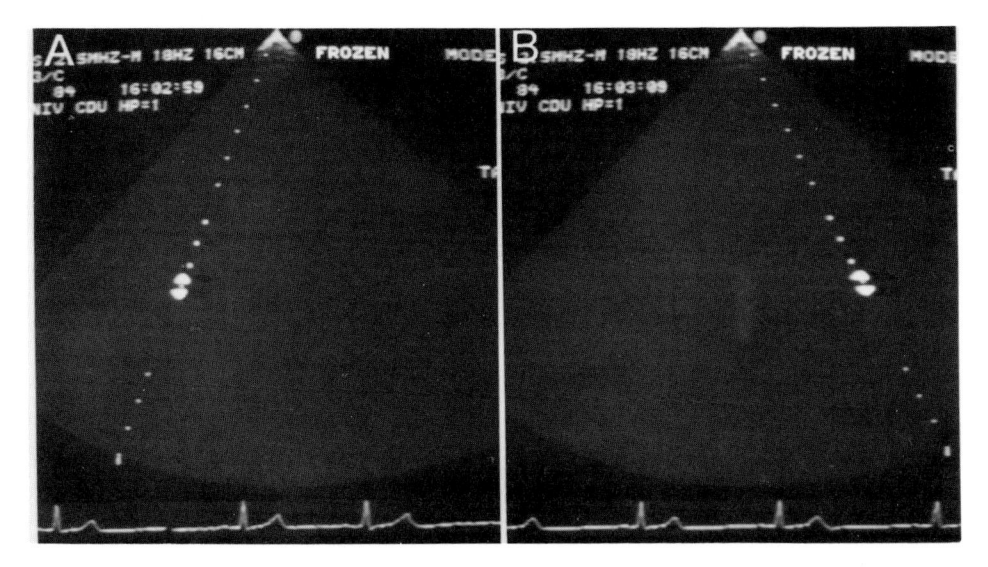

FIG. 4.15. (A) Placement of the Doppler cursor on the left side of the two-dimensional sector and (B) placement to the right side of the two-dimensional sector are shown.

gate (Fig. 4.18). This capability makes the detection of small jets easier and also provides a mechanism to inspect flow across the entire diameter of a vessel. However, as the gate is increased in length, there is a decrease in the ability of the system to measure higher velocities. Most users of pulsed Doppler will leave this gate in some midposition for routine scanning and decrease or

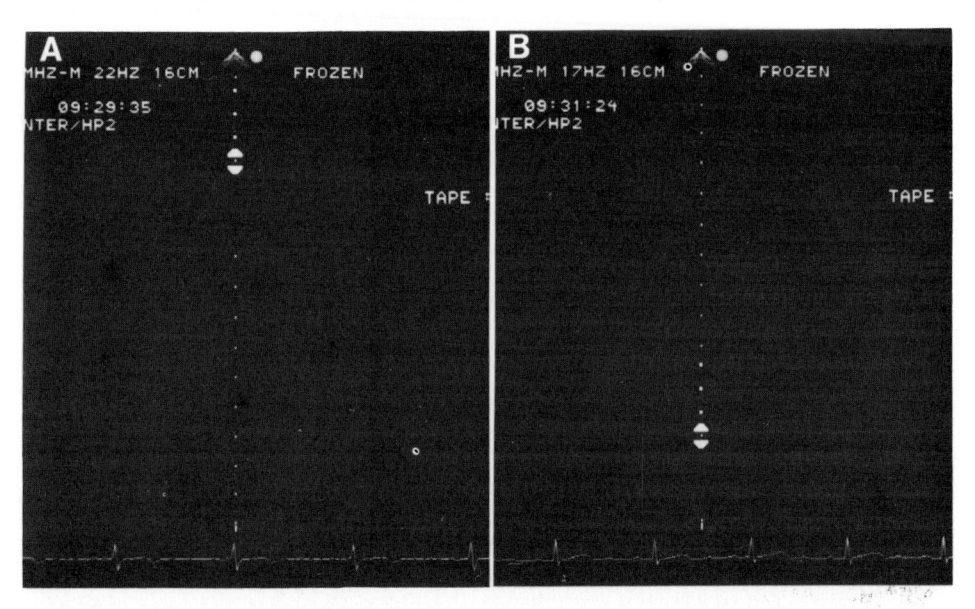

FIG. 4.16. The pulsed Doppler sample volume may be located at any depth along the cursor by operator selection.

60 BASIC DOPPLER ECHOCARDIOGRAPHY

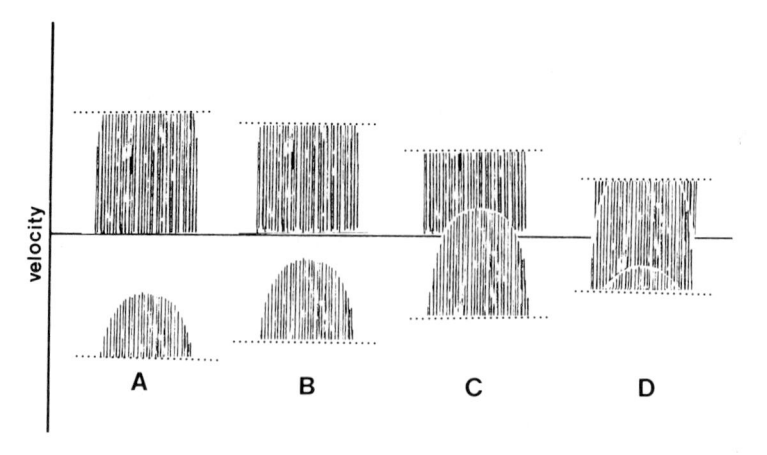

FIG. 4.17. Progressive degrees of aliasing will occur for any given jet as sample volume is placed deeper and deeper into the heart. For details see text.

increase the size of the gate, depending upon the clinical situation.

There is a complex interplay between sample volume size and its range position into the heart. Since the size of any ultrasound beam increases farther into the tissues, there will be an automatic and progressive increase in sample volume size with increases in depth location. This is very important to remember since the size of the pulsed sample volume will appear the same size on the two-dimensional display whether located at a depth of 4 or 15 cm. Failure to recognize this fact will result in an operator thinking that a given jet found

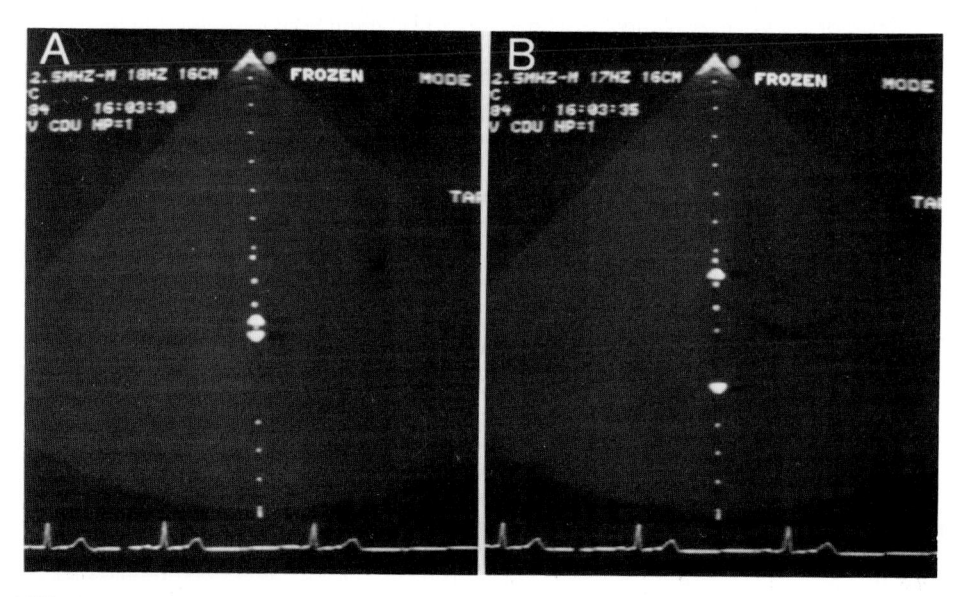

FIG. 4.18. (A) The pulsed Doppler sample volume at its smallest size. (B) The sample volume at its widest size.

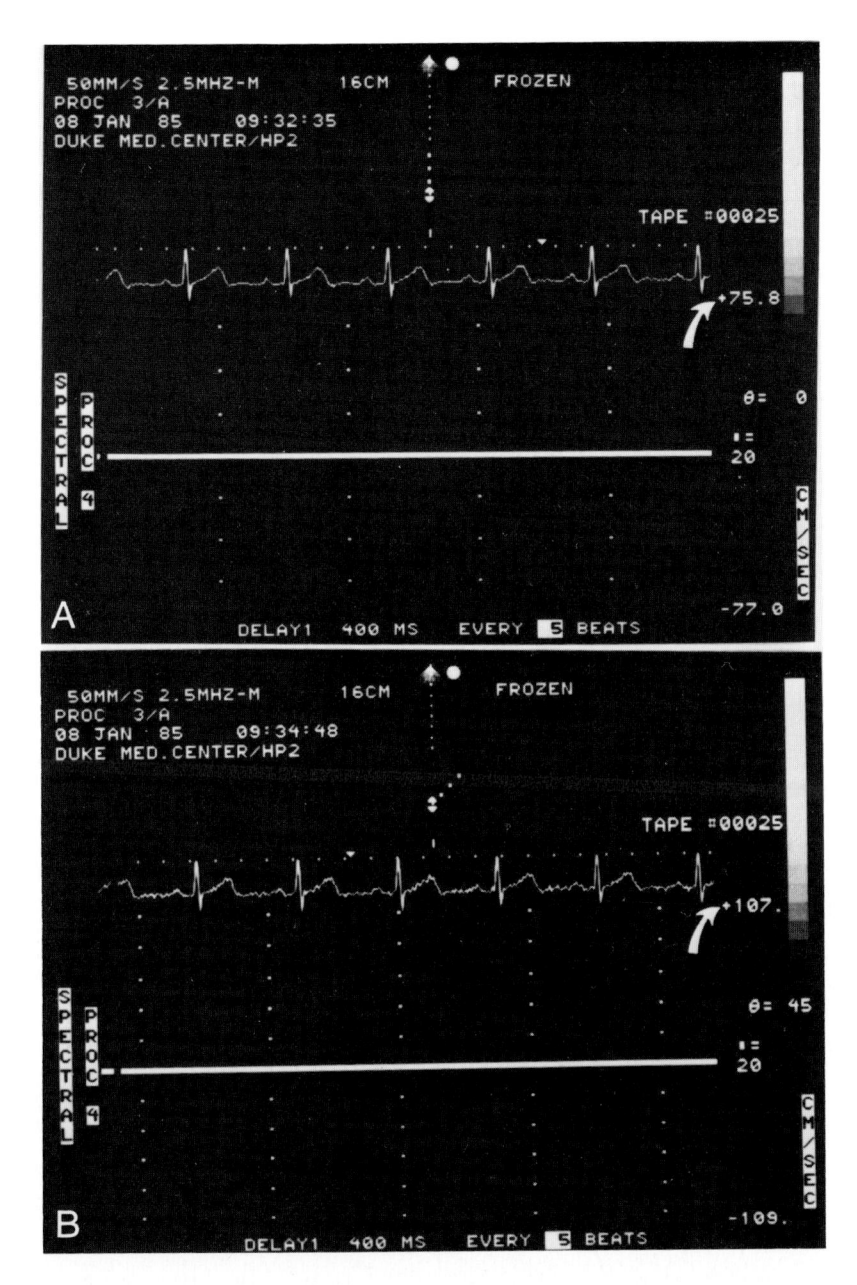

FIG. 4.19. (A and B) The effect of moving the angle correction arm to compensate for not being parallel to blood flow is demonstrated. The machine will calculate this new angle θ, and the scale factors change.

at far ranges can precisely be localized. The farther into the tissues a sample volume is placed the less precise our ability to localize a jet becomes.

PULSED ANGLE CORRECTION

Most pulsed Doppler systems have some angle correction mechanism (Fig. 4.19). The purpose and effect of this control may be very confusing to beginners in Doppler echocardiography. When the operator recognizes that the Doppler beam and sample volume are not actually parallel to flow, the angle correction arm may be positioned into the estimated direction of flow. As previously indicated, the Doppler equation is very sensitive to the angle of the beam in relationship to the direction of flow.

Although seemingly quite useful, in reality the use of this control only serves to make minor adjustments in the scale factor of the display. Note that when the arm is aligned with the cursor (Fig. 4.19A), the maximum velocity in either channel is approximately 75 cm/sec. When rotated in some other direction, the scale is increased to 107 cm/sec. The use of this control does not actually change the direction of the Doppler beam, and its use does not alter the quality of either the audio output or the spectral recording. In actual practice, it is better to realign the position of the transducer as parallel to perceived flow as possible than to depend upon this angle correction mechanism. This control is best left unused.

5 The Doppler Examination

DAVID ADAMS
DANIEL B. MARK
JOSEPH KISSLO

There are no standardized methods for the conduct of a Doppler examination such as exist for two-dimensional echocardiography.[1] We have evolved a partially systematic approach in our laboratory that begins after the imaging part of the examination is completed. Performing the two-dimensional examination first is very helpful in familiarizing the operator with the spatial positioning of the chambers and valves to be examined by Doppler.

BEAM ORIENTATION

It is critical that the operator remember that the best Doppler information is obtained when the Doppler beam is oriented so that it lines up as close to parallel to blood flow as possible (Fig. 5.1). This will ensure that the strongest Doppler signals are reflected back to the transducer and that maximum peak velocities are obtained. When using a combined two-dimensional and Doppler machine, the novice must bear in mind the fact that the best two-dimensional pictures usually will not be achieved from exactly the same window that yields the best Doppler tracings. In order to achieve the goal of a small intercept angle to blood flow (as required by the Doppler equation), the operator must not be afraid to try a wide variety of acoustic windows, some of which are not used for standard M-mode or two-dimensional examinations.

In patients with valvular disease, we routinely begin a Doppler examination from the apical window. In this view the beam is most likely to be positioned parallel to flow through the mitral, tricuspid, and aortic valves. Alternative starting positions may be selected for evaluation of certain specific disorders. For example, initial use of the left parasternal window may be most fruitful when the presence of a ventricular septal defect is suspected.

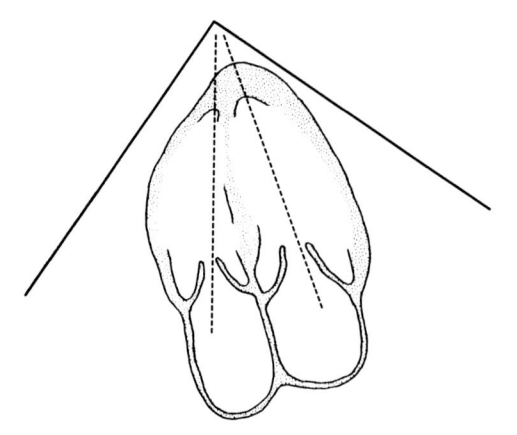

FIG. 5.1. The best Doppler signal is obtained when the beam is oriented parallel to flow. This orientation may result in a suboptimal two-dimensional image.

AUDIO OUTPUT

The audio output is critical for locating the presence and direction of an abnormal jet. The operator should never assume that the direction of abnormal blood flow is parallel through a valve or within a vessel. Therefore, the operator should always optimize the Doppler signal by concentrating carefully on the characteristics of the audio output.

For example, using the apical four-chamber view, a beginner with pulsed Doppler may simply position the sample volume directly behind the mitral valve when examining for the presence of mitral insufficiency. Although this may provide the best image possible, the abnormal jet may be directed very eccentrically and in any direction rather than straight back. By concentrating on the Doppler audio output rather than the two-dimensional view at this point, the operator will be able to fine-tune the alignment of the ultrasound beam, thereby avoiding the natural tendency to keep the two-dimensional picture on axis while doing the Doppler examination.

The same principle holds true for continuous wave Doppler examinations. For example, using an apical window a beginner may simply position the beam along the expected course of flow in a patient with both aortic stenosis and insufficiency. However, this will often produce a suboptimal Doppler recording, since the stenotic jet may be aimed predominantly in one direction or along one axis and the regurgitant jet may be directed along a different axis (Fig. 5.2).

The anatomical knowledge gained through the use of two-dimensional images should only be considered a rough guideline for the Doppler examination. When valves are thickened and narrowed, the resultant jet of blood may be directed in an unpredictable fashion.

COMBINED ECHO-DOPPLER

Beginners in Doppler echocardiography usually find it easier to acquire initial experience with this technique using an "add-on" Doppler system. This combi-

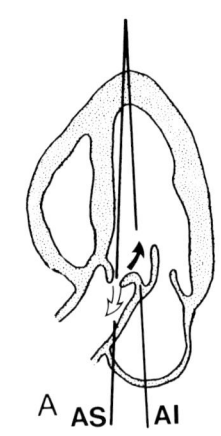

FIG. 5.2. (A) Schematic diagram of the orientation of the systolic and regurgitant aortic valve jets in relation to the CW beam. (B) The transducer must be moved, in this case from the best spectral recording of aortic stenosis (AS, open arrow) to a position to best record the aortic insufficiency (AI, closed arrow).

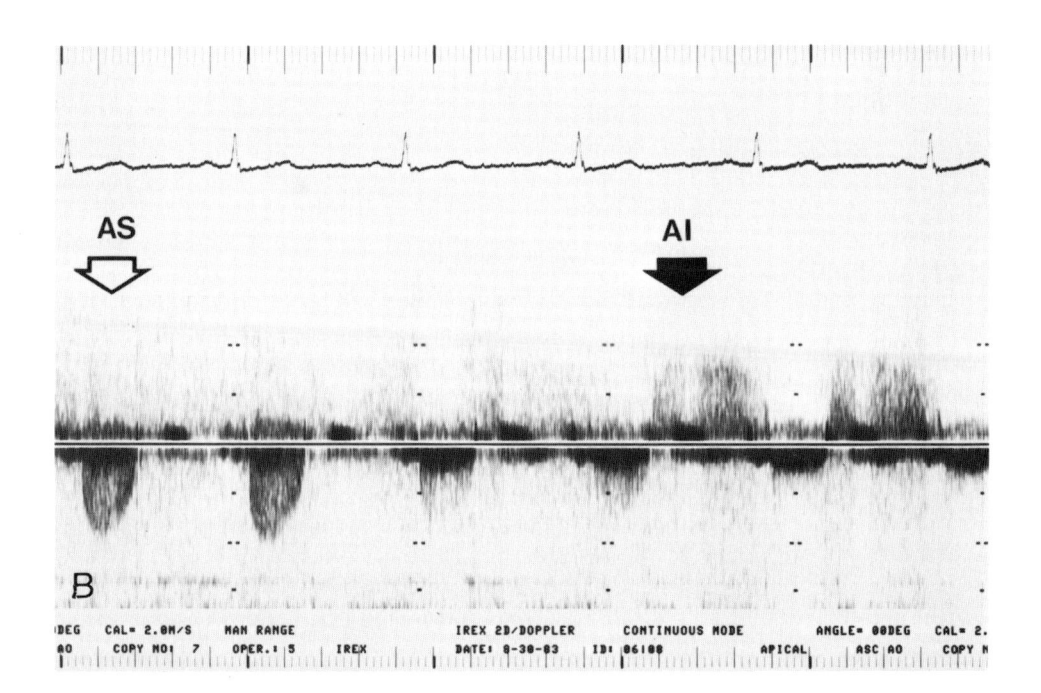

nation of Doppler and imaging capabilities helps in achieving an appreciation for the relationship of normal and abnormal flows within cardiac structures.

As was discussed in detail in Chapter 3, the operator should remember that the best Doppler tracings are obtained when in a dedicated Doppler mode, and the best two-dimensional recordings are made in a dedicated imaging mode. When any form of combined Doppler and imaging is attempted, some sacrifices in quality of one or both must be made.

66 BASIC DOPPLER ECHOCARDIOGRAPHY

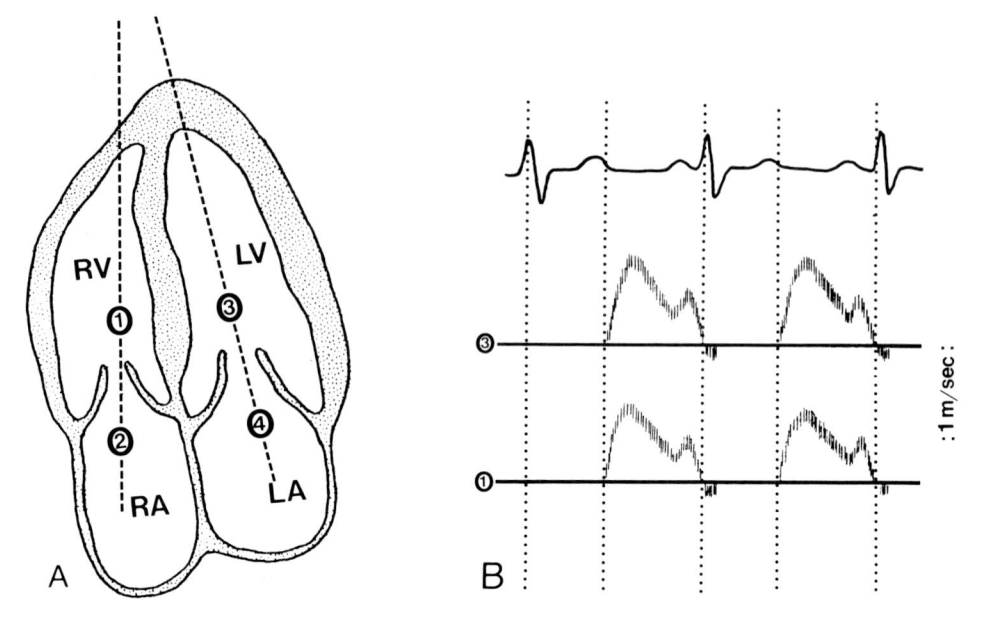

FIG. 5.3. (A) An apical four-chamber view with PW sample sites on either side of the atrioventricular valves. (B) A schematic spectral recording of normal mitral (site 3) and tricuspid (site 1) diastolic flow. Note that peak tricuspid velocity is normally lower than mitral.

Operators should begin by becoming familiar with the Doppler-imaging time-sharing arrangements in their imaging systems. Despite the varied arrangements of imaging and Doppler in the available commercial systems, certain general comments can be made. For mechanical imaging systems, transducer motion must almost always be stopped to switch into the pulsed Doppler mode. Thus, the Doppler cursor can be moved and the sample volume positioned during imaging, but the image must be frozen to acquire the Doppler information. Unless the operator has a very steady hand, some transducer movement will occur after a few beats and the location of the Doppler sample volume on the frozen image will not indicate its true position. The operator must therefore manually switch back and forth between imaging and Doppler to confirm the position of the sample volume.

For phased-array imaging systems, the solution to the time-sharing problem is a bit different. These systems allow automatic image updating by means of some gating system. The operator switches into pulsed Doppler mode and is required to set the image gate to update the image every few beats. Thus, for a pulsed Doppler to operate at full capacity and deliver the highest PRF possible, the imaging capability must be stopped and held in memory. Switching between these two modes is done manually when a mechanical transducer is being used and can be done automatically with a phased-array system.

For continuous wave (CW) Doppler, the examination must always be conducted in a blind fashion and without assistance of the two-dimensional image.

THE DOPPLER EXAMINATION 67

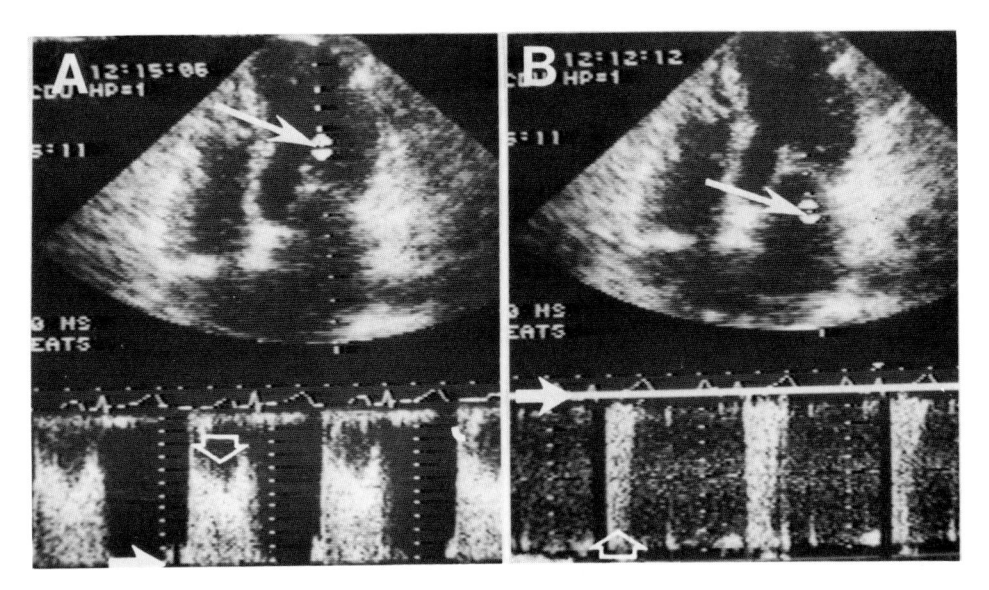

FIG. 5.4. Two-dimensional stop-frame and spectral pulsed recordings from a patient with mitral stenosis and insufficiency. (A) Location of the sample volume on the ventricular side of the mitral valve (arrow). The baseline of the spectral tracing is at the bottom, and the diastolic jet is toward the transducer (open arrow). (B) Location of the pulsed sample volume on the atrial side of the valve. The baseline is at the top of the spectral recording, and the systolic regurgitant jet is away from the transducer.

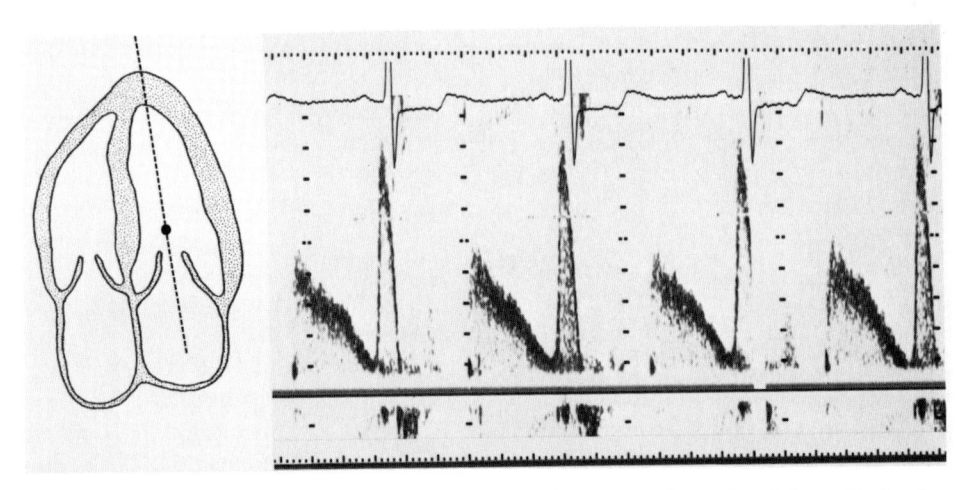

FIG. 5.5. Pulsed wave spectral recording from the ventricular side of the mitral valve. Note that flow is laminar. The diastolic *a* wave is peaked as a result of left ventricular hypertrophy and reduced diastolic compliance.

Although some commercial systems provide CW capabilities with a two-dimensional display, the operator should remember that this results from some compromises in both the Doppler and imaging data, as was discussed in Chapter 3.

Once experience is gained with combined imaging and Doppler systems, the beginner will find the use of "stand-alone" Doppler much easier. The major advantage of these latter systems is that they allow transducer and signal-processing capabilities wholly dedicated to Doppler and usually result in superior Doppler quality.

APICAL WINDOW

For routine Doppler examination of patients with suspected valvular heart disease, it is usually best to begin by using the apical window. For pulsed wave echocardiography this provides some image guidance for positioning of the sample volume and allows selective orientation of the Doppler beam as parallel as possible to the direction of assumed flow through the mitral and tricuspid valves. This allows the largest Doppler shift to be recorded and the strongest signals to be reflected back to the Doppler transducer.

The imaging mode of the system may be used to acquire an apical four-chamber view as seen in Fig. 5.3. The pulsed Doppler sample volume can then be positioned on the atrial or ventricular sides of the mitral or tricuspid valves. Figure 5.3B shows schematic representations of the normal spectral outputs through the mitral (sample site 3) and tricuspid valves (sample site 1).

In most normal individuals, whether the sample volume is on the atrial or ventricular sides of the mitral and tricuspid valves results in spectral flow outputs that are quite similar. In the presence of valvular disease, however, markedly different flow patterns are encountered, depending upon sample volume position. Figure 5.4 shows recordings made from a patient with combined mitral valve disease with the resultant spectral outputs from the sample volume positioned on the ventricular and then atrial sides of the mitral valve. There is turbulent diastolic flow on the ventricular side of the valve that shows a slowed early diastolic descent. On the atrial side of the valve the very high-velocity systolic regurgitant jet is detected moving in a negative direction, away from the transducer.

Abnormalities of flow are not always related to the presence of valvular disease. Figure 5.5 shows the pulsed sample volume located on the ventricular side of the mitral valve in a patient with severe left ventricular hypertrophy. There is a high-velocity late diastolic blood flow produced by contraction of the left atrium into the noncompliant left ventricle.

When in the apical four-chamber view, slight superior angulation of the scan plane will allow the operator to encounter the left ventricular outflow tract (Fig. 5.6). An operator can almost always obtain Doppler flow data from the ventricular side of the aortic valve. In some patients data may also be obtained from the aortic root side.

THE DOPPLER EXAMINATION 69

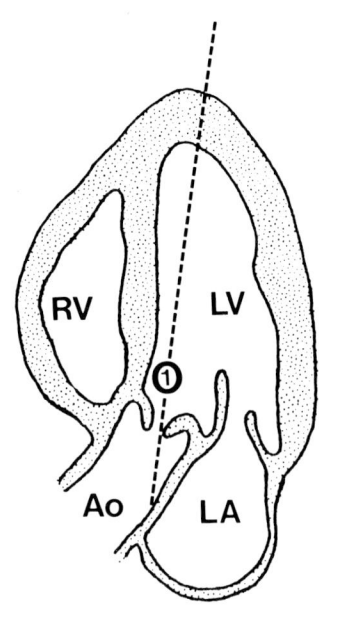

FIG. 5.6. Schematic drawing of superior angulation of the apical four-chamber view to encounter the left ventricular outflow tract.

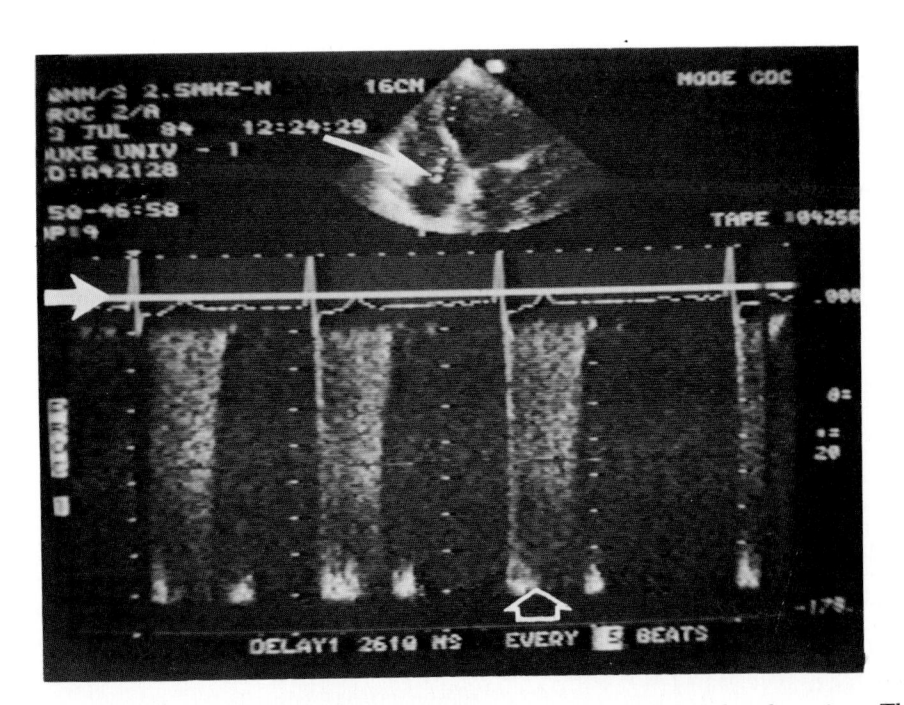

FIG. 5.7. Stop-frame two-dimensional image in the apical four-chamber view. The pulsed sample volume (arrow top) is located just on the atrial side of the tricuspid valve. The baseline of the spectral recording is at the top, and the systolic tricuspid regurgitant jet is away from the transducer.

70 BASIC DOPPLER ECHOCARDIOGRAPHY

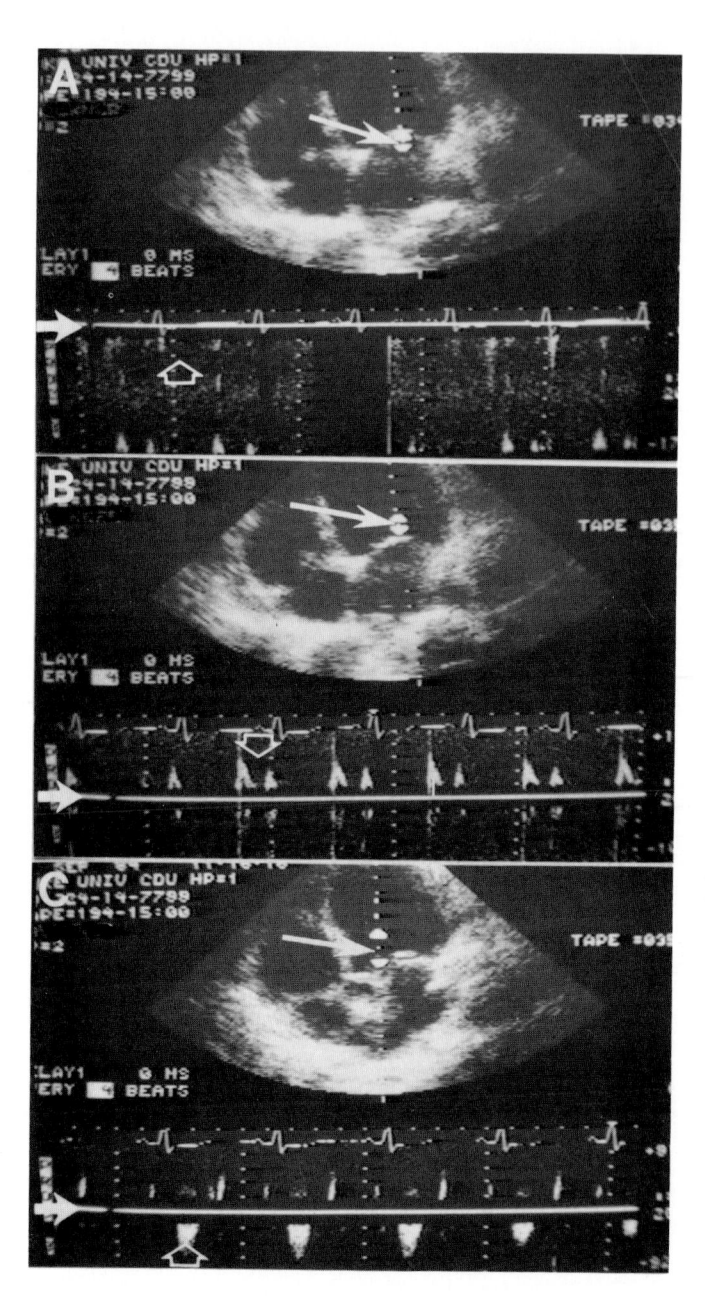

FIG. 5.8. Stop-frame images of the apical four-chamber view with progressive movement of the pulsed sample volume on the atrial (A, top arrow) and then ventricular (B, top arrow) side of the mitral valve, with final positioning in the left ventricular outflow tract (C, top arrow). The position of spectral baselines is indicated by the solid arrow at the left. See text for details.

During the conduct of an actual examination, the operator should routinely begin with the apical four-chamber view, and then position the sample volume on the ventricular and atrial sides of the mitral and tricuspid valves to detect normal or abnormal flow. Figure 5.7 demonstrates the positioning of the sample volume just behind the tricuspid valve in a patient with tricuspid insufficiency. The abnormal flow away from the transducer in systole is displayed across the full-velocity spectrum.

A complete pulsed Doppler evaluation would continue with movement of the sample volume from place to place such as shown in Fig. 5.8. Here, there is progressive positioning of the sample volume on the atrial and then ventricular side of the mitral valve and then eventually just below the aortic valve with superior angulation and cursor repositioning. When positioned behind the mitral valve, there is no abnormal flow detected in systole (Fig. 5.8A, open arrow). Normal mitral diastolic flow is encountered with repositioning the sample volume on the ventricular side of the mitral orifice (Fig. 5.8B, open arrow). Finally, movement of the sample volume to the ventricular side of the aortic valve demonstrates normal systolic flow away from the transducer (Fig. 5.8C, open arrow).

Continued practice repositioning the pulsed wave (PW) cursor and sample volume in the various portions of the cardiac chambers accessible from the apical four-chamber view will eventually provide the novice operator with an appreciation of the spatial locations and directions of normal and abnormal flows. The heart chambers are actually three-dimensional structures, and an abnormal flow jet may be directed anywhere within this three-dimensional structure. An experienced operator will be able to track an abnormal jet even if it is directed out of a standard two-dimensional plane.

The apical window is also an excellent position for obtaining some initial experience with continuous wave Doppler. Placing the CW transducer directly over the apical impulse (located by palpation) and angling the beam somewhat leftward and posteriorly will usually result in a typical mitral flow profile (Fig. 5.9). It is wise for the beginner to practice locating flow through the mitral valve as the flow profile resembles the appearance of the mitral valve on M-mode and is readily recognized.

Marked medial redirection of the CW beam from the apex will result in a flow profile through the tricuspid valve. Figure 5.10 shows the abnormal systolic profiles away from the transducer typical of tricuspid and mitral insufficiencies in the same patient. These two different abnormal flow signals were easily obtained by angling medially and then laterally through each atrioventricular valve. Because pressures are higher on the left side of the heart, velocities are generally higher on the left when compared with the right in normal and diseased states. Exceptions to this rule are encountered in severe pulmonary hypertension and pulmonic stenosis.

The ranges of normal flow velocities are shown in Table 5.1. Notice that the normal flows are slightly higher in children than adults and slightly higher on the left side of the heart in comparison with the right.

This angulation back and forth from mitral to tricuspid valve from the apical

72 BASIC DOPPLER ECHOCARDIOGRAPHY

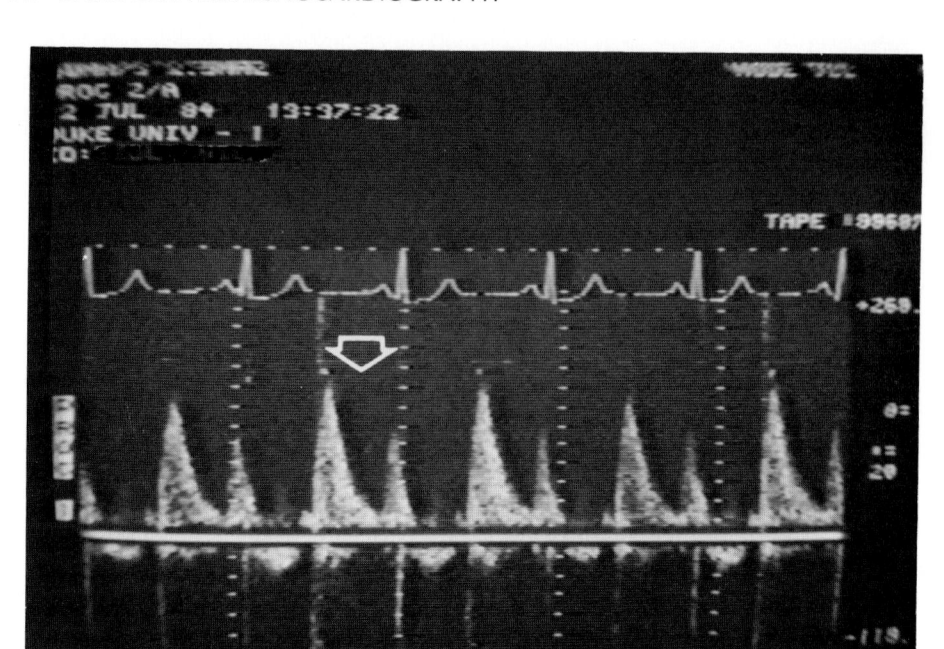

FIG. 5.9. CW recording from the apex in a normal individual. Note that diastolic flow is toward the transducer. No two-dimensional image is possible in full CW mode.

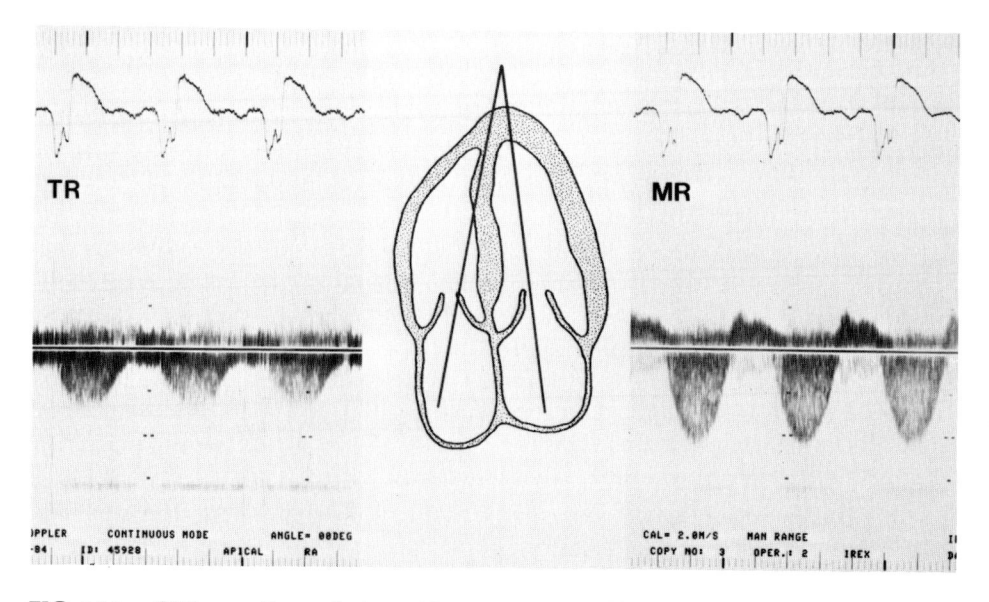

FIG. 5.10. CW recordings of tricuspid regurgitation (TR) and mitral regurgitation (MR) from the apical window. The central schematic diagram shows the relative positions of the valves. The regurgitant velocity is higher on the left heart side.

TABLE 5.1 Normal Doppler Velocities

Flow	Children (m/sec)	Adults (m/sec)
Mitral diastolic	1.00 (0.7–1.4)	0.92 (0.6–1.4)
Tricuspid diastolic	0.62 (0.5–0.9)	0.58 (0.4–0.8)
Pulmonary systolic	0.84 (0.6–1.2)	0.72 (0.5–0.9)
Aortic systolic	1.52 (1.2–1.7)	1.40 (0.9–1.8)

window may also be practiced in normals. Normal mitral diastolic velocity is slightly higher than through the tricuspid valve, and the operator can then differentiate the two atrioventricular valve flows.

Since a CW examination is done without benefit of image guidance, continued practice is required. Sometimes the abnormal jet moves through the Doppler beam with the phases of the cardiac cycle making a full-spectral recording difficult. Figure 5.11 shows the continuous wave Doppler of a patient with mitral insufficiency. The spectral trace is that of turbulent high-velocity flow away from the transducer. In midsystole the jet moves out of the interrogating beam (closed arrow), causing a dropout in the recording of the very highest velocities (open arrow). This occasionally happens no matter what the transducer beam to jet orientation is attempted. The goal in the Doppler examination is, obviously, to attempt to record full cardiac cycle profiles such as shown in Fig. 5.12. This figure also shows a patient with mitral insufficiency, but here there are complete velocity profiles identified during systole and diastole.

An experienced user will ultimately be able to move the CW beam quickly and precisely from a somewhat superior direction that intercepts the left ventricular outflow tract to one that intercepts mitral inflow. Note the apparent similarity of the patterns of aortic insufficiency and mitral stenosis recorded when this maneuver is utilized in Fig. 5.13.

There are differences in the quality of the spectral recordings from these two lesions. Turbulence is encountered that results in the detection of many different velocities. This results in what is called "spectral broadening" in the recording from both the aortic insufficiency (first two complexes) and the mitral stenosis (last two complexes). The spectral recordings are, however, remarkably different since the tracings from the mitral stenosis appear darker than those from aortic insufficiency. This reflects the fact that the darker portions of this spectral tracing mean that a higher number of red cells are moving at the given velocity than are present in the lighter tracing.

Figure 5.14 shows an additional example of the use of CW to examine the left-sided heart valves. At first, the beam is directed superiorly to encounter aortic insufficiency and stenosis (Fig. 5.14A). The insufficiency is directed toward the transducer and appears on the spectral display in diastole. The aortic stenosis flow moves away from the transducer in systole. The CW is then

74 BASIC DOPPLER ECHOCARDIOGRAPHY

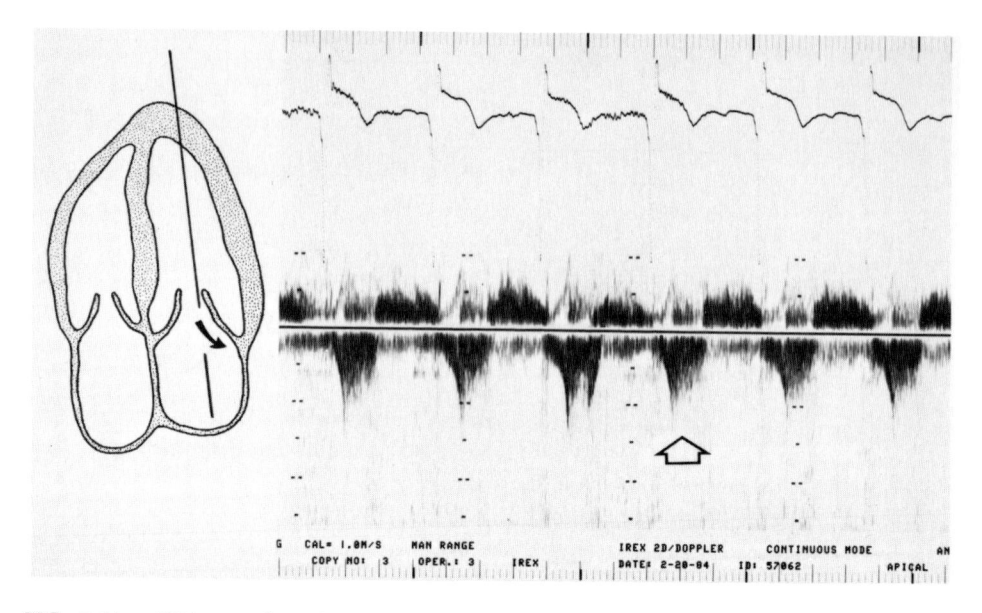

FIG. 5.11. CW recording from the apex that intercepts a mitral regurgitant jet that moves through the beam in systole (closed arrow, left). Note the lack of the complete spectral profile (open arrow).

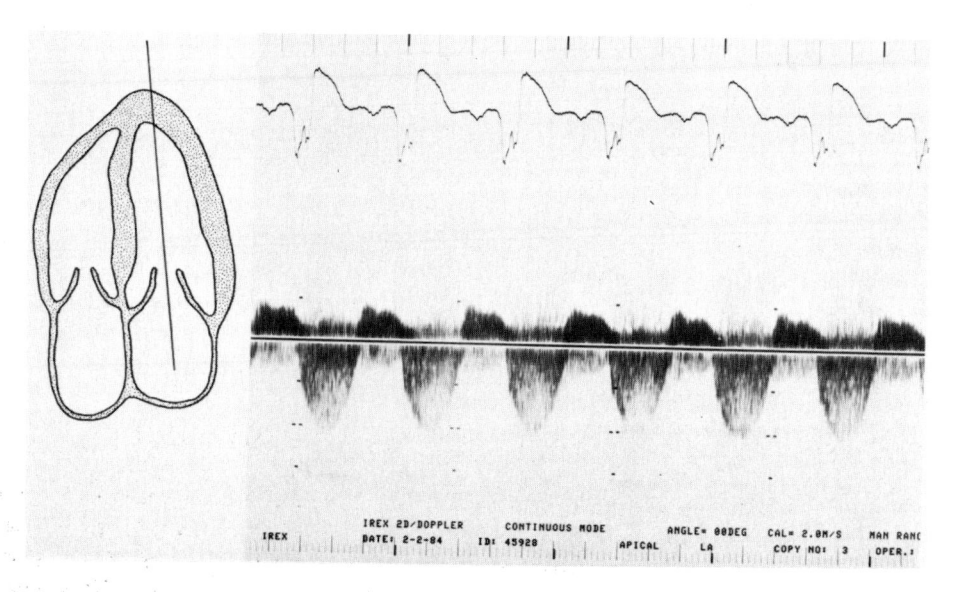

FIG. 5.12. CW full-spectral recording of both diastolic mitral flow and regurgitant flow in systole away from the transducer.

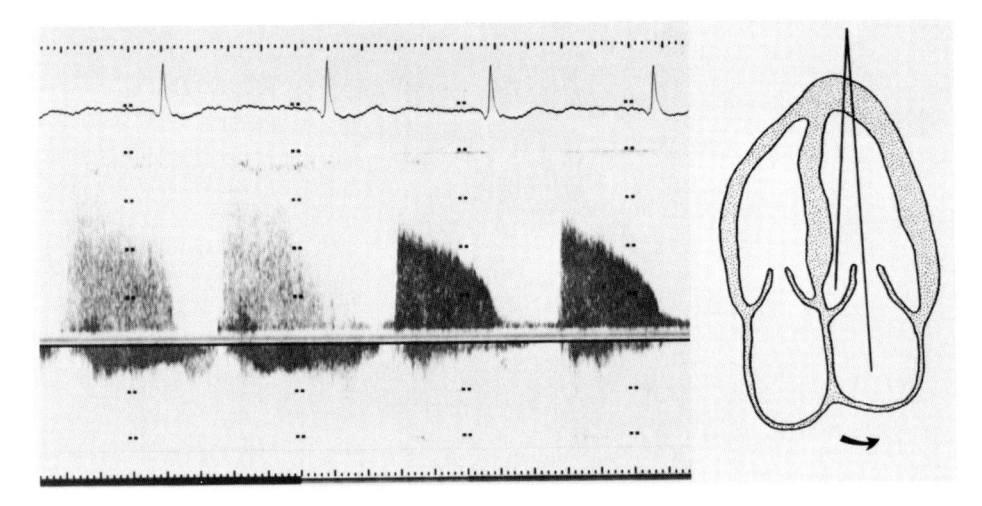

FIG. 5.13. CW spectral recording of aortic insufficiency (first two beats) and mitral stenosis (last two beats) resulting from slight transducer beam movement. For details see text.

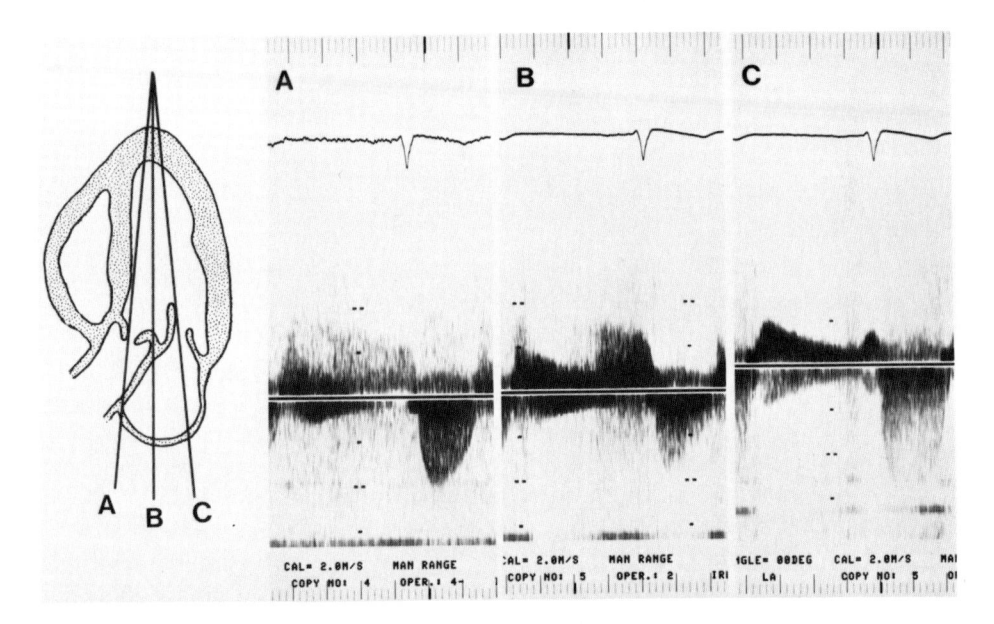

FIG. 5.14. CW velocity spectral recording from three apical transducer beam positions (A, B, and C). (A) Aortic insufficiency and stenosis is shown. Slight movement of the beam begins to mix the aortic insufficiency with diastolic flow through a mildly stenotic mitral valve. (C) Pure mitral diastolic flow and mitral regurgitation is demonstrated.

76 BASIC DOPPLER ECHOCARDIOGRAPHY

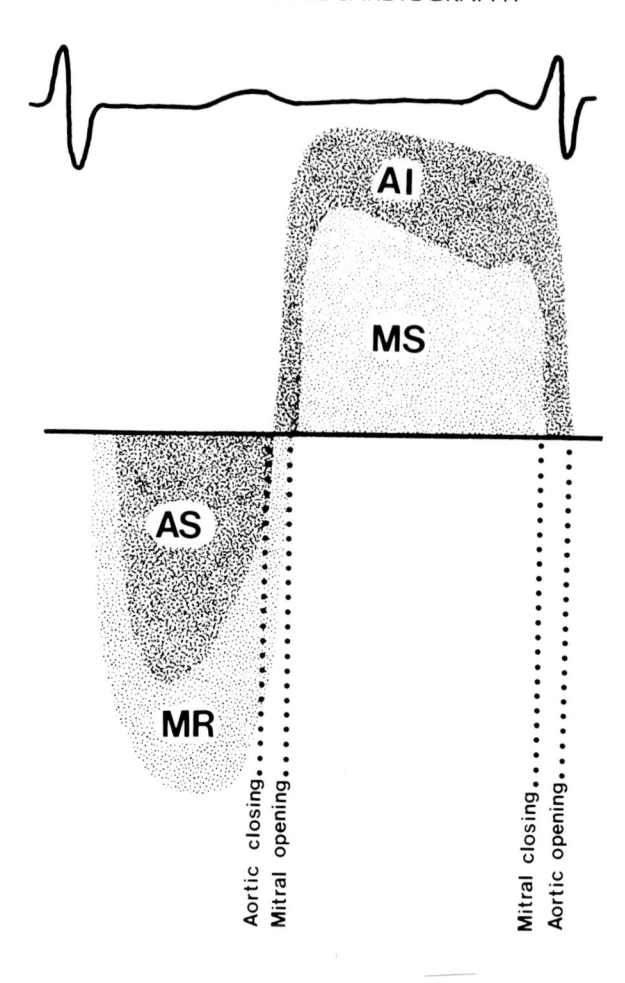

FIG. 5.15. Relationships of abnormal systolic and diastolic flows. For details, see text.

angled midway between ventricular outflow and inflow (Fig. 5.14B) and encounters a mixed diastolic profile with mitral inflow superimposed on the aortic insufficiency. Progressive angulation through the mitral valve demonstrates a pure mitral inflow in diastole with mitral insufficiency in systole (Fig. 5.14C).

The problem of recording flow across mitral and aortic valve simultaneously (Fig. 5.14B) results partly from the fact that the ultrasound beam width is large enough to detect more than one jet. Failure to appreciate this may lead the unwary beginner to diagnose mitral stenosis, for example, when only aortic regurgitation is present.

At first, it may appear that the spectral profiles of aortic stenosis resemble mitral insufficiency and those of aortic insufficiency resemble mitral stenosis. These various disease profiles may be differentiated by a knowledge of the various timing relationships of left-sided valvular opening and closing. Figure 5.15 shows the relationships between these various abnormal spectral velocities. The duration of mitral insufficiency is generally longer than that of aortic

THE DOPPLER EXAMINATION 77

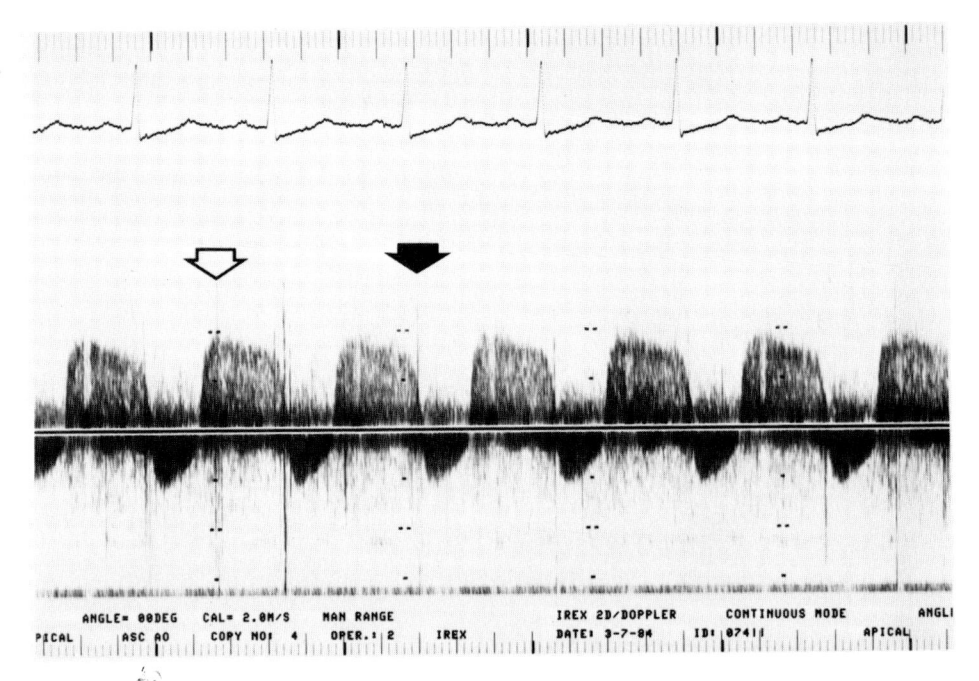

FIG. 5.16. CW spectral trace from the apex in a patient with aortic insufficiency showing valve opening spike (closed arrow). Other, poorly explained, spikes may occasionally occur (open arrow).

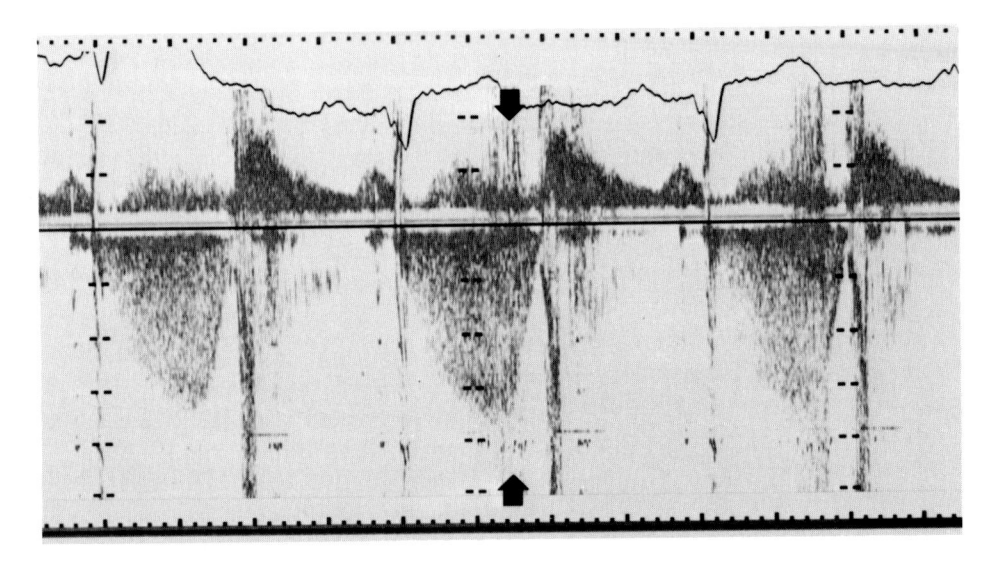

FIG. 5.17. CW spectral velocity recording from the apex in a patient with mild mitral stenosis and severe mitral insufficiency. Many valve opening and closing clicks are noted. A late systolic spike is noted and was caused by a hyperdynamic ventricular apical beat interfering with the acoustic gel-transducer interface.

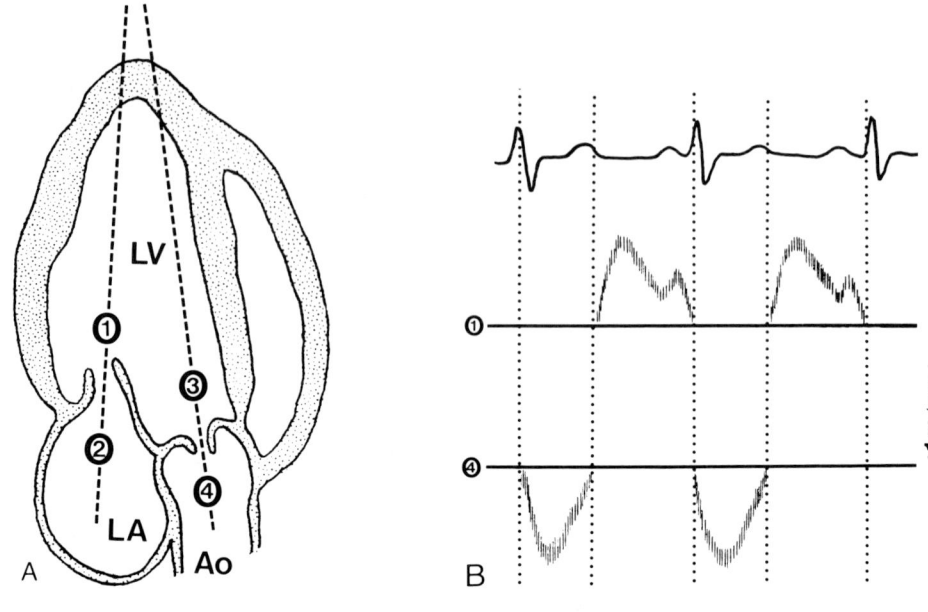

FIG. 5.18. (A) An apical two-chamber view with PW sample sites on either side of the mitral and aortic valves. (B) A schematic spectral recording of normal mitral diastolic (site 1) and aortic systolic (site 4) flow.

stenosis, in part because the time from mitral valve closing to mitral valve opening is longer than from aortic valve opening to closing. Similarly, the duration of aortic insufficiency is longer than mitral stenosis because the time from aortic closing to aortic opening is longer than from mitral opening to closing. Similar relationships are true of the pulmonic and tricuspid valves on the right side of the heart. Those experienced in phonocardiography will realize the advantage of using this technique to assist in the identification of the various valve profiles.

Occasionally the various valve movements such as closure may be recorded in the spectral outputs and usually appear as spikes. In Fig. 5.16 (solid arrow) the spike of aortic valve opening is noted. More difficult to explain are similar spikes located during the midphases of the cardiac cycle (open arrow). Sometimes artifacts are induced from extracardiac sources. Figure 5.17 demonstrates a continuous wave spectral output obtained from the apical window in a patient with severe mitral insufficiency. As the recording was being made, the hyperactive ventricular apical beat was moving the interface gel back and forth, resulting in the artifact (solid arrow).

The apical window also supplies an opportunity for examination of left-sided flow with pulsed Doppler echocardiography by movement of the imaging plane to the apical two-chamber view (Fig. 5.18). This view is obtained by rotating the two-dimensional transducer counterclockwise and 90° from the apical four-chamber view and is particularly suited for examination of both

THE DOPPLER EXAMINATION 79

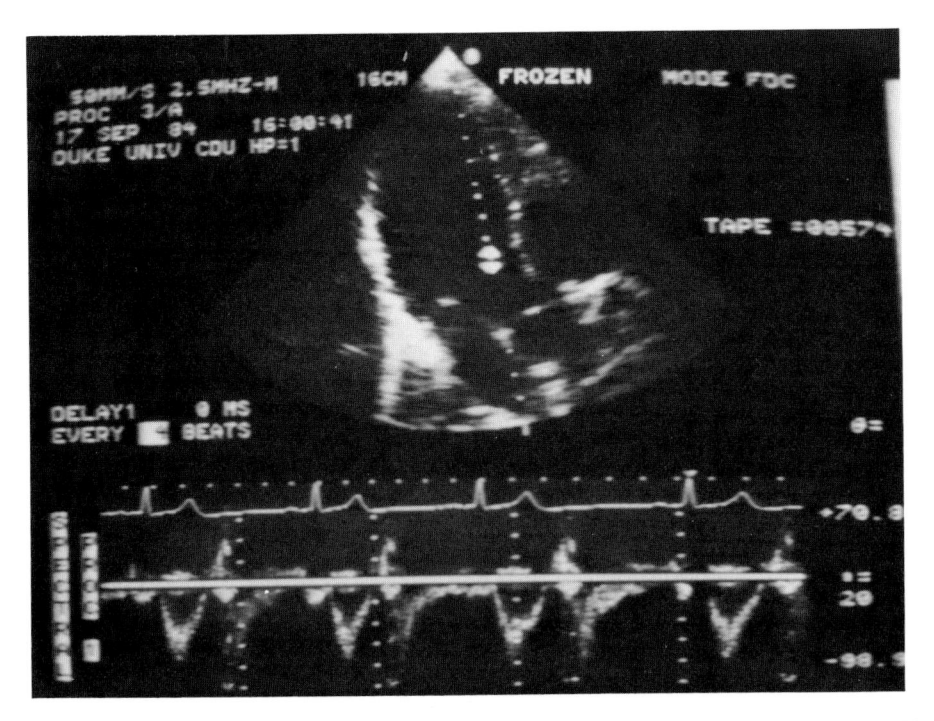

FIG. 5.19. Stop-frame two-dimensional image in the apical two-chamber view. The pulsed sample volume is located just on the ventricular side of the aortic valve. The spectral recording shows normal systolic aortic flow away from the transducer.

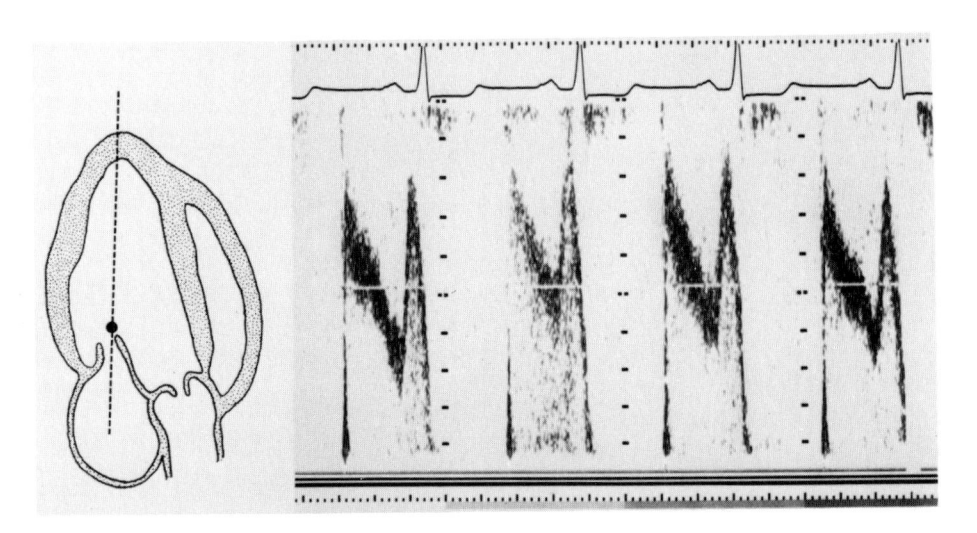

FIG. 5.20. Pulsed spectral velocity tracing from just on the ventricular side of the mitral valve obtained in the apical two-chamber view.

80 BASIC DOPPLER ECHOCARDIOGRAPHY

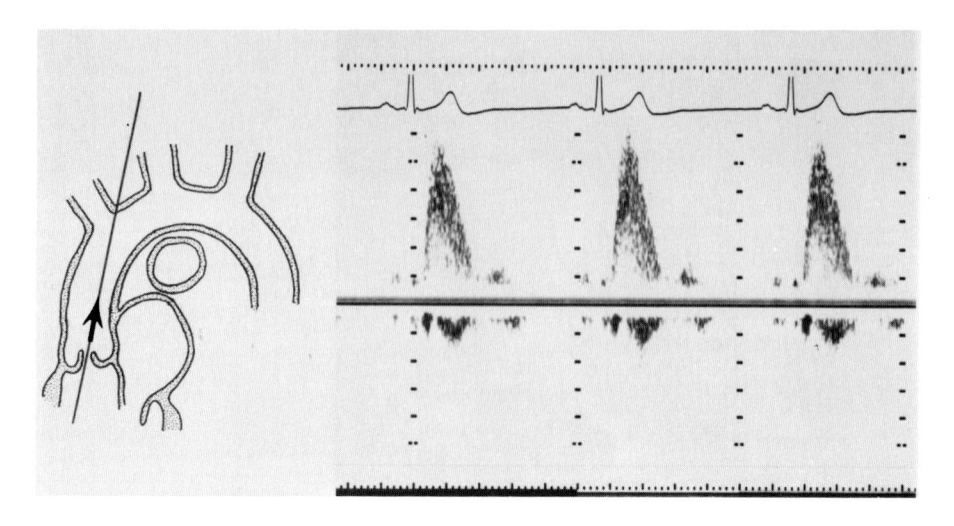

FIG. 5.21. CW spectral recording of normal aortic flow toward the transducer from the suprasternal window.

left ventricular inflow (sample sites 1 and 2) and outflow (sample sites 3 and 4).

Flow-velocity profiles through the mitral valve resemble those obtained in the apical four-chamber view and are directed toward the transducer in diastole (Fig. 5.18B). In our experience, we are able to position and hold the pulsed sample volume on the aortic side of the aortic valve a bit easier using the two-chamber approach rather than the four chamber with extreme superior angulation.

Normal left ventricular systolic outflow is seen in Fig. 5.19 using the apical two-chamber view for cursor guidance. Notice that the sample volume is located

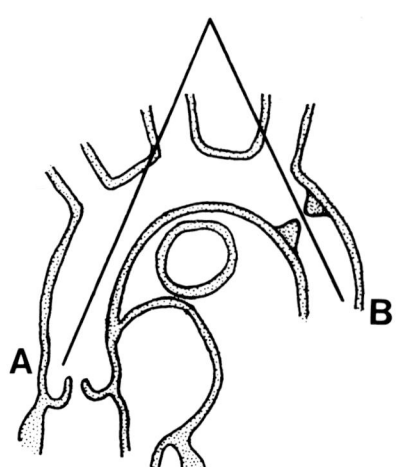

FIG. 5.22. Schematic representation showing direction of the CW beam from the suprasternal window into the ascending aorta (A) and descending aorta (B) in a patient with coarctation of the aorta.

in the left ventricular outflow tract. Sometimes, opening the cursor sample very wide may enhance the operator's ability to detect small disturbances of flow. It is also important to remember (see also Chapter 3) that the farther the sample volume is positioned from the transducer, the larger it will become.

Figure 5.20 shows a normal mitral flow velocity on an expanded scale in relation to the apical two-chamber approach. When an abnormal jet, such as mitral insufficiency, is located in one of these apical views by pulsed Doppler, we recommend rotation into the other view to confirm its presence and location. Use of these alternating views helps an operator to practice tracking a given jet and also aids in developing a three-dimensional sense of jet direction.

SUPRASTERNAL WINDOW

Another window which provides an opportunity for the Doppler beam to be directed parallel to flow is the suprasternal. Placement of the PW or CW transducer in the suprasternal notch allows easy access to systolic flow toward the transducer in the ascending aorta (Fig. 5.21) and systolic flow away from the transducer in the descending aorta. Positioning a large mechanical or phased-array transducer in the suprasternal notch is frequently difficult, and we have

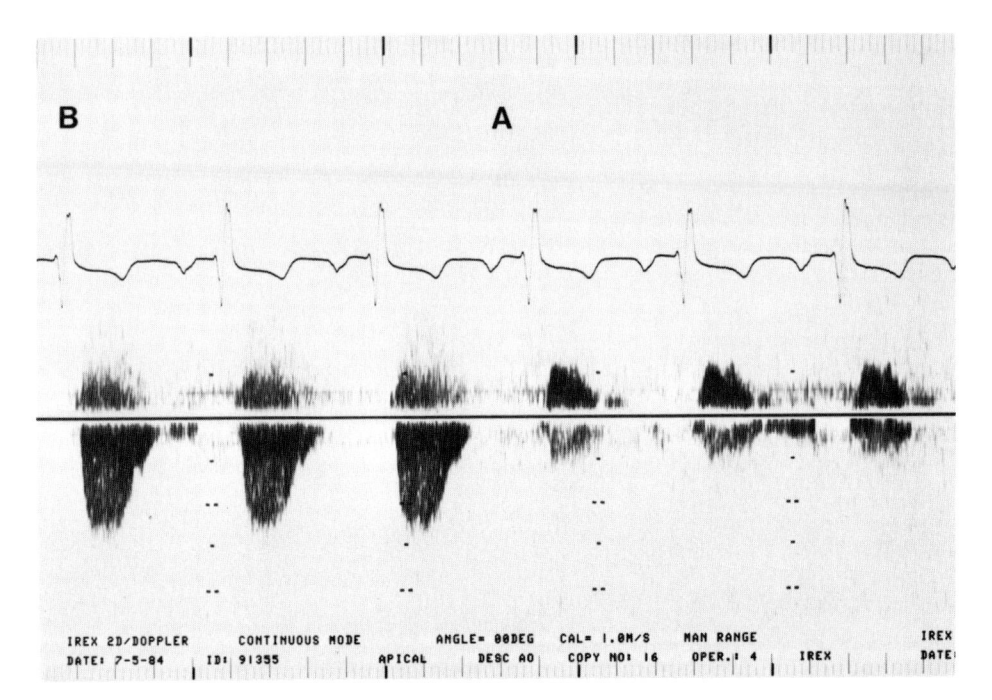

FIG. 5.23. CW spectral velocity recording from the patient in Fig. 5.22. When angled into the descending aorta (B), high-velocity flow is encountered moving away from the transducer. Angling into the ascending aorta produces normal-velocity flow toward the transducer. Calibration marks are 1 m/sec.

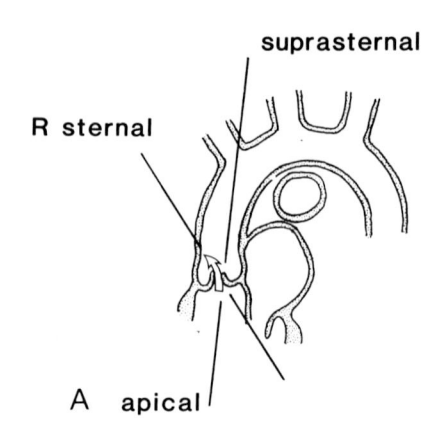

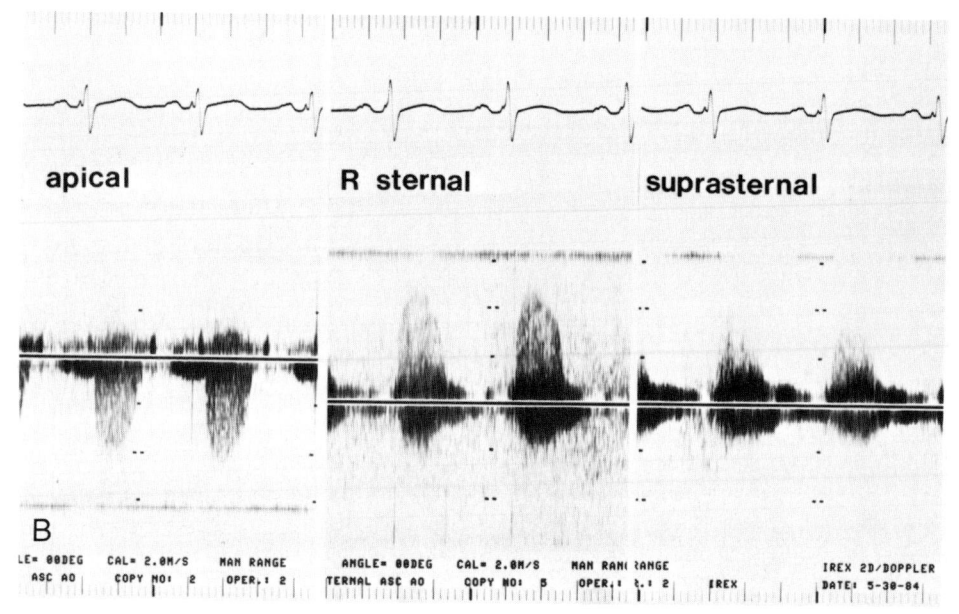

FIG. 5.24. (A) An aortic stenotic jet in relationship to possible viewing directions using CW Doppler. (B) CW spectral velocity tracings from each respective window. The best recording is from the right sternal window. Calibration marks are 2 m/sec.

learned to depend upon CW for this window because the transducer is small and easily maneuvered.

Figure 5.22 shows how a CW beam can be angled from the descending aorta (position B) to the ascending aorta (position A) in a patient with coarctation of the aorta. Notice that in the companion spectral recording (Fig. 5.23) the systolic velocity in the descending aorta is directed away from the transducer (B), and the peak is much higher than the positive flow in the ascending aorta (A).

THE DOPPLER EXAMINATION   83

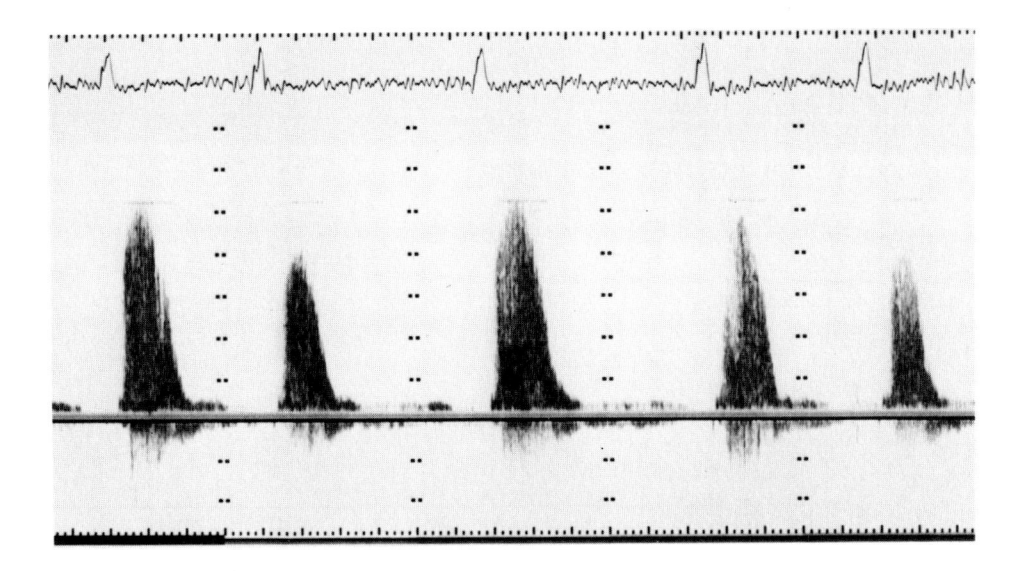

FIG. 5.25. CW spectral velocity recording from the suprasternal window into the ascending aorta from a patient with severe aortic stenosis. Notice the varying peak velocities with varying R-R interval of the EKG. Calibration marks are 1 m/sec.

The suprasternal window is used for interrogating systolic aortic flow for quantitative purposes. As we shall see in Chapter 8, certain quantitative flow measures, such as cardiac output, may be obtained using this approach. This view is preferred for quantitative purposes since a Doppler beam directed down the ascending aorta from the suprasternal notch may be assumed to be parallel to flow in most individuals with no evidence of aortic stenosis.

In patients with aortic valve disease and stenosis no such assumption as to direction of systolic aortic flow can be made. In this case, we are most interested in recording the highest peak systolic velocity present. As previously pointed out, the most faithful representation of flow will be obtained when the beam is parallel. The use of multiple positions for the recording of peak systolic aortic velocity is very important in aortic stenosis since this jet may be directed in a wide variety of orientations. Figure 5.24A demonstrates one such direction of flow and its relationship to various transducer positions for CW recording. In this case (Fig. 5.24B) peak flow was best recorded by CW from the right sternal approach rather than from the suprasternal notch. The velocity profile from the apex seems adequate but is just a bit lower than the right sternal recording. The recording from the suprasternal notch is grossly inadequate and is without a fully formed profile. When examining for aortic stenosis, all available acoustic windows should be utilized.

There will be times when the changing appearance of the spectral trace is not the result of an improper beam direction or misadjustment of system controls. Figure 5.25 shows a continuous wave recording from the suprasternal

84   BASIC DOPPLER ECHOCARDIOGRAPHY

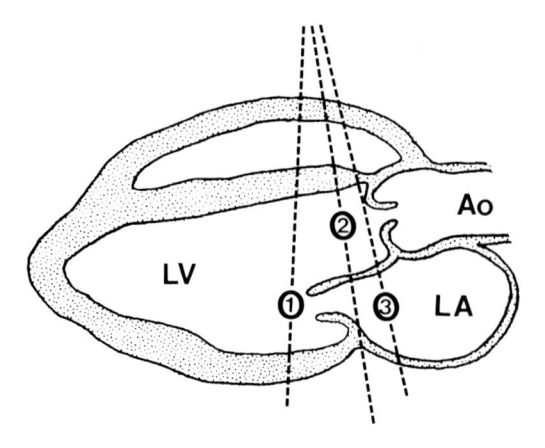

FIG. 5.26. Schematic representation of possible pulsed sample sites in the long axis of the left ventricle when using the left parasternal window. Notice that the Doppler beam is usually not parallel to flow through the mitral and aortic valves.

notch with the beam directed toward the ascending aorta. The differing appearances of the velocity profiles are a result of an irregular heart rate which leads to beat-to-beat changes in stroke volume and, consequently, gradient.

PARASTERNAL WINDOWS

The right and left parasternal windows may also be utilized for Doppler echocardiography. We have just demonstrated a case in Fig. 5.24 where the maxi-

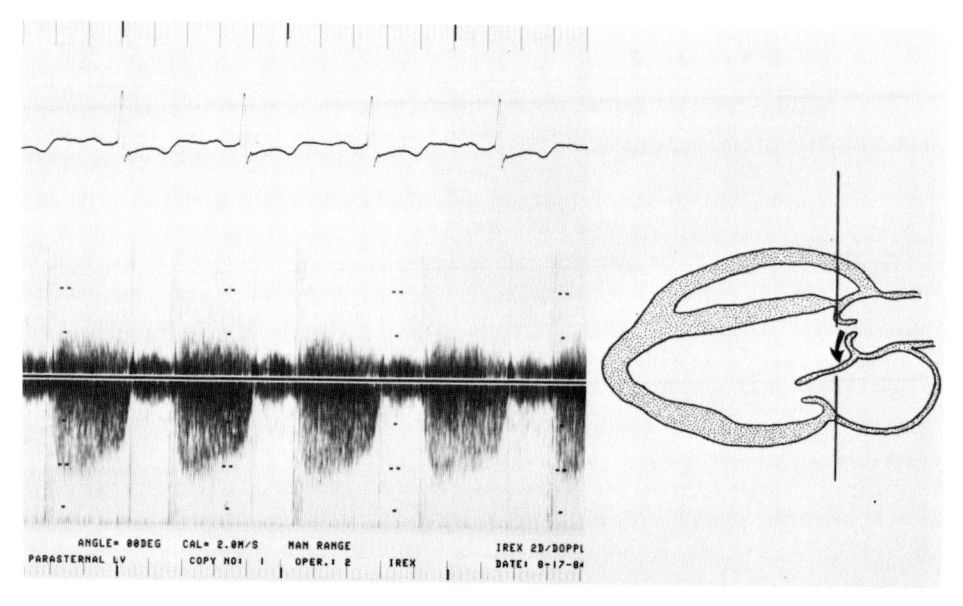

FIG. 5.27. CW spectral velocity recording from the left parasternal window encountering an aortic diastolic jet directed eccentricly and away from the transducer.

mum systolic aortic velocity in aortic stenosis was obtained from the right sternal approach. This is certainly not a conventional view for echocardiographic imaging but is frequently useful for interrogating the ascending aorta by Doppler. This view is best obtained by rotating the patient into a right lateral decubitus position and placing the patient's right hand behind the head to open the intercostal spaces. In the beginning, it is usually helpful to place the two-dimensional imaging transducer at the second or third right intercostal spaces and angle medially to intercept the ascending aorta. Practice with concomitant imaging will help in spatially orienting the beginner to the location of the ascending aorta. In our experience, it is just a short time before one can easily interrogate the ascending aorta from the right sternal approach by using CW mode alone.

The left parasternal window is usually not the best for recording valvular flows through the left heart. As seen in Fig. 5.26, where the left parasternal long axis is represented, it is difficult to orient the Doppler beam parallel to flow through the aortic or mitral valves. This is not to imply that such a view is useless for Doppler as we frequently use this view to confirm the orientation of a given jet in combination with the other views previously mentioned.

The course of any given Doppler beam from the left parasternal approach intercepts flow through the mitral and aortic valves more perpendicular than is desirable. For this reason, the amplitude of the velocity recordings is usually very low. Since continuous wave Doppler has no ability to discriminate in range and the beam would cross low-amplitude flows through both aortic and mitral valves at any one time the routine use of CW in this position for a beginner is generally unrewarding. This deserves specific mention since the first reaction of most individuals when confronted with a new imaging machine is to orient the transducer into the left parasternal long-axis view.

When using the left parasternal approach for interrogation of the aortic and mitral valves, it is frequently most profitable to use pulsed wave Doppler in order to provide some range information for interpreting the low-amplitude signals. When experience is acquired, one may find this view helpful in specifically localizing turbulence and tracking the spatial orientation of any given jet. Occasionally, the direction of an abnormal jet such as aortic insufficiency will be posteriorly, making it easiest to record from the left parasternal window (Fig. 5.27).

The left parasternal window does have very important use for examining the interventricular septum for ventricular septal defects (Fig. 5.28). Flow through a ventricular defect is generally parallel to the interrogating Doppler beam from the left parasternal window. The technique of searching for a ventricular septal defect involves moving the sample cursor along the right ventricular side of the interventricular septum until abnormal flow is detected. Flow through a ventricular septal defect is generally of high enough velocity to alias, despite the close position of the sample volume to the transducer. Once localized by pulsed wave, the full profile signal may be searched for using continuous wave (Fig. 5.29). Most users of Doppler echocardiography will con-

86 BASIC DOPPLER ECHOCARDIOGRAPHY

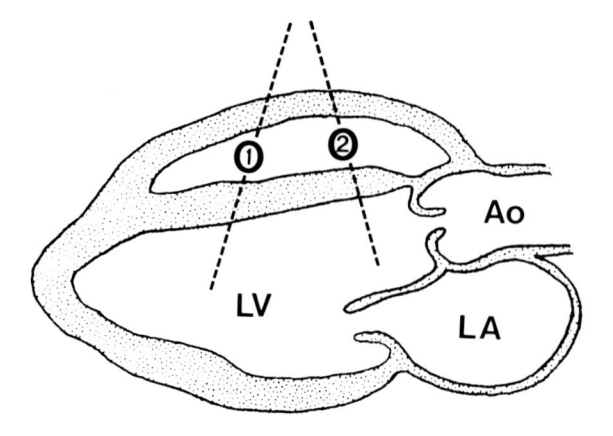

FIG. 5.28. Schematic drawing in the left parasternal long-axis view showing possible pulsed sample sites for exploration for ventricular septal defects.

firm the great utility of this approach for the detection of ventricular septal defects.

The left parasternal window is also ideal for detecting flow through the pulmonic and tricuspid valves. Using pulsed Doppler, it is best to start with a short-axis view at the level of the aortic root (Fig. 5.30). This shows that Doppler beams directed at the tricuspid or pulmonic valves are parallel to blood flow and will result in a strong Doppler signal. Sample volumes may be positioned on either side of these valves, and the flow profiles resemble

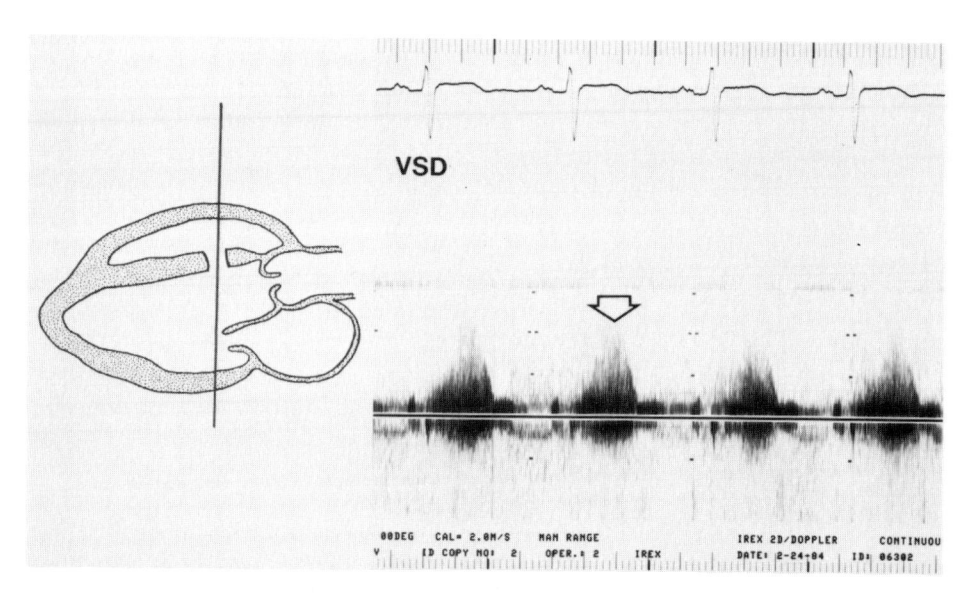

FIG. 5.29. CW spectral velocity recording through a ventricular septal defect. The systolic profile is toward the transducer indicating a left-to-right shunt during systole (arrow).

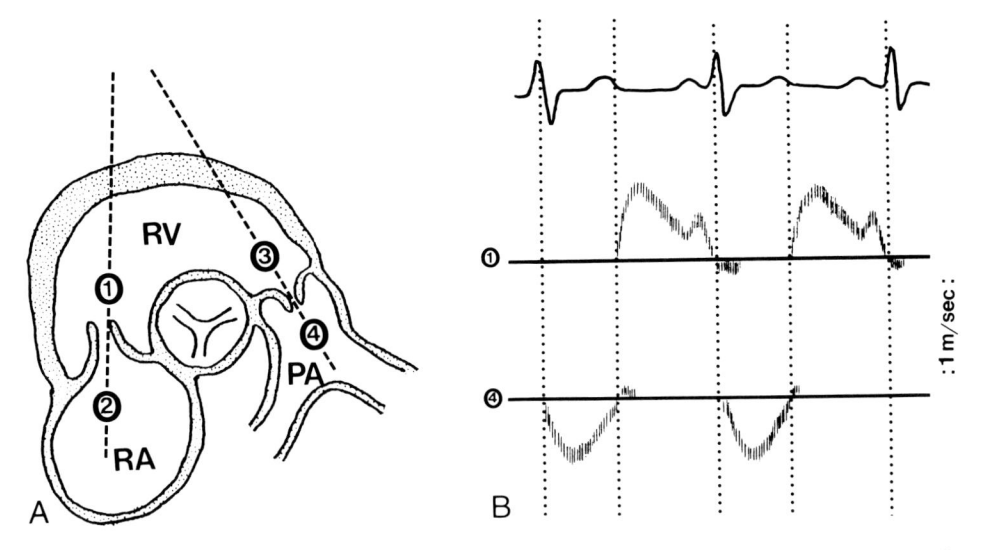

FIG. 5.30. (A) A parasternal short-axis view at the level of the aorta with PW sample sites on either side of the tricuspid and pulmonic valves. (B) Schematic spectral recording of normal tricuspid diastolic (site 1) and pulmonic systolic (site 4) flows.

the configuration of their left-sided counterparts, except that the velocities are a bit lower (Fig. 5.30B).

In some patients the left parasternal view may be the only one where intelligible flow is detected through the pulmonic valve. Beginners will find the use of pulsed Doppler for detection of flow easiest (Fig. 5.31). Note that normal systolic flow in the pulmonary artery is away from the transducer in this position. As the operator gains experience, he or she will also feel comfortable

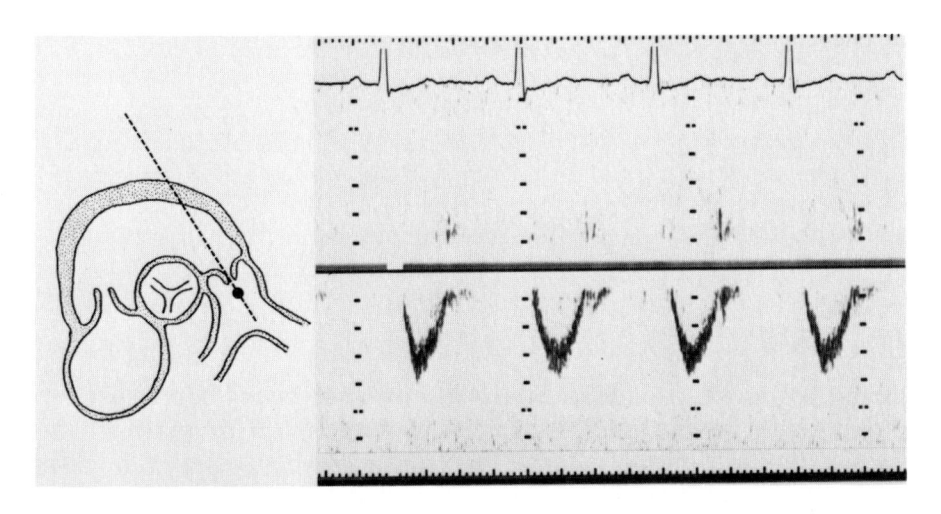

FIG. 5.31. PW spectral trace of normal pulmonic flow away from the transducer obtained from the parasternal short-axis orientation at the level of the aorta.

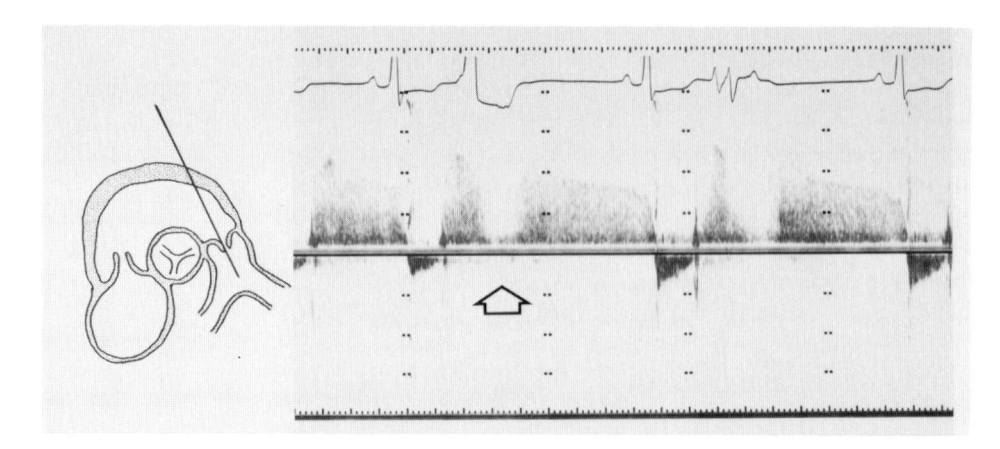

FIG. 5.32. CW spectral velocity recording from the parasternal window in a patient with pulmonic insufficiency. Note the diastolic flow toward the transducer. Due to the PVC, no systolic flow is noted on some beats (arrow).

using continuous wave Doppler for recording the full spectral profile of abnormal jets (Fig. 5.32). Note the similarity in appearance of pulmonic insufficiency with the preceding examples of aortic insufficiency. This example also shows the absence of systolic flow into the pulomonary artery (arrow) following a premature ventricular contraction.

Skill in examining flow through the pulmonary valve is most useful in the study of congenital heart disease. As we shall see in Chapter 9, much information can be obtained through study of differential flow rates through the aorta and pulmonary arteries.

OTHER WINDOWS

As will be pointed out in future examples, it is important note that all other available windows may be used for differing purposes. These include the lower left parasternal, subcostal, and many intermediate windows. We have described a few windows in detail to provide a means for beginners to familiarize themselves with the easiest, and generally most productive, transducer positions and beam directions.

THE DOPPLER EXAMINATION

Using this sequential window approach is not the only way to conduct a methodical Doppler examination, but it has appeared to us to be very helpful to those with little, or no, Doppler experience. When conducting a Doppler examination, the operator should remember that these studies may be very difficult to interpret for an individual not present during the actual examination. A poor-quality echocardiographic image of cardiac structures may be possible to identify by an experienced observer, but a poor-quality Doppler tracing may be impossible to identify and interpret.

For this reason, we believe that sonographers and physicians interested in acquiring skills in Doppler echocardiography should conduct the examinations jointly during the learning period. We also highly recommend that each laboratory develop an annotation system so that sonographers may convey key orientation information to an interpreting physician not actually present during the examination. This may be accomplished on almost every commercial system by voice labeling (or commenting) on the audio track of the tape recording of the video or audio record information concerning window used, probable beam orientation, and suspected lesion encountered. We also suggest written annotation on the graphic recorder hard-copy paper output of similar information.

REFERENCES

1. Henry WL, DeMaria A, Gramiak R, King DL, Kisslo JA, Popp RL, Sahn DJ, Schiller NB, Tajik A, Teichholz LE, Weyman AE: Report of The American Society of Echocardiography Committee on Nomencalture and Standards in Two-Dimensional Echocardiography. American Society of Echocardiography Publisher, Raleigh, N.C., 1979

6 Doppler Evaluation of Valvular Regurgitation

DANIEL B. MARK
JEFFERY H. ROBERTSON
DAVID ADAMS
JOSEPH KISSLO

CHARACTERISTICS OF REGURGITANT JETS

Valvular regurgitation (or insufficiency) is loosely defined as the presence of backward, or retrograde, flow across a given closed cardiac valve. It is clinically assumed that there is normally no flow backward into the ventricles through the aortic or pulmonic valves in diastole. Similarly, there is no flow backward into the atria across the mitral or tricuspid valves in systole. Thus, the first effect of regurgitation on blood flow through the heart is a change in direction. Figure 6.1 demonstrates the abnormal direction of flow in the left heart for mitral and aortic regurgitation. Given the ability of Doppler echocardiography to detect the direction of blood flow, it seems ideally suited for assessment of valvular insufficiencies.

The second effect of regurgitation on cardiac blood flow is the creation of turbulence. Most valvular regurgitation is associated with some abnormality of leaflet coaptation. Regurgitant jets originate from small, irregular openings. They may be directed quite eccentrically, and they are almost always turbulent. Regurgitant jets are made up of many different velocities and complex flow patterns. These features are represented on the Doppler recording as spectral broadening, which is the graphic equivalent of turbulent flow.

The third factor that characterizes the abnormal flow of a regurgitant jet is an increase in velocity, which is a result of a pressure gradient that exists across a regurgitant valve. For example, normal systolic pressure in the left ventricle is over 100 mmHg. At the same time, the pressure in the left atrium is very low and ranges from 2 to 12 mmHg. When mitral regurgitation is present, there is an abnormal communication between the left ventricle and

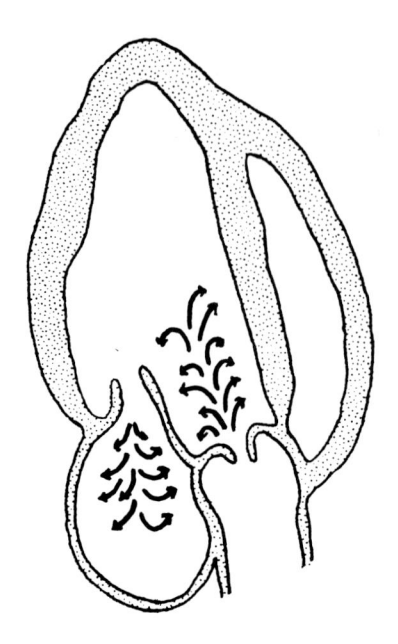

FIG. 6.1. Schematic diagram showing the direction of aortic insufficiency in diastole and mitral regurgitation in systole. Valvular regurgitation results in turbulence and an increase in velocity.

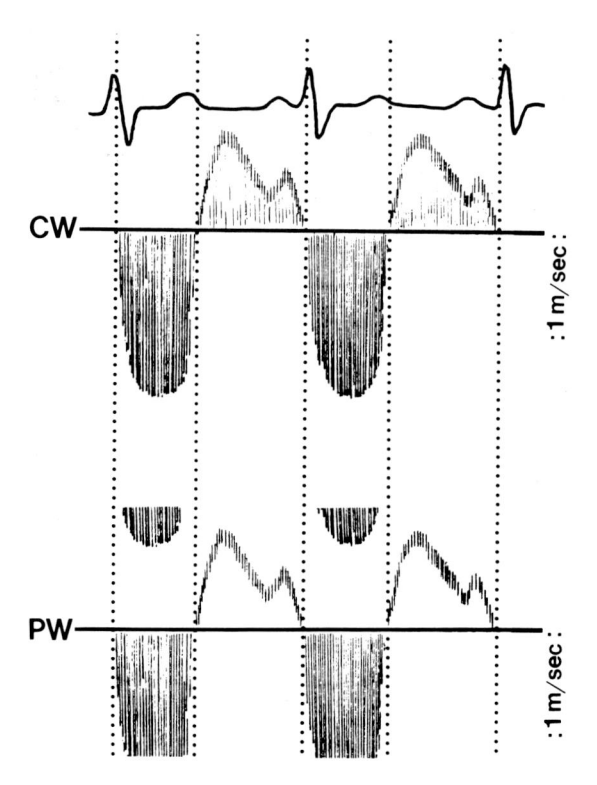

FIG. 6.2. Schematic diagram of a mitral regurgitant jet recorded from the apex. The flow is away from the transducer, and there is spectral broadening. Most regurgitant jets result in velocities that exceed 1.5 m/sec and require CW Doppler to record the full-spectral velocity profile. PW recordings are almost always aliased.

FIG. 6.3. Left panel demonstrates that regurgitant jets may be eccentrically directed in any direction. Right panel demonstrates that regurgitant jets also have size, from small to large.

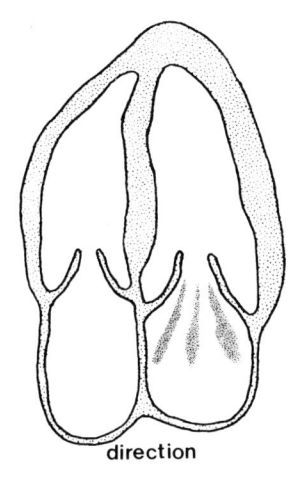

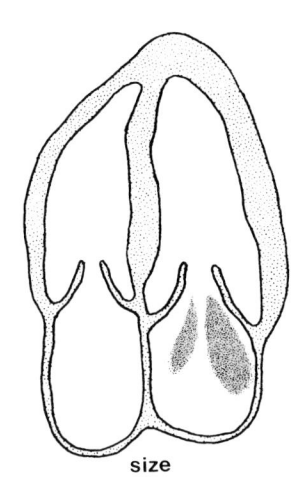

left atrium in systole, and a pressure gradient of 85 mmHg or more produces retrograde flow into the left atrium. This flow takes the form of a high-velocity regurgitant jet, as predicted by the Bernoulli principle (see Chapter 3). One important practical effect of high velocities on Doppler recordings is that in pulsed wave mode aliasing is almost always produced. This is shown in Fig. 6.2. In this idealized drawing, the top panel shows systolic turbulent flow moving away from the transducer, which is positioned at the apex. The full profile is recorded by continuous wave Doppler. When the same jet is interrogated by pulsed wave Doppler, aliasing occurs.

Appreciation of the three main features of regurgitant jets described above (i.e., abnormal direction, turbulence, and high velocity) is crucial to the success of the Doppler beginner. He or she should realize that a regurgitant jet may be directed anywhere within the spatial volume of the receiving chamber (Fig. 6.3, left). The jet may vary in size from small to large, and its spatial location and general magnitude are best assessed using pulsed wave Doppler echocardiography (Fig. 6.3, right). During assessment with pulsed Doppler, however, aliasing invariably occurs as a result of the high velocities encountered (Fig. 6.4). This makes recognition of the complete abnormal flow profile of a regurgitant jet almost impossible by pulsed Doppler alone. In the pulsed spectral tracing of aortic insufficiency shown, the spectral recording is filled from top to bottom in diastole, and recognition of the complete spectral profile is quite difficult. Thus, continuous wave Doppler must be used to record the full contour of the abnormal regurgitant profile in this same patient (Fig. 6.5). Continuous wave Doppler, in turn, has the disadvantage of lack of depth resolution and is therefore not suitable for localizing areas of turbulent flow in the heart.

DOPPLER-ANGIOGRAPHIC COMPARISONS

The first Doppler echocardiographic studies of valvular regurgitation were focused outside the heart. In 1971, Tunstall Pedoe demonstrated that retrograde blood flow could be detected during diastole in the subclavian arteries of pa-

94 BASIC DOPPLER ECHOCARDIOGRAPHY

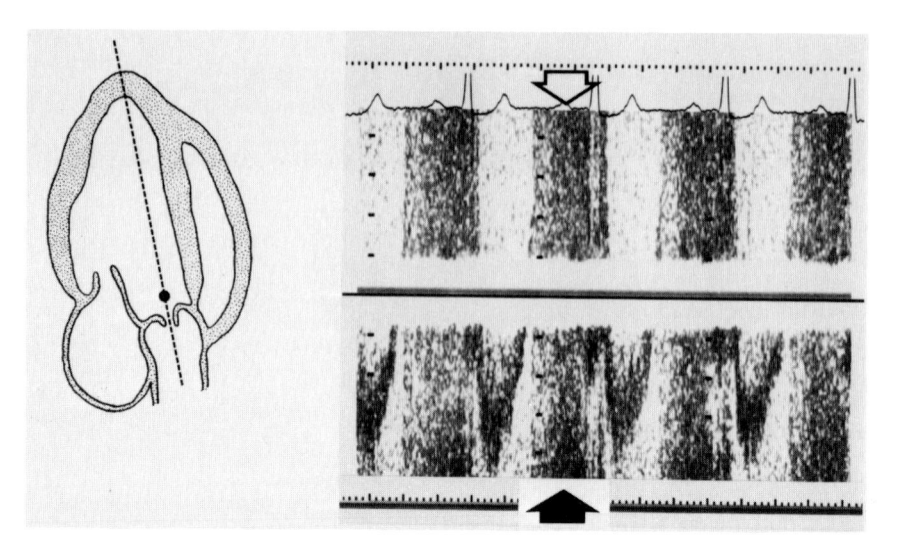

FIG. 6.4. Pulsed Doppler spectral recording of aortic insufficiency. Flow is toward the transducer, and aliasing occurs (open arrow) with placement of the higher velocities at the bottom of the spectral tracing (closed arrow). Almost all regurgitant jets reach velocities that alias with standard pulsed Doppler. Scale marks are 20 cm/sec.

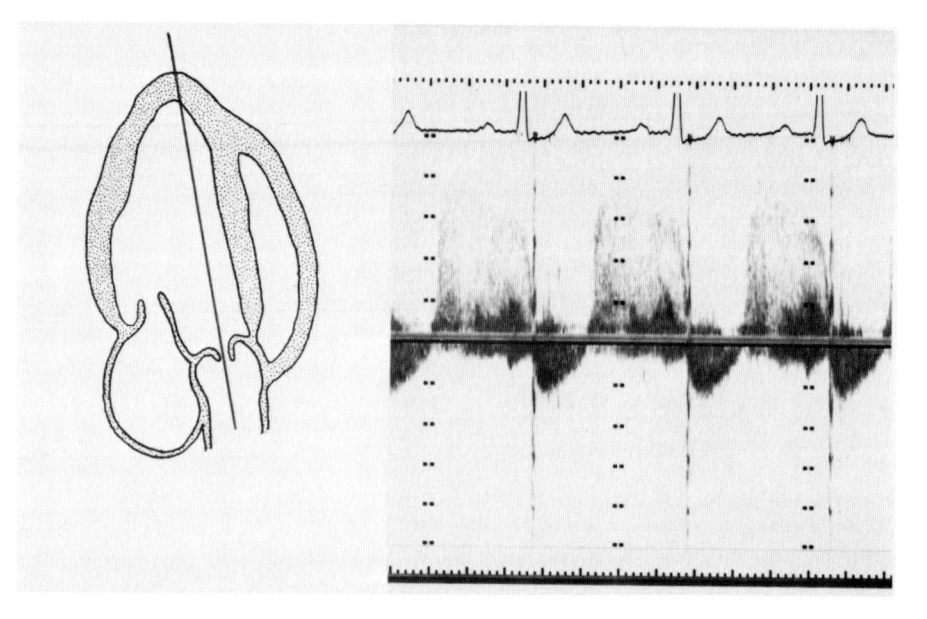

FIG. 6.5. CW spectral velocity recording from the apex of the same patient as Fig. 6.4. The full abnormal profile of aortic insufficiency is easily recorded toward the transducer (positive shift). Scale marks are 1 m/sec.

tients with aortic insufficiency.[1] At the same time, Kalmanson and colleagues reported on the flow abnormalities detected in the jugular veins of patients with tricuspid insufficiency.[2] Since then there have been many studies using direct evaluation of the heart valves for insufficiency, and it is now becoming generally accepted that Doppler is a fairly sensitive and specific method for the detection of valvular insufficiency.

The beginning student of Doppler, however, should not be misled by assuming that previous reports have absolutely established that Doppler echocardiography is both 100 percent sensitive and specific for the detection of valvular insufficiency. The only currently acceptable standard for comparison of Doppler data is cineangiography. However, catheterization is not an ideal "gold standard." When small regurgitant jets are directed into enlarged chambers, the resulting dilution of the angiographic contrast agent may render the regurgitation undetectable. Angiographic evaluation of right-sided lesions is particularly difficult, since catheters must be placed across the valve being evaluated, causing at least some degree of iatrogenic insufficiency (Fig. 6.6). Furthermore, the angiographic grading scheme for insufficiency used in most catheterization labo-

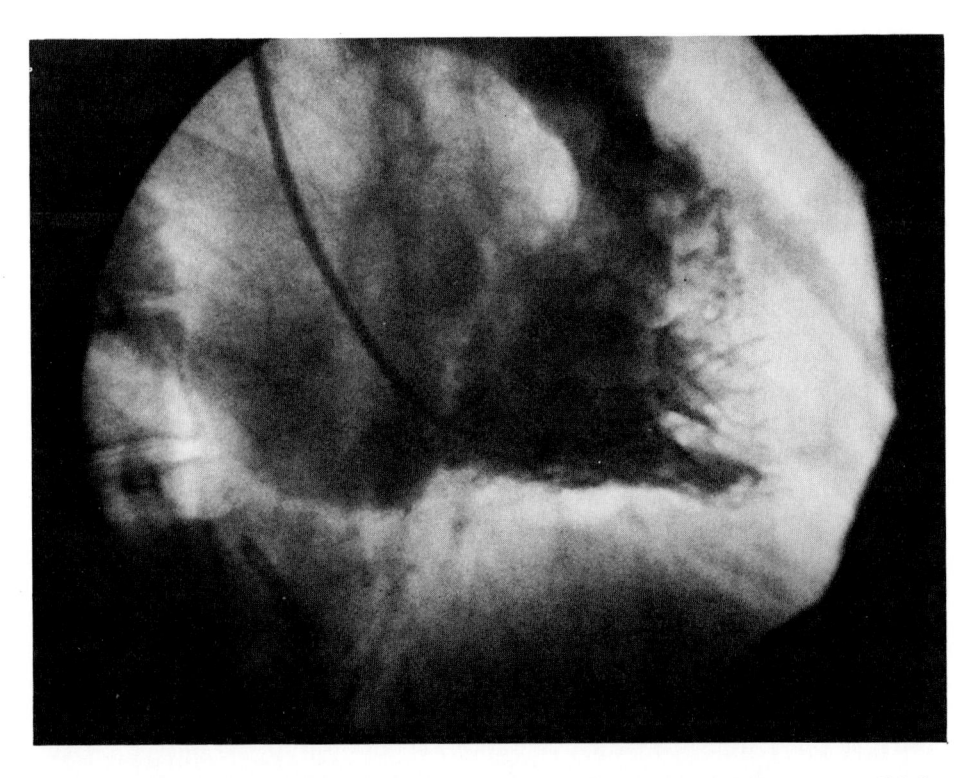

FIG. 6.6. Right ventricular angiogram in slight right anterior oblique view. With a catheter across the tricuspid valve, some degree of tricuspid regurgitation almost always results.

ratories (0 to 4+) is based on subjective interpretation, and there is general agreement that this method is not very accurate relative to quantitative methods.

Most Doppler-angiographic comparisons have involved small numbers of catheterized patients and, in some cases, the criteria for patient selection have not been specifically stated. Almost all studies have involved patients with sufficient disease of the valve to warrant catheterization, and the very favorable results reported might not apply to larger groups of patients with less advanced disease. Some studies have even included Doppler evaluations performed after the angiograms by operators who may have been influenced by the angiographic results.

Our experience with Doppler is that Doppler-angiographic comparisons yield a sensitivity and specificity approaching 100 percent when significant (2+ or greater) angiographic regurgitation is present.[3] When there is little or no angiographic regurgitation present (0 or 1+), the two techniques are somewhat less likely to agree. As we shall see, Doppler may detect the presence of valvular regurgitation in patients without any evidence of a cardiac murmur. Indeed, there are surprisingly high rates of detectable lesions such as tricuspid and pulmonic insufficiencies in normal patients.[4] Thus, it must be recognized that even experienced operators will detect regurgitant jets which cannot be documented by angiography and will miss some small jets recognized by angiographic methods. It is clearly best for beginners with Doppler echocardiography to perform some Doppler-angiographic comparisons of their own in order to establish the level of reliability in their own laboratories.

AORTIC REGURGITATION

Pulsed wave Doppler has been reported to have a sensitivity ranging between 86 and 100 percent[5-8] for the detection of aortic regurgitation. Pulsed Doppler examinations for this lesion are best begun using the apical window with the apical two- or four-chamber two-dimensional views for operator guidance. Note that in the normal subject some low-frequency diastolic sounds are encountered which the novice may mistake for evidence of aortic insufficiency (Fig. 6.7). Careful searching just on the ventricular side of the aortic valve in abnormal patients reveals the high-frequency sounds and diastolic spectral pattern typical of aortic insufficiency (Fig. 6.8). Almost all regurgitant jets are severely aliased, and the top of the spectral trace appears cut off and placed at the bottom of the display.

Sometimes these regurgitant jets are very small, and slight movement of the sample volume will result in the loss of the originally detected jet (Fig. 6.9). Note that the zero baseline of the spectral display has been moved to the bottom of the display, as described in Chapter 5, in an attempt to eliminate the aliased diastolic signal and to provide as much display of the spectral profile as possible. Even with this maneuver, the top of the aliased signal is still missing. Although it does not appear that there has been a major change in the position of the sample volume (Fig. 6.9B), there is a major change in

DOPPLER EVALUATION OF VALVULAR REGURGITATION 97

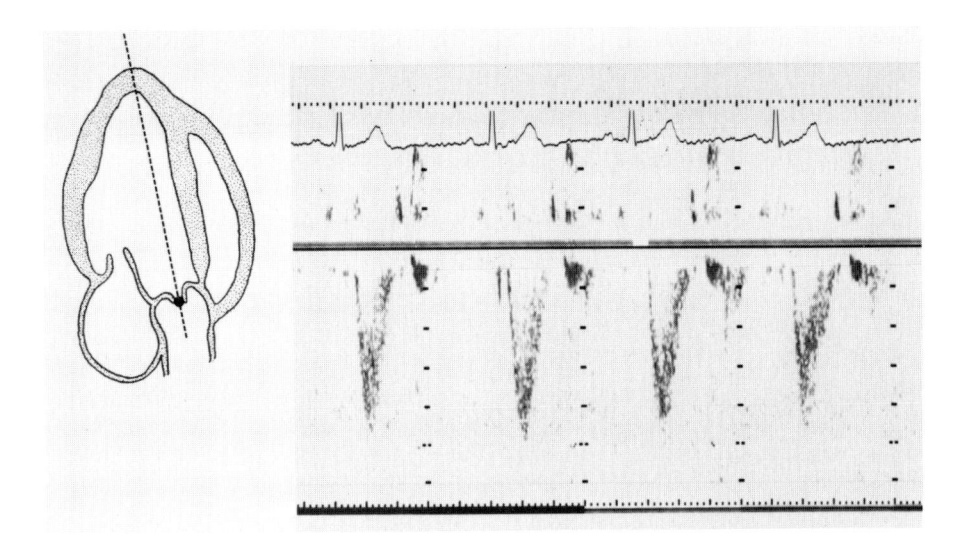

FIG. 6.7. Normal pulsed Doppler spectral recording. Systolic flow is away from the transducer, and the velocity shift is negative. Some apparent "abnormalities" are usually recorded in diastole. Scale marks are 20 cm/sec.

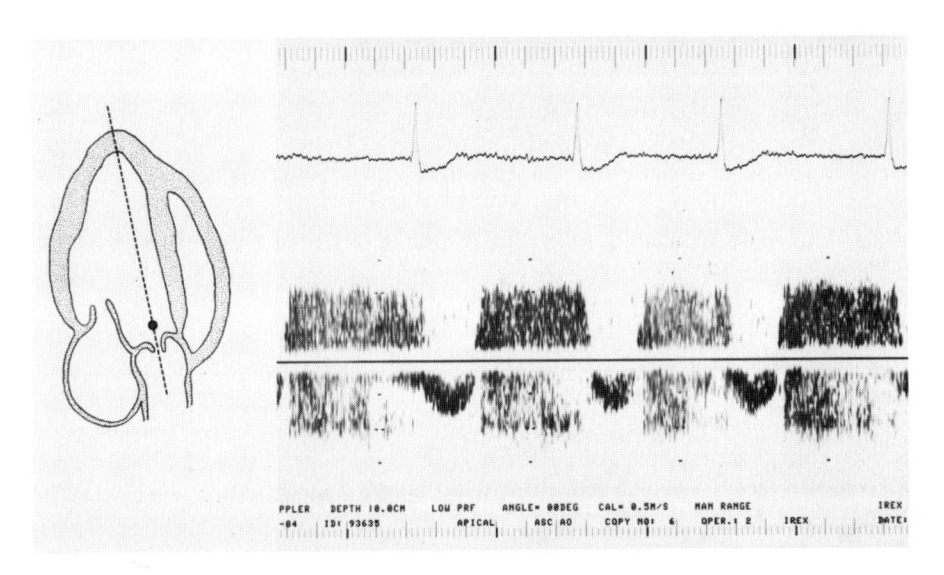

FIG. 6.8. Pulsed Doppler recording of aortic insufficiency with severe aliasing. Scale marks are 0.5 m/sec.

98 BASIC DOPPLER ECHOCARDIOGRAPHY

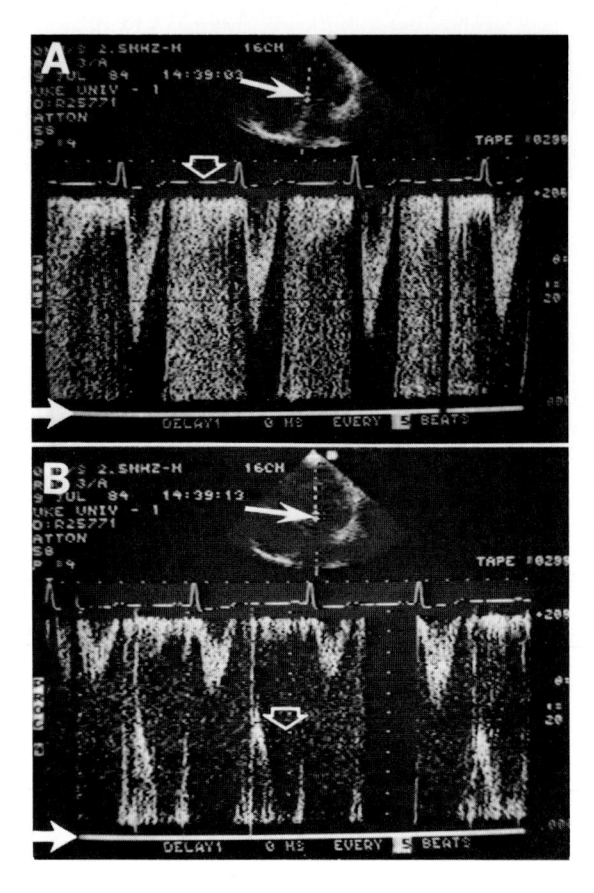

FIG. 6.9. (A) Pulsed spectral recording of aortic insufficiency with the sample volume located just below the aortic root (top arrow). Aliasing is seen (open arrow). (B) Normal mitral diastolic flow (open arrow) encountered with only slight movement of the sample volume. Arrows locating baselines are at left. Scale marks are 20 cm/sec.

the appearance of the spectral display. Note the typical mitral inflow profile on Fig. 6.9B.

Similarly, the best window for the evaluation of aortic insufficiency with continuous wave Doppler is the apical window. Using this approach, aortic insufficiency appears as a holodiastolic high-frequency turbulent jet with spectral broadening and flow toward the transducer (Fig. 6.10). The resultant spectral shift is positive (i.e., above the baseline).

It is usually of interest to beginners with Doppler echocardiography who are familiar with auscultation that the Doppler spectrum in aortic insufficiency has a holodiastolic duration, and its duration does not vary with severity. This example serves to highlight the differences between the audible sounds generated by the Doppler shift device and those heard by auscultation. Using the latter approach, the typical murmur of aortic insufficiency is early diastolic and decrescendo.

The operator should keep in mind some possible causes for false-positive or false-negative examinations when evaluating patients with suspected aortic insufficiency (Table 6.1). One very common reason for a false-positive test is confusion with mitral valve diastolic inflow. Figure 6.11 shows a continuous

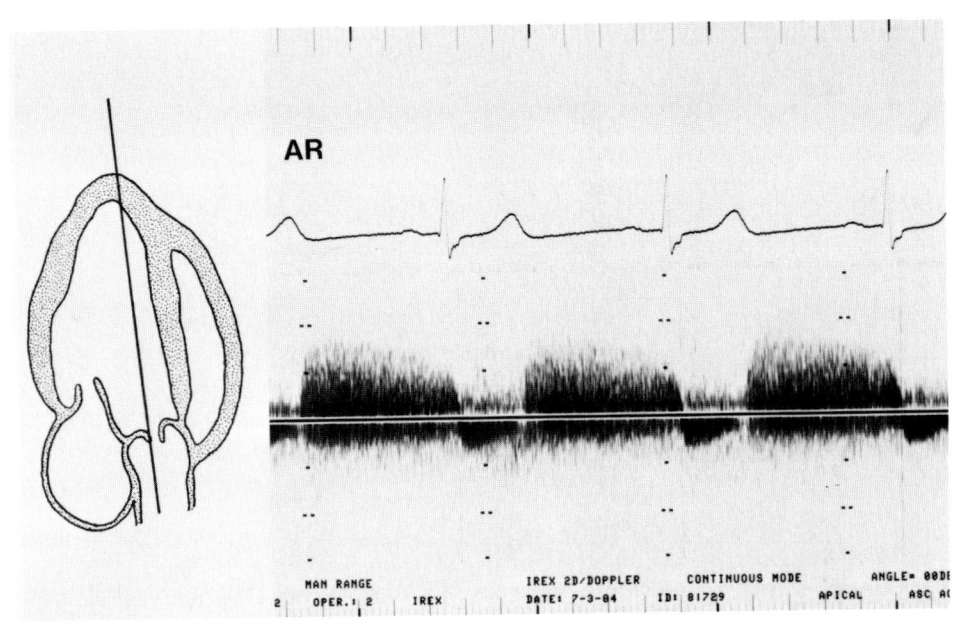

FIG. 6.10. CW spectral velocity recording of aortic insufficiency. Abnormal flow is positive and toward the transducer. Scale marks are 2 m/sec.

wave recording taken from the apical window in a patient with aortic valve disease. Note the different timing of the aortic diastolic jet and the mitral inflow signal. The duration of diastole is longer in aortic insufficiency than mitral inflow. Confusion with mitral inflow is particularly a problem when mitral stenosis is present. Note the similar contours of these two lesions in Fig. 6.12. Note also that the spectral distribution of both abnormal jets is wide, but much less intense in aortic insufficiency when compared with mitral stenosis. Recognition of the different features of the spectral display in these two lesions plus a thorough examination of the location of the suspected abnormal diastolic jet using the pulsed wave approach should allow the operator to reliably separate aortic insufficiency and mitral stenosis in most cases.[8]

It is also possible that a false-positive recording of aortic insufficiency may result from inadvertent detection of coronary blood flow. Although coronary flow is mostly diastolic and the size of the Doppler beam is usually large at remote distances from the transducer, it seems unlikely that this is a very frequent cause of false positives in clinical practice.

It is worthwhile to keep in mind that detection of aortic regurgitation by Doppler with a negative cardiac catheterization may not necessarily constitute a false-positive study. However, the amount of regurgitation in this situation is likely minimal.

The most likely reason for a false-negative diagnosis of aortic insufficiency is that the jet is small and not easily detected with either pulsed or continuous wave Doppler. Not only may the jet be small, it may move through the interro-

TABLE 6.1 Common Reasons for Misidentification of Aortic Insufficiency

False positive	Confusion with mitral inflow, particularly mitral stenosis
	Pulmonic insufficiency
	Coronary blood flow
False negative	Small jet missed by inadequate examination
	Dominant mitral inflow obscures small aortic-insufficiency jet
	Moving jet

gating beam with the phases of the cardiac cycle, making it difficult to record a full profile (Fig. 6.13). Figure 6.14 shows a pulsed wave recording of aortic insufficiency with incomplete recording of the diastolic jet on some beats.

This phenomenon also may occur due to the respiratory cycle (Fig. 6.15). Here the full profile of aortic insufficiency is recorded on some beats and not on others. In this situation, the operator should try different transducer positions and angulations to record as much of the suspected abnormal profile as possible.

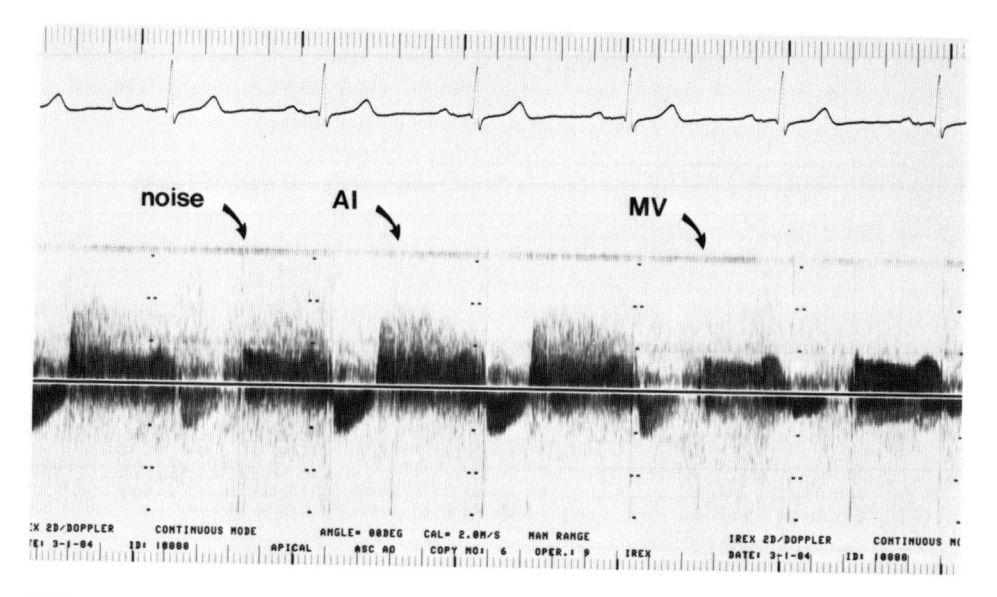

FIG. 6.11. Changing CW spectral patterns encountered when moving the direction of the transducer (at the apex) from aortic outflow where aortic insufficiency (AI) is noted to mitral valve (MV) inflow. Note the mitral profile superimposed on the AI spectra. Range marks are 2 m/sec.

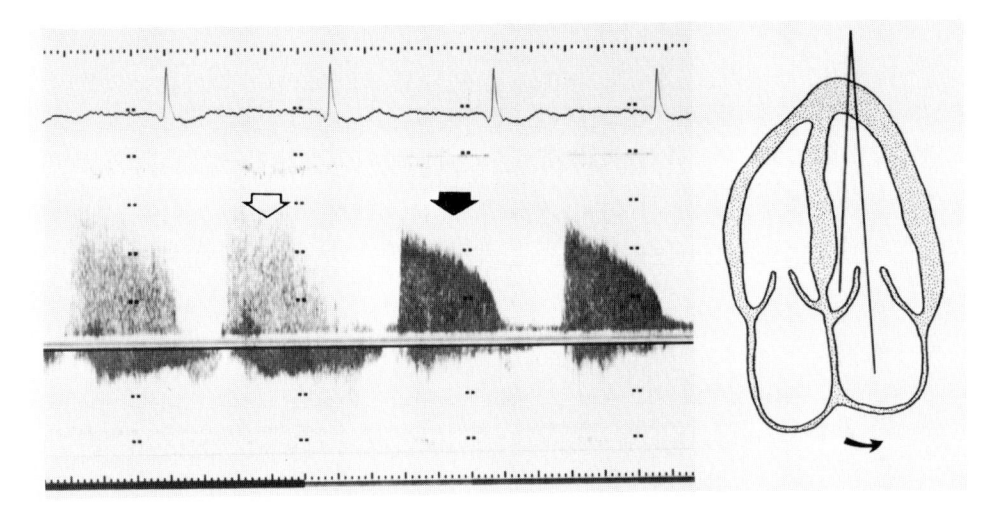

FIG. 6.12. Similar spectral patterns of aortic insufficiency (open arrow) and mitral stenosis (closed arrow) occurring with slight movement of the Doppler beam. For details, see text. Scale marks are 1 m/sec.

Some jets may be so small as to require interrogation from slightly different transducer positions to record the full profile. Figure 6.16 is not a continuous-strip recording but, rather, a five-panel demonstration of the diastolic appearance of aortic insufficiency from five slightly different apical positions in a patient with aortic insufficiency. The only way to overcome this problem is

FIG. 6.13. Regurgitant jets may move eccentrically during the cardiac cycle and cross the Doppler beam.

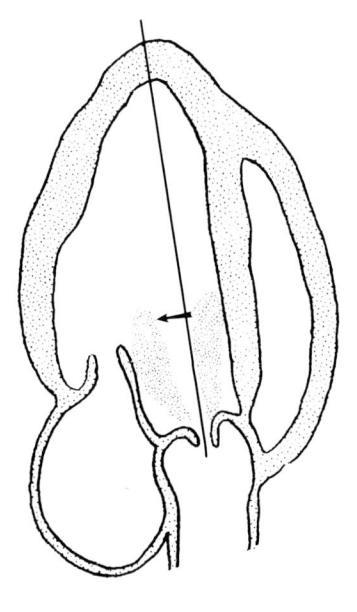

102 BASIC DOPPLER ECHOCARDIOGRAPHY

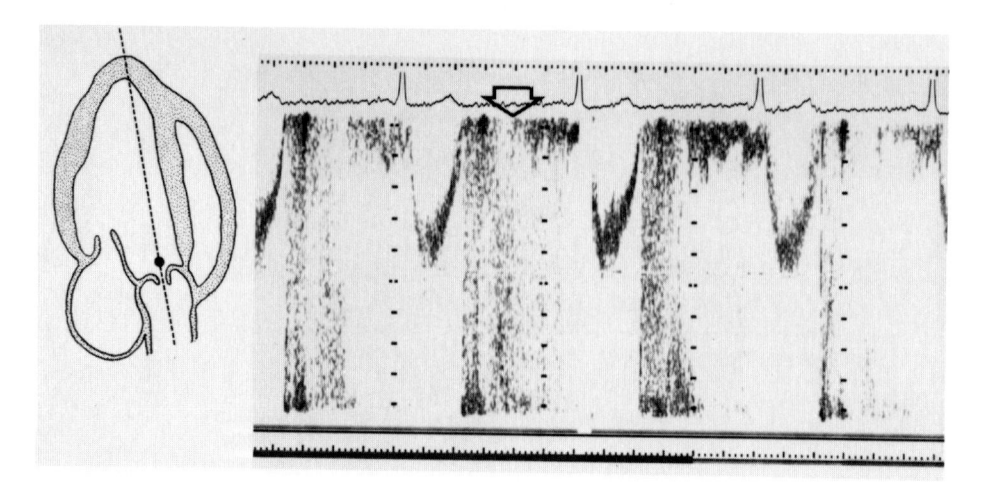

FIG. 6.14. Pulsed Doppler recording of changing patterns of an incompletely visualized aortic regurgitant jet that is encountered from slightly different angles from beat to beat. Range marks are 20 cm/sec.

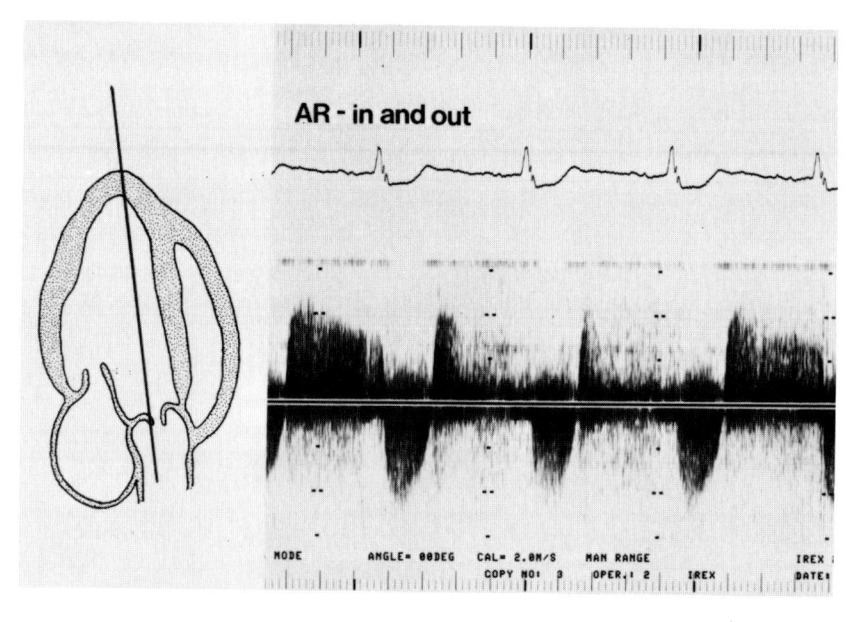

FIG. 6.15. CW spectral recording of aortic regurgitation from apex where the regurgitant jet moves in and out of the beam. Scale marks are 2 m/sec.

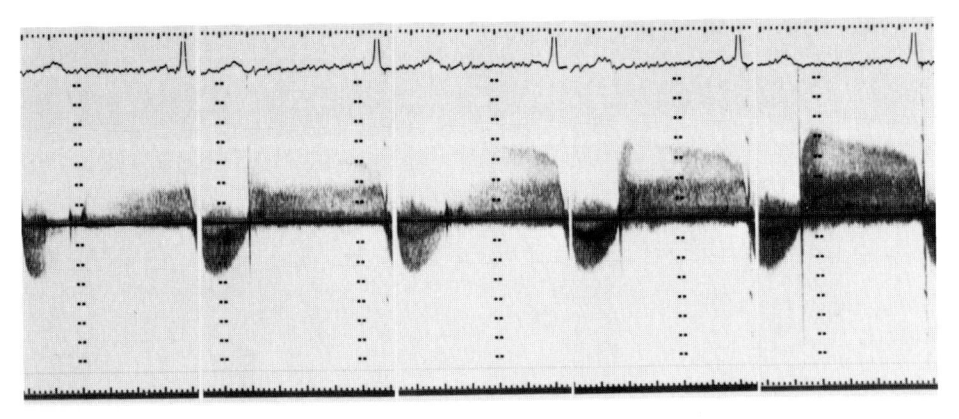

FIG. 6.16. Five panels showing differing appearances of aortic regurgitation from five slightly different positions near the apex using CW Doppler. The best spectral profile is at right. Scale marks are 1 m/sec.

to be assured that every possible area has been adequately interrogated for aortic insufficiency during the Doppler examination.

Although the apical approach is the most profitable window for the detection of aortic insufficiency, it is worth keeping in mind that some jets are directed eccentrically and may be detectable only from some other window such as the left parasternal (see Fig. 5.27). Caution should be used, however, when using continuous wave Doppler from parasternal windows since it might be possible to mistake pulmonic insufficiency (which can be recorded in many subjects) for that of aortic valve insufficiency.

Some information as to left ventricular end-diastolic pressure may be gained in the setting of aortic insufficiency. Since the velocity of any jet relates to the pressure drop across the valve, there exists a pressure gradient between the aorta and left ventricle at end-diastole. This pressure gradient may be estimated by measuring the velocity of the aortic regurgitant jet at end-diastole (Fig. 6.17) using the simplified Bernoulli equation (see Chapter 3). Subtracting this pressure from diastolic blood pressure (as measured by cuff at the time of the Doppler examination) provides an estimate of left ventricular end-diastolic pressure.[9] In the example shown, the end-diastolic velocity is 1.9 m/sec, which corresponds to a pressure gradient of 14 mmHg. This patient had severe aortic insufficiency, and the measured diastolic blood pressure was 55 mmHg by cuff. This resulted in an end-diastolic pressure estimate of 41 mmHg. At catheterization, the actual measured pressure was 38 mmHg.

It should be noted, however, that this approach only shows satisfactory correlations in patients with severe (3+ to 4+) angiographic aortic insufficiency. Application of this method to individuals with lesser degrees does not yield good correlations with catheterization measurements of left ventricular end-diastolic pressure.

104 BASIC DOPPLER ECHOCARDIOGRAPHY

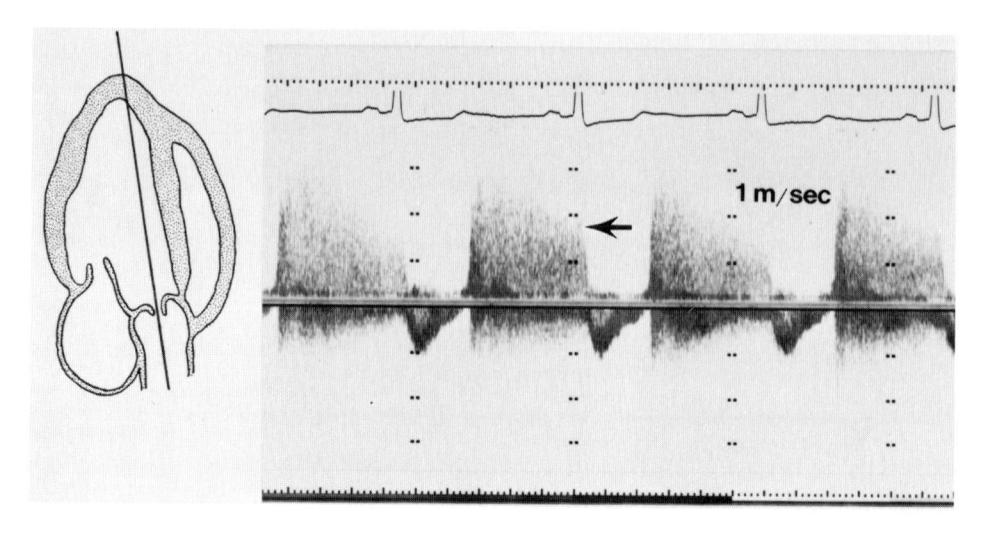

FIG. 6.17. CW spectral recording of aortic insufficiency used in measurement of end-diastolic pressure gradient. Scale marks are 1 m/sec.

MITRAL REGURGITATION

A number of studies have shown that Doppler echocardiography is both very sensitive and very specific for the detection of mitral regurgitation when compared with cardiac catheterization.[10-13] Using pulsed wave Doppler, most cases of mitral regurgitation can be detected with the transducer at the apex and the sample volume located in the left atrium just behind the mitral valve

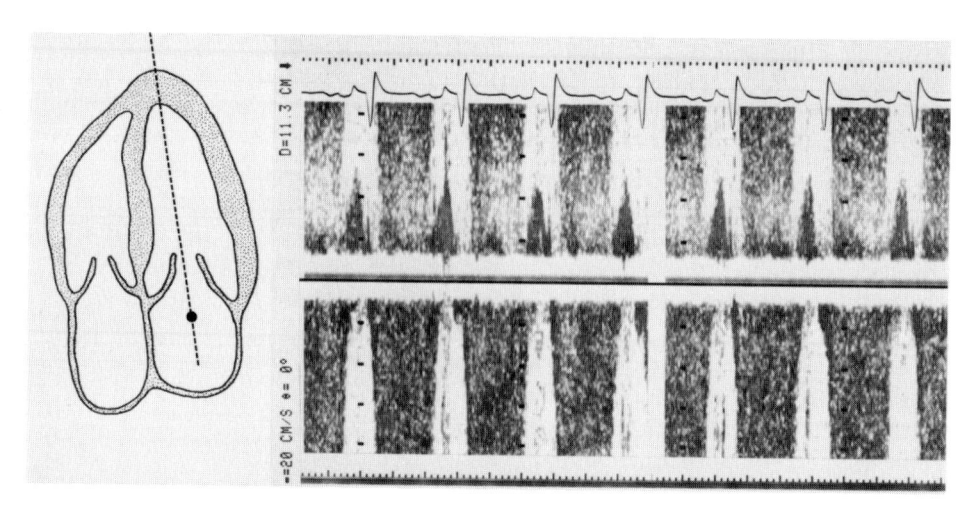

FIG. 6.18. Pulsed Doppler spectral analysis of mitral insufficiency with the sample volume located in the left atrium. The high velocities encountered in mitral insufficiency produce aliasing. Scale marks are 20 cm/sec.

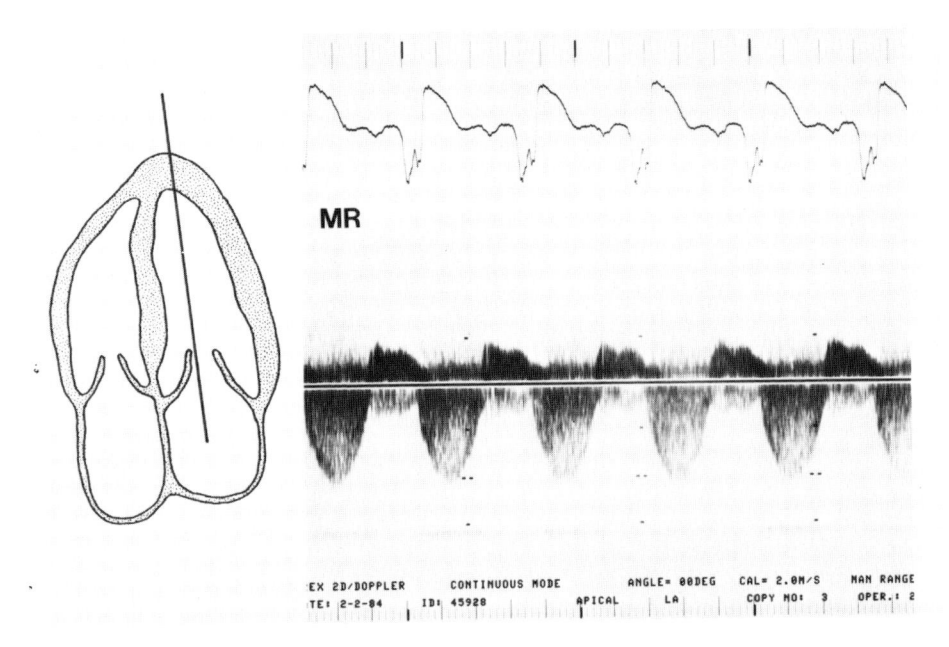

DOPPLER EVALUATION OF VALVULAR REGURGITATION 105

FIG. 6.19. CW Doppler recording of typical mitral regurgitation from apex. The jet is away from the transducer in systole and is usually symmetric in shape. Scale marks are 2 m/sec.

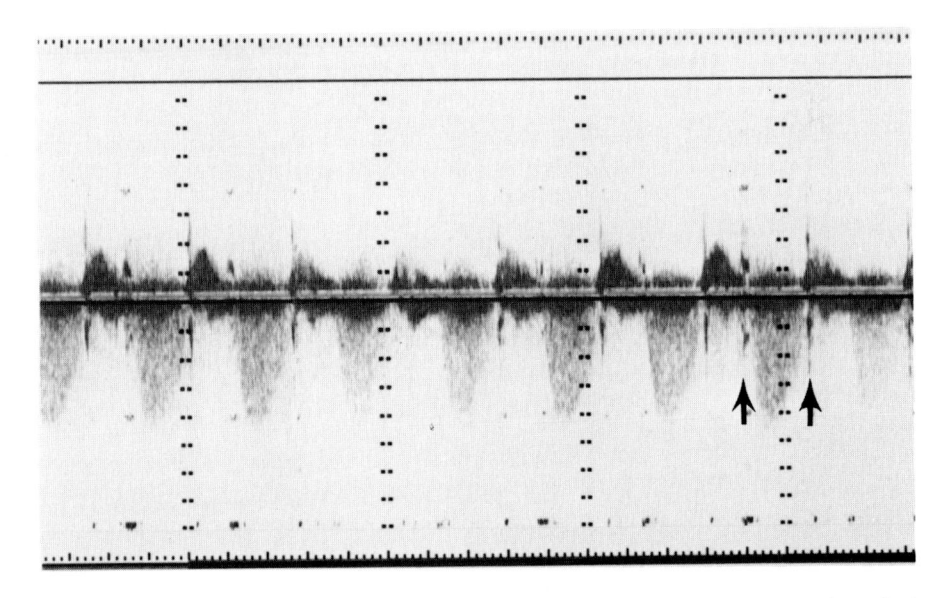

FIG. 6.20. CW spectral recording of typical mitral regurgitation. Note valve closing and opening spikes. Scale marks are 1 m/sec.

106   BASIC DOPPLER ECHOCARDIOGRAPHY

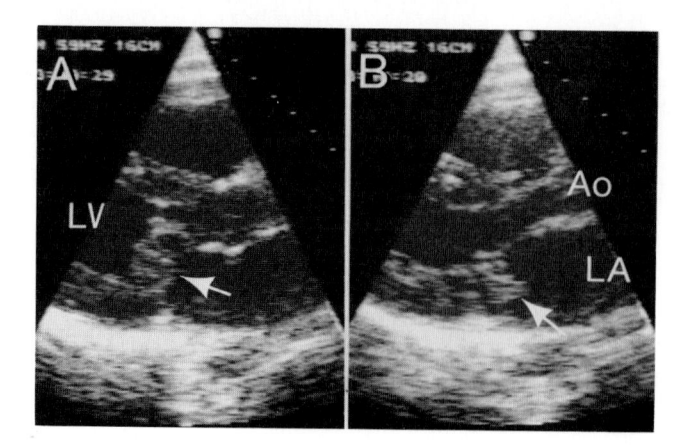

FIG. 6.21. Video stop-frames in the parasternal long axis in diastole (A) and systole (B) in a patient with a large vegetative mass lesion (arrows).

(Fig. 6.18). Because of the high velocities of the regurgitant jet and the distance from the transducer to the jet, aliasing of the mitral regurgitant jet invariably occurs. As with all regurgitant lesions, location of the abnormal turbulence is done in pulsed Doppler mode, and continuous wave Doppler is then used to record the full-spectral profile (Fig. 6.19).

The full-spectral profile of mitral regurgitation commonly reaches peak velocities between 3 and 6 m/sec and is usually quite symmetric, as seen in Figs. 6.19 and 6.20. Mitral regurgitation associated with endocarditis, ruptured chordae tendineae, and/or partial leaflet flail (Fig. 6.21) is frequently associated with loud clicking noises and high-frequency spikes on the spectral recording created by rapid movements of the diseased target through the field of view (Fig. 6.22). Occasionally, the systolic profile of mitral regurgitation peaks slightly early, as is seen in this patient with endocarditis.

Figure 6.23A shows combined aortic insufficiency with aortic outflow tract

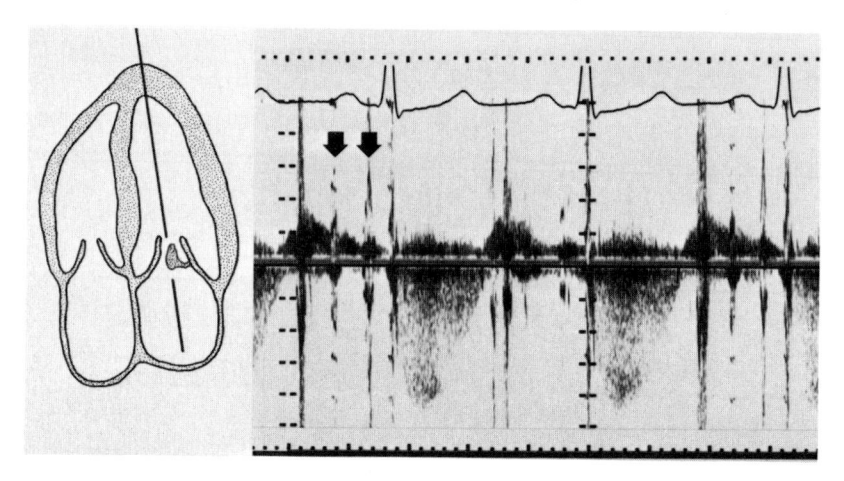

FIG. 6.22.   High-velocity diastolic spikes (arrows) on the CW recording of mitral regurgitation made by vegetation movement.

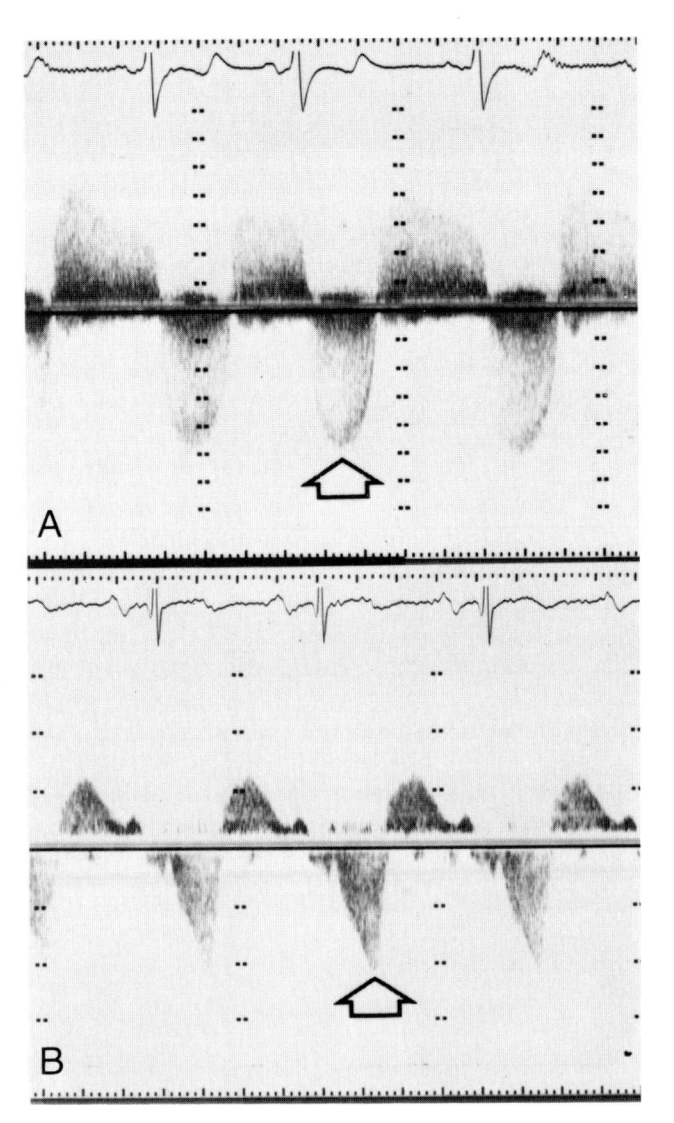

DOPPLER EVALUATION OF VALVULAR REGURGITATION   107

FIG. 6.23. (A) Typical recording of aortic insufficiency and obstruction. Note how the aortic outflow tract turbulence resembles mitral insufficiency (arrow top). (B) Actual late systolic mitral insufficiency (bottom arrow) with CW beam angled through the mitral orifice. Scale marks are 1 m/sec.

obstruction. This tracing was obtained from an individual with hypertrophic cardiomyopathy and a resting outflow tract gradient. Note that the systolic peak velocity approaches almost 5 m/sec. Interrogation of the mitral valve (Fig. 6.23B) shows a clear late systolic profile typical of the late systolic mitral regurgitation seen in this disorder.

False-positive examinations for mitral regurgitation do occur, and some common explanations are listed in Table 6.2. One common reason for a false-positive examination is confusion of the aortic outflow signal with that of mitral regurgitation. Figure 6.24 shows the similarity in the systolic flow profile away from the transducer in mitral regurgitation and aortic stenosis. As previously mentioned, the longer duration of mitral systole may help to differentiate

108 BASIC DOPPLER ECHOCARDIOGRAPHY

TABLE 6.2 Common Reasons for Misidentification of Mitral Regurgitation

False positive	Confusion with aortic outflow, particularly aortic stenosis
	Confusion with tricuspid regurgitation
	Valve slap
False negative	Small jet missed by inadequate examination
	Dominant aortic stenotic jet obscures small mitral regurgitant jet directed adjacent to aortic root
	Moving jet
	Intermittent jet

these two lesions. In addition, it is usual to see mitral diastolic flow in the same spectral recording with mitral insufficiency.

Even though the use of pulsed Doppler may help to locate the systolic turbulent jet in the left atrium rather than the aortic outflow tract, it is important to remember that the size of the sample volume becomes larger at remote distances from the transducer. For example, when the sample volume is positioned in the left atrium from an apical transducer location, the sample volume is almost always larger than it appears on the two-dimensional display (because of the diverging shape of the ultrasound beam). For this reason, it is best to use caution when a negative jet within the left atrium can be detected only in the vicinity of the aortic root since it may very well reflect aortic outflow (Fig. 6.25) rather than mitral regurgitation.

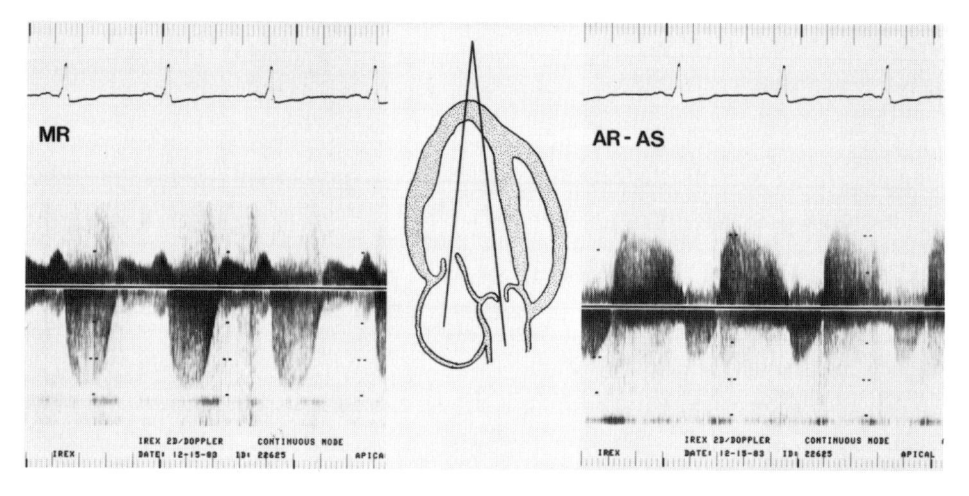

FIG. 6.24. With a transducer located at the apex, both mitral regurgitation (MR) and aortic stenosis (AS) appear as systolic movement in a negative direction. Note that mitral systole is longer in duration than aortic. Aortic regurgitation (AR) is also present. Scale marks are 2 m/sec.

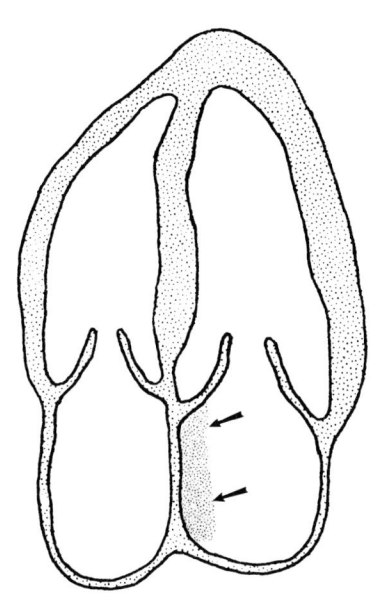

FIG. 6.25. A Doppler sample volume is large in the far field and, when placed in the left atrium in areas near the aortic root, may cause spurious evidence for mitral regurgitation.

It is also possible to confuse tricuspid with mitral regurgitation. This is more of a problem with continuous wave than with pulsed wave echocardiography for a beginner, and the use of pulsed wave with concurrent imaging aids in recognizing this error. Another reason for false positives is the interpretation of a loud systolic closure sound of the mitral valve leaflets, commonly known as "valve slap," as partial recording of the early profile of a moving mitral regurgitation jet (Fig. 6.26).

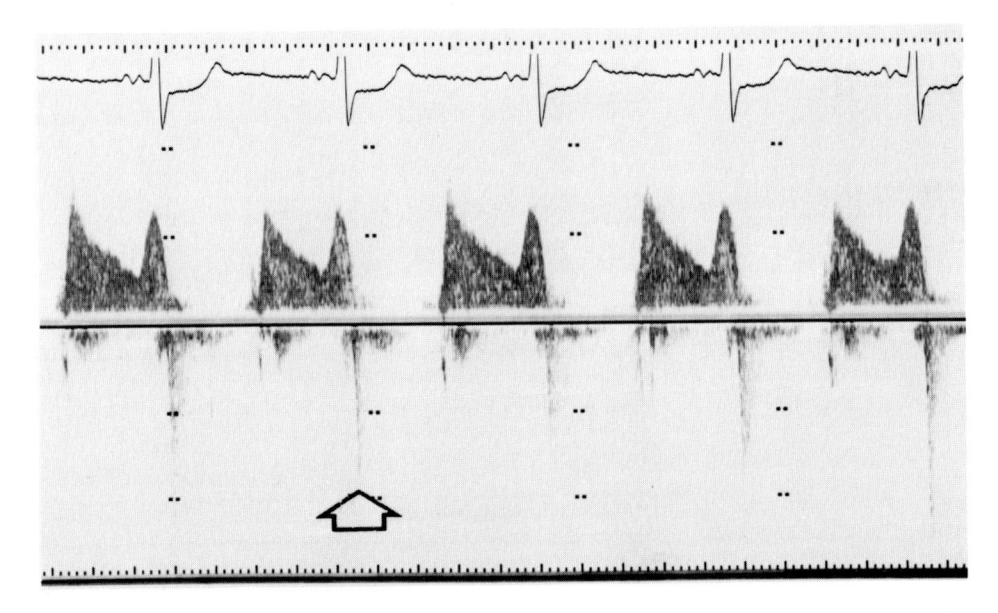

FIG. 6.26. CW spectral recording from patient with valve slap (arrow) that may be wrongly interpreted as an incomplete recording of mitral regurgitation.

110   BASIC DOPPLER ECHOCARDIOGRAPHY

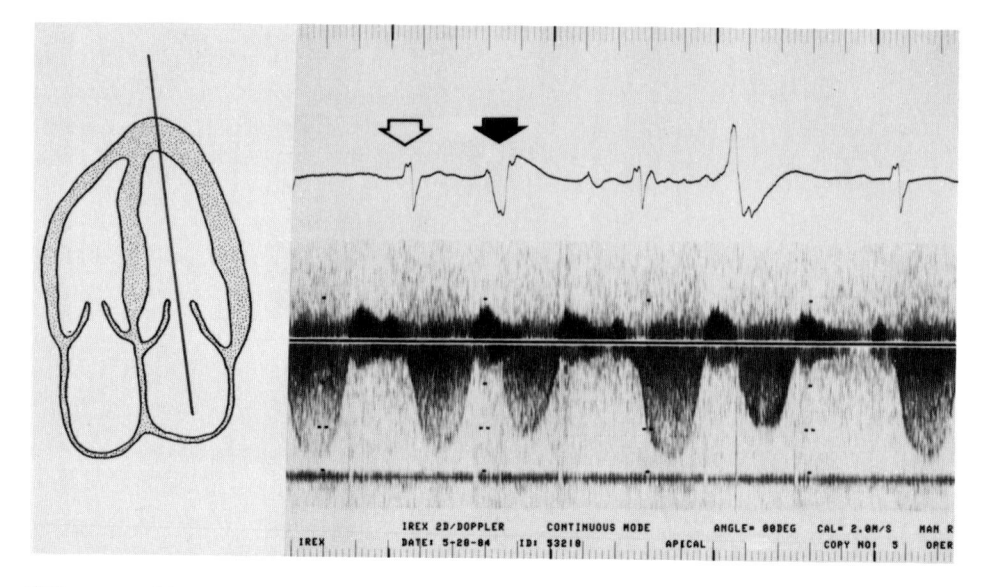

FIG. 6.27. Varying appearance of mitral insufficiency with arrhythmias. A smaller profile follows the PVC (closed arrow) than the normal beat (open arrow). Scale marks are 2 m/sec.

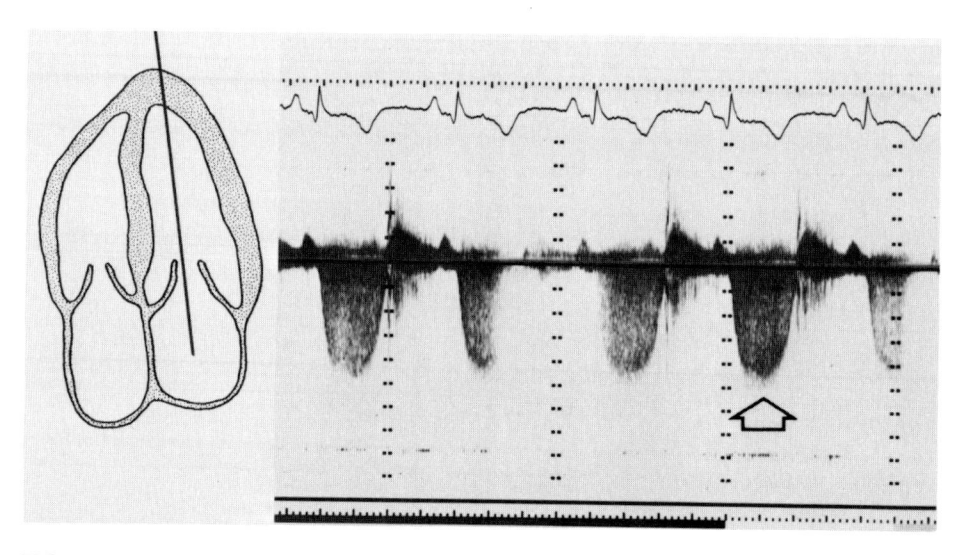

FIG. 6.28. The jet of mitral regurgitation is incompletely recorded due to movement of the jet in and out of the beam. The best spectral profile is at the arrow. Scale marks are 1 m/sec.

Detection of mitral regurgitation when it is not present by angiography is very uncommon, especially when an apical transducer position is used. It is, however, possible that a very small amount of regurgitation may be detected by Doppler and yet fail to be seen on left ventriculography, particularly if there is poor opacification of the left ventricle with contrast.

False-negative evaluations for mitral insufficiency also may occur and are probably most frequently due to a small jet that was missed on examination. A moving jet may also be encountered but is, as mentioned, frequently difficult to differentiate from valve slap (Fig. 6.26). Mitral insufficiency jets may also vary in appearance with arrhythmias (Fig. 6.27), change their spatial relationships to the Doppler beam with respiration (Fig. 6.28), or be obscured by very significant aortic stenotic lesions.

Mitral regurgitant jets, like others, are often eccentrically directed, and it is important to examine the left atrium from all available windows. Besides the apical window, the left parasternal region is very useful for this purpose.

TRICUSPID REGURGITATION

Tricuspid regurgitation is also best evaluated from the apical window. The left parasternal right ventricular inlet view is another useful position. In tricuspid insufficiency, systolic turbulence is detected just behind the tricuspid valve leaflets. The contour of the flow profile is very similar to that of mitral regurgitation. As with other regurgitant jets, continuous wave Doppler is usually needed to obtain an unaliased recording of the full spectrum (Fig. 6.29).

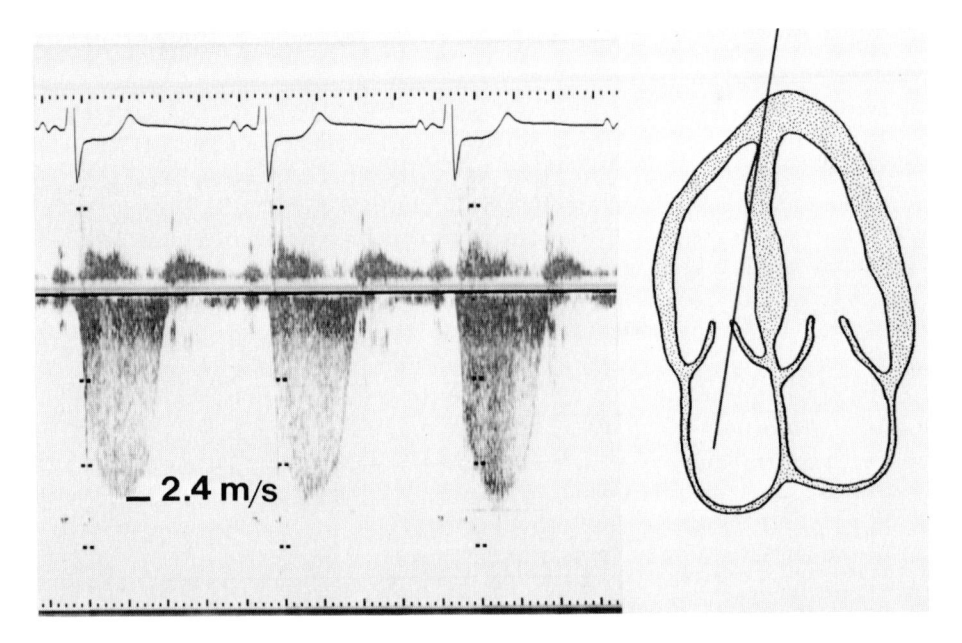

FIG. 6.29. Typical CW spectral recording of tricuspid regurgitation from the apex. The peak velocity in the jet measures 2.4 m/sec. Scale marks are 1 m/sec.

We frequently detect tricuspid regurgitation by Doppler in otherwise normal individuals and find that even beginning operators of Doppler instruments will readily record this entity in well over half of their patients. Wise et al.[14] found a similar, frequent systolic reversal of flow in normal individuals using contrast echocardiography of the inferior vena cava. Recently, Yock et al.[4] demonstrated that 96 percent of normal volunteers had Doppler evidence of true valvular tricuspid regurgitation and that this flow signal was not due to coronary sinus systolic flow.

These findings indicate that Doppler evidence for tricuspid regurgitation is extraordinarily common and presents an interpretive dilemma for echocardiographers. It is clear to us that the physical findings of tricuspid regurgitation are extraordinarily insensitive and are usually seen only when the regurgitation is severe. There is no widely accepted standard method for reporting this lesion. Currently, we prefer not to report tricuspid regurgitation if it is localized just behind the tricuspid leaflets, but we do report it if the regurgitant jet can be found to extend at least halfway between valve leaflets and the posterior wall of the right atrium by pulsed Doppler.

A tricuspid regurgitant jet may be used to estimate right ventricular systolic pressure (RVSP) in millimeters of mercury.[15] This method is, like all Doppler pressure estimates, based on the modified Bernoulli equation ($\Delta P = 4V^2$) discussed in Chapter 3. Using this method, one first estimates mean jugular venous pressure (JVP) in centimeters by inspection of the jugular venous pulse with the patient at a 45° angle. Right atrial pressure (RAP) is estimated by adding 5 cm to the venous pressure measurement and then converted to millimeters of mercury by dividing by 1.3. This is then added to the transtricuspid systolic gradient estimated from the peak tricuspid velocity. The formula is:

$$(JVP + 5)/1.3 + (\text{peak systolic velocity}^2 \times 4) = RVSP$$

The patient pictured in Fig. 6.29 has a peak systolic velocity of 2.4 m/sec, which is equivalent to a peak transtricuspid gradient of 23 mmHg. Since the jugular venous pulse was estimated at 15 cm, the right atrial pressure would be 20 cm of water (or 15 mmHg). Using the above equation, we would predict a right ventricular systolic pressure of 38 mmHg. Yock and Popp[15] have reported these Doppler-catheterization correlations for measurement of right ventricular systolic pressure to be very close ($r = .93$).

One frequently observes respiratory variation in tricuspid insufficiency Doppler spectra, as noted in Fig. 6.30, and with various arrhythmias, as seen in Fig. 6.31, in a patient with atrial fibrillation.

As with left-sided valves, there are reasons for the detection of false-positive and false-negative results (Table 6.3) that are similar to those previously discussed. One interesting difficulty that may result from excessive upward angulation of the interrogating beam is interception of aortic flow, rather than tricuspid. Figure 6.32A demonstrates the proper direction for CW interrogation of the right atrium. With slight superior angulation, the beam may actually intercept the ascending aorta. Figure 6.32B shows such a maneuver in a patient with both tricuspid regurgitation and aortic stenosis.

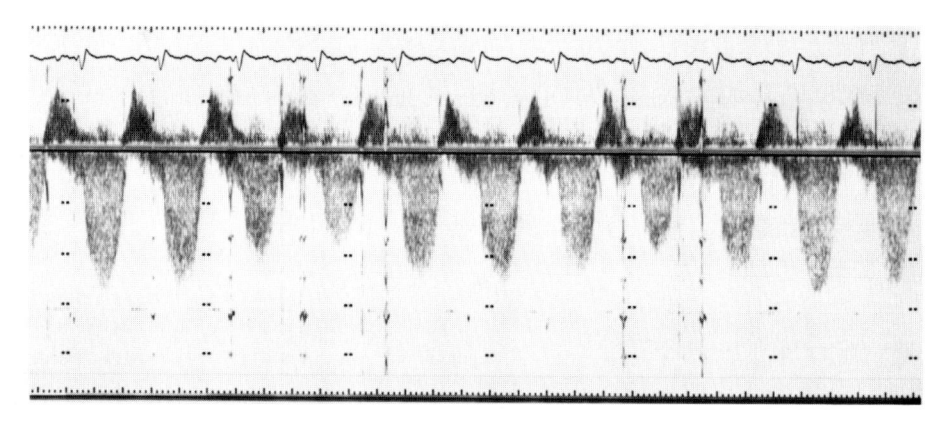

FIG. 6.30. Varying configuration of tricuspid insufficiency with respiration. Scale marks are 1 m/sec.

PULMONIC INSUFFICIENCY

The diastolic pattern of pulmonic insufficiency greatly resembles that of aortic insufficiency (Fig. 6.33). This lesion is best detected from the left parasternal window, as shown in Fig. 6.34. As with tricuspid regurgitation, this abnormal pattern is found in a surprisingly high number of otherwise normal individuals (Table 6.4). Yock et al.[4] have indicated it occurs in as many as 40 percent of normal volunteers.

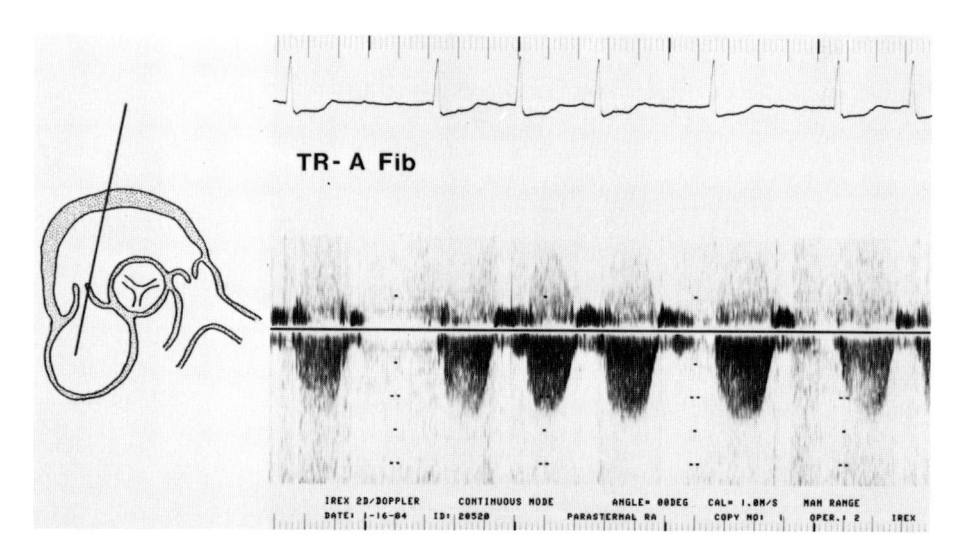

FIG. 6.31. Varying appearance of tricuspid regurgitation with atrial fibrillation. Scale marks are 1 m/sec.

114 BASIC DOPPLER ECHOCARDIOGRAPHY

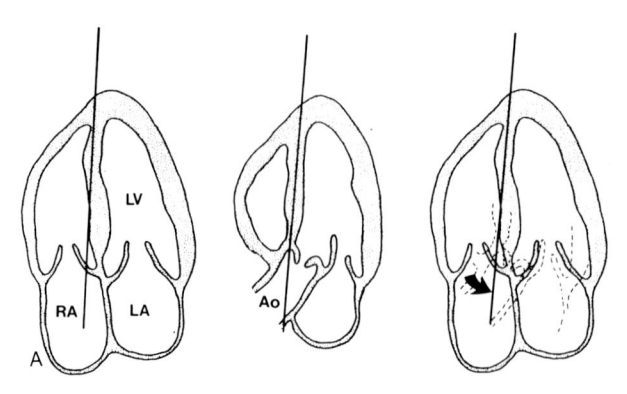

FIG. 6.32. (A) Schematic diagram of CW beam direction for detection of tricuspid regurgitation (left); if angled a bit too superiorly, the beam will actually intercept the aortic root (middle and right). Thus, aortic outflow may be a reason for false-positive tricuspid regurgitation (arrow). (B) A maneuver from the tricuspid valve to aortic is shown.

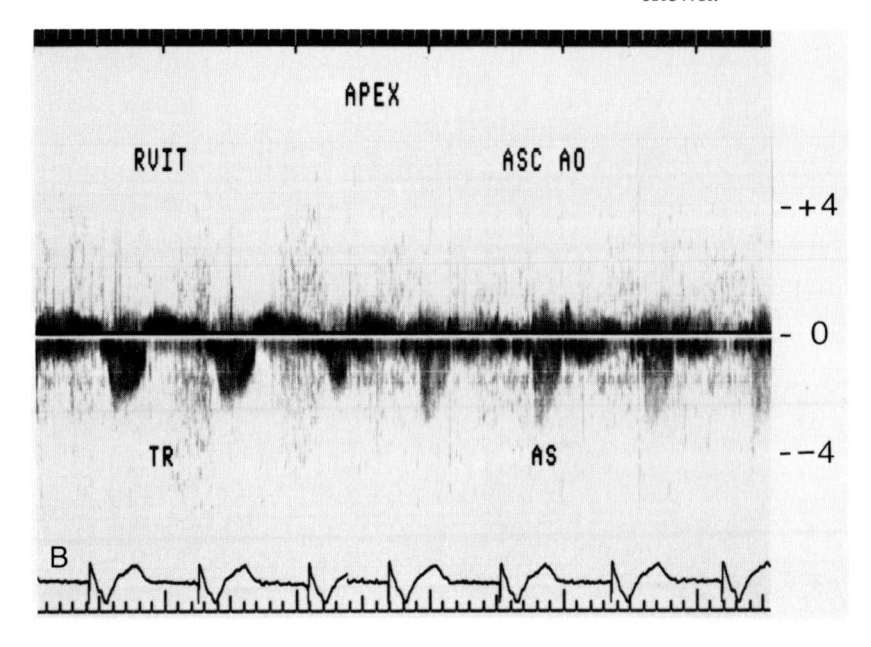

TABLE 6.3 Common Reasons for Misidentification of Tricuspid Regurgitation

False positive	Confusion with aortic outflow, particularly aortic stenosis
	Confusion with mitral regurgitation
	Valve slap
	Normal finding
False negative	Small jet missed by inadequate examination
	Moving jet
	Intermittent jet, particularly with respiration

DOPPLER EVALUATION OF VALVULAR REGURGITATION **115**

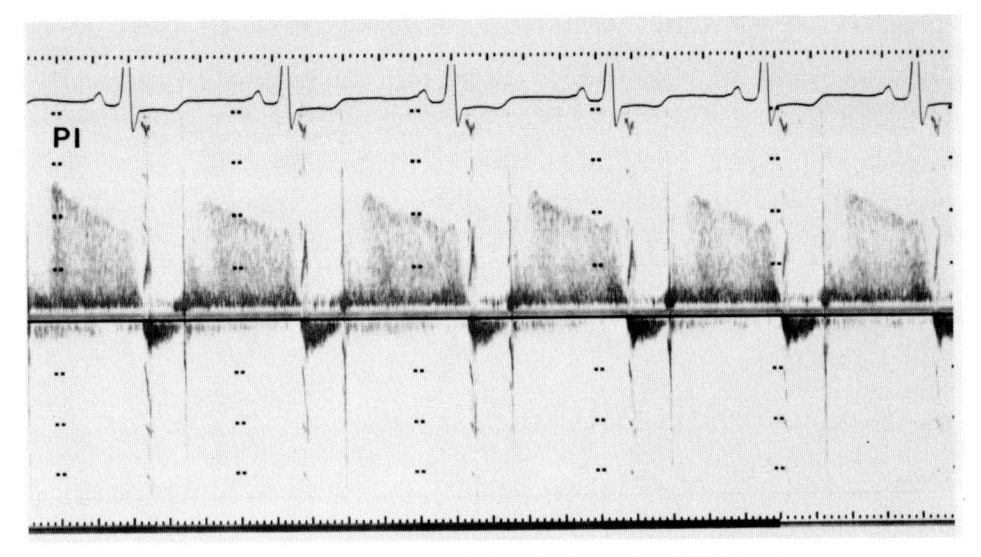

FIG. 6.33. Typical pulmonic insufficiency by CW Doppler.

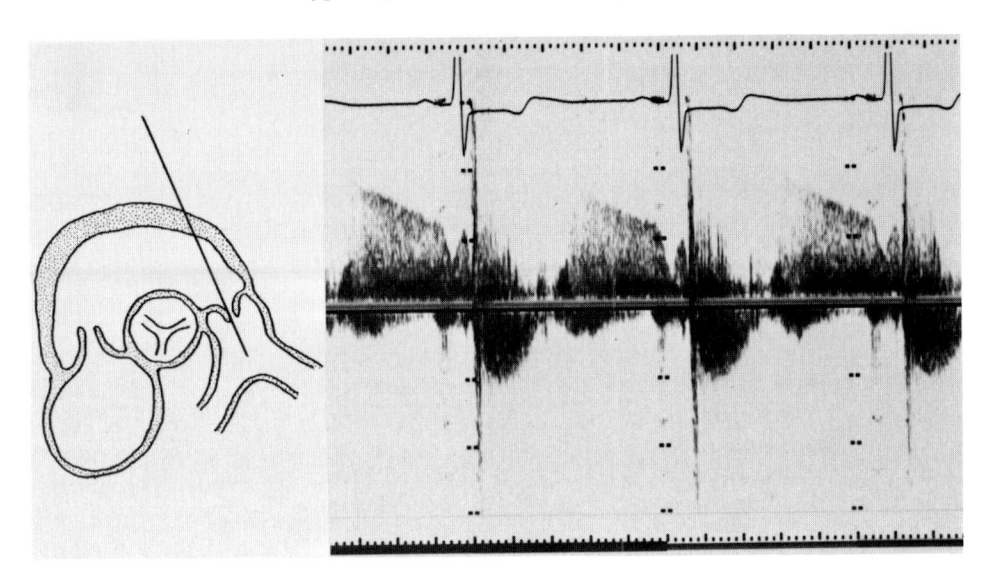

FIG. 6.34. The left parasternal window is excellent for interrogation of the pulmonic valve.

TABLE 6.4 Common Reasons for Misidentification of Pulmonic Insufficiency

False positive	Confusion with aortic insufficiency
	Normal finding
False negative	Small jet missed by inadequate examination
	Moving jet

QUANTITATION OF VALVULAR INSUFFICIENCY

Doppler assessment of the severity of valvular regurgitation has been moderately successful in comparison with angiographic techniques. The invasive gold standard for quantitation of valvular insufficiency is the volume of regurgitant blood flow calculated by subtracting the total cardiac output, calculated angiographically, from the forward output, calculated by the Fick principle. The regurgitant volume divided by the total angiographic stroke volume (i.e., the sum total of blood ejected forwards and backwards out of the left ventricle with each systole) is referred to as the regurgitant fraction. The other commonly used measure of severity is a subjective grading (usually 0 to 4+) based on a visual evaluation of the amount of regurgitation seen by contrast angiography. Both methods have limitations, and there is only a rough correlation between them.[16] Thus, it has been difficult to find a suitable gold standard for comparison with Doppler methods.

Three general approaches have been used to quantitate regurgitant lesions with Doppler. One method relies on the use of pulsed wave Doppler to map the size and distribution of the regurgitant jet within a cardiac chamber. Another is based upon the relationship of forward to reverse flow, and the last attempts to quantitate the absolute flow through each valve orifice and then use these flow volumes to calculate the regurgitant fraction. The latter two methods are more complex and not easily performed by beginners in Doppler echocardiography.

Even though mapping is the most straightforward approach to the evaluation of severity of valvular regurgitation, it can be a very difficult and time-consuming process. It is important to keep in mind the three-dimensional geometry of the chamber being studied and the fact that regurgitant jets may be directed anywhere within the chamber. Simply using a single, standard two-dimensional view without angling the transducer around to examine the whole chamber may result in significant underestimation of severity.

The mapping technique can only be performed with pulsed wave echocardiography and requires some experience with the Doppler technique plus facility with two-dimensional imaging, since the sample volume has to be systematically located in various places, sampling for valvular regurgitation. The interrogating two-dimensional plane in the frozen or periodic updated image must be kept constant as each area is sampled until one view has been completely evaluated. Keep in mind that the mapping technique only provides rough estimates of the severity of valvular insufficiency, and further comparisons with standards such as carefully validated angiographic volume measurements must still be done to assess the value of the technique.

Figure 6.35 shows an example of multiple areas sampled (circles) by the pulsed Doppler sample volume while in the apical two-chamber view. In Fig. 6.35A, the pulsed Doppler detects aortic insufficiency only on the ventricular side of the aortic valve leaflets (closed circles), and this corresponds to mild aortic insufficiency. Figure 6.35B demonstrates the areas where aortic insufficiency was detected (closed circles) much deeper into the left ventricle, and

FIG. 6.35. Various sample sites for mapping the severity of aortic regurgitation (circles). (A) Positive detection of regurgitation just below the aortic valve (closed circles). (B) Broader distribution compatible with more severe disease. Sampling near the mitral orifice will invariably detect mitral inflow (arrow).

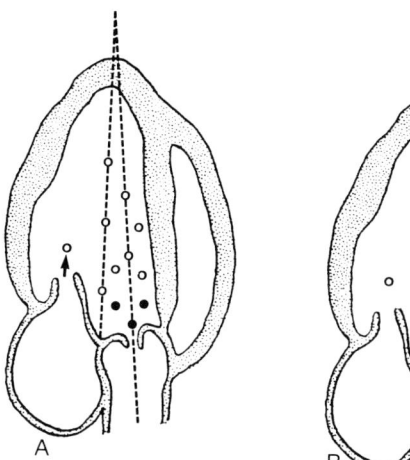

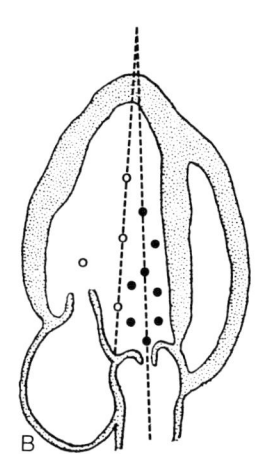

this corresponds to severe aortic insufficiency. Sampling directly in the mitral orifice (arrow) will almost always detect mitral diastolic flow that may be interpreted incorrectly as aortic insufficiency, particularly when there is associated mitral stenosis.

Figure 6.36 gives the general areas where turbulent flow would be found in mild, moderate, and severe aortic regurgitation. An actual case where mapping was employed is pictured in Fig. 6.37. In Fig. 6.37A, the sample volume is located on the ventricular side of the aortic valve with the two-dimensional image in the apical four-chamber view (top arrow). Aortic insufficiency is easily detected (open arrow). When the sample volume is moved to the area near the tip of the mitral valve (Fig. 6.37B), aortic insufficiency is still encountered (open arrow). Aortic insufficiency was not detected deeper into the ventricle.

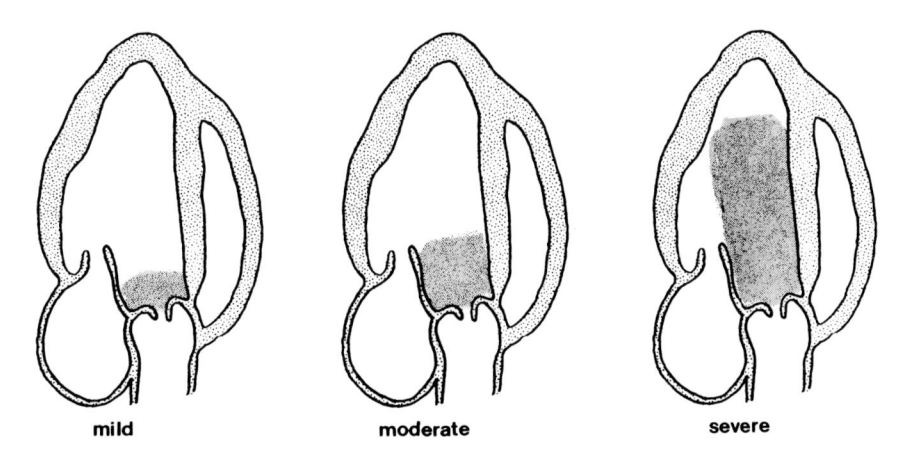

FIG. 6.36. General areas for detecting mild, moderate, and severe aortic insufficiency by pulsed Doppler mapping.

118 BASIC DOPPLER ECHOCARDIOGRAPHY

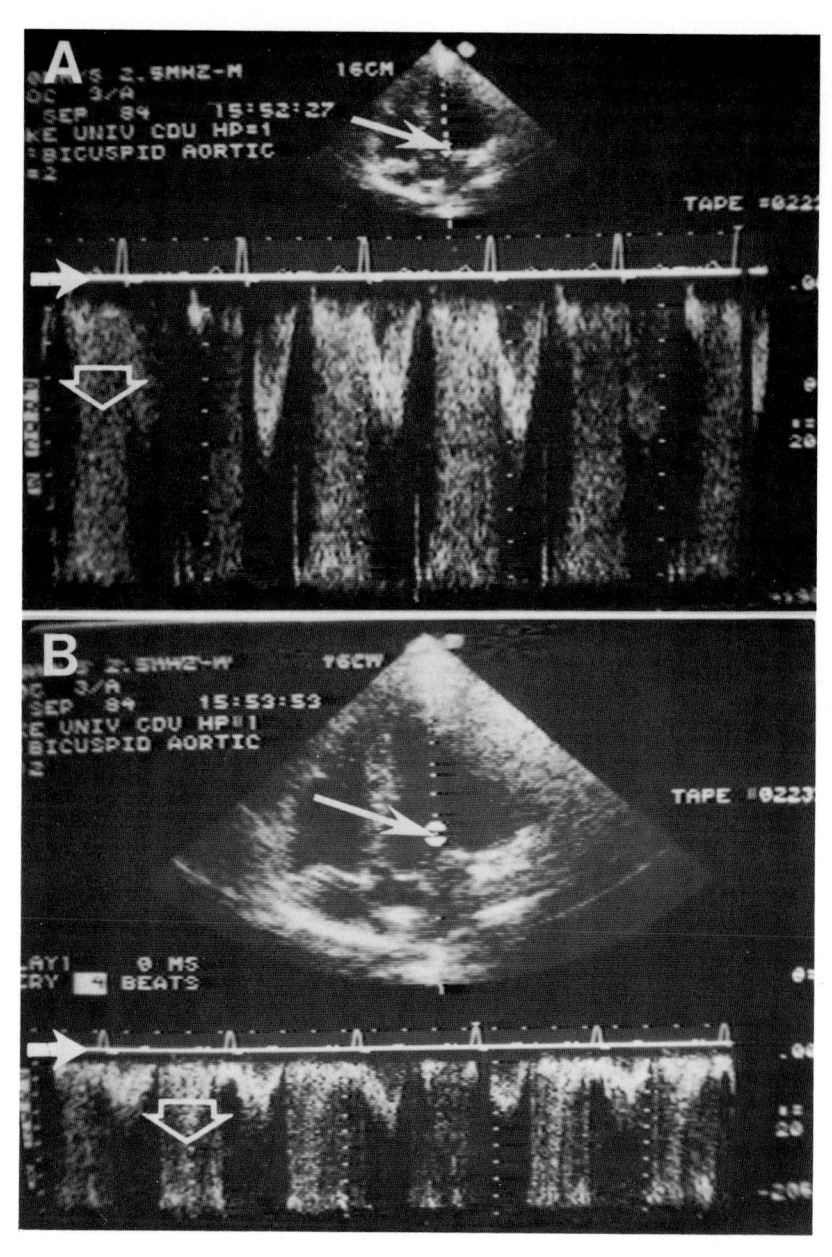

FIG. 6.37. (A) Pulsed Doppler sample volume (top arrow) is shown just below aortic valve in apical four-chamber view. Aortic insufficiency is detected (open arrow). (B) Movement of the sample volume toward the tip of the mitral valve is shown and insufficiency is still detected (open arrow). Baselines are indicated by arrows at left. Scale marks are 20 cm/sec.

For mitral regurgitation, the process is similar, and mapping of the left atrium may be done either from the parasternal long-axis window or from an apical window. We generally prefer to begin with the apical window and then add further spatial information about the size and direction of the regurgitant jet using additional apical and parasternal views. Figure 6.38 shows multiple placements of the pulsed Doppler sample volume (circles). In Fig. 6.38A, regurgitation is detected only on the atrial side of the mitral leaflets, a finding consistent with mild mitral regurgitation (closed circles). Figure 6.38B shows abnormal flow detected almost all over the atrium, and this corresponds to severe valvular regurgitation (closed circles). If higher-velocity flows are detected only medially, this may be due to aortic outflow because the sample volume is relatively large at this depth. Interception of aortic outflow signals can present a particular problem in patients with aortic stenosis since this lesion, like mitral regurgitation, produces high-velocity flow away from the transducer. A schematic diagram of the general distribution of mild, moderate, and severe mitral regurgitation is seen in Fig. 6.39.

Similar methods are available for mapping tricuspid regurgitation, which involve movement of the sample volume in various areas of the right atrium (Fig. 6.40). A schematic representation of mild, moderate, and severe tricuspid regurgitation is seen in Fig. 6.39.

The other approaches to the estimation of severity of valvular regurgitation are more complex. The first attempts were indirect in assessing the amount of regurgitant flow in mitral regurgitation. Nichol et al.[17] used continuous-wave Doppler to study systolic velocity in the descending aorta. They divided the area under the velocity curve into two halves and compared the ratio of the two (first half of systole/second half) in 18 normal subjects and 16 mitral regurgitation patients. They found that in mitral regurgitation patients more blood was ejected in the first half of systole. Their ratio showed a good correlation with the regurgitant fraction measured at cardiac catheterization. More

FIG. 6.38. Schematic diagrams showing many possible pulsed Doppler sample volume sites (circles). (A) Positive detection of mitral regurgitation just near the valve, consistent with mild disease (closed circles). (B) Wider distribution of positive sample sites compatible with more severe regurgitation. Sampling near the aortic root (arrow) may bring interference from the ascending aorta.

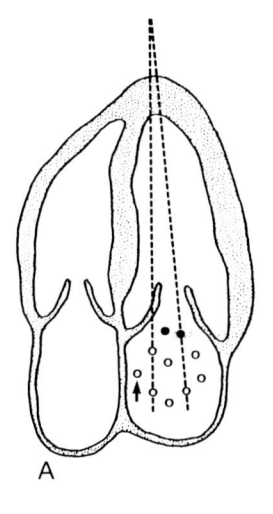

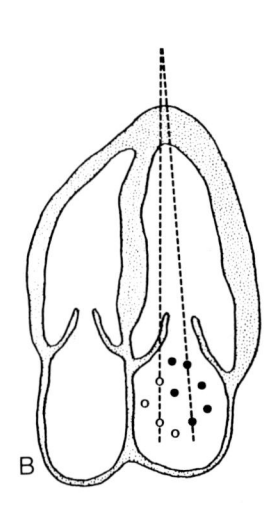

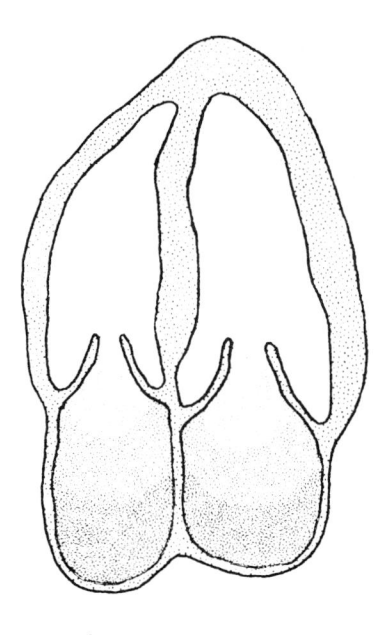

FIG. 6.39. General areas for detection of mild (light stipple), moderate (medium stipple), and severe (heavy stipple) mitral and tricuspid regurgitations.

recently, some investigators have explored the use of direct volume of flow measurement with Doppler (described in Chapter 8) to directly calculate the regurgitant volume and regurgitant fraction.[18] More work will be needed to assess the clinical utility of this approach.

The first attempt at direct quantitation of regurgitant flow in aortic insufficiency was reported by Thompson et al.[19] in 1970. Using CW Doppler aimed at the ascending aorta from the suprasternal notch, they compared the area under the forward and reverse flow curves and made a ratio of retrograde to forward flow. This ratio was compared with direct measurements made at operation using an electromagnetic flowmeter. Boughner[20] used a similar ap-

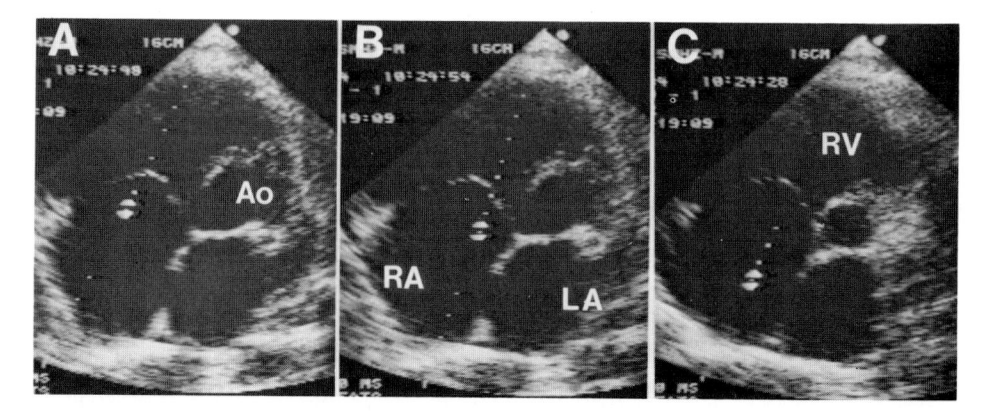

FIG. 6.40. Modified apical four-chamber view showing different positions for placing the pulsed sample volume within the right atrium for evaluating tricuspid regurgitation.

proach but studied flow in the descending aorta and compared his results with the regurgitant fraction measurement by cardiac catheterization. He found an excellent agreement between Doppler and catheterization estimates. A number of other workers have obtained similar results in small groups of patients.[21]

GENERAL GUIDELINES

As seen from the many examples described in this chapter, there are several major points to keep in mind when examining patients for the presence of valvular insufficiency. One practical point not previously emphasized is that the audible output may be more sensitive than the spectral display. It is not infrequent that a given lesion is heard by audio but cannot be adequately recorded on the spectral hard copy. Interpretation in these cases is often difficult and, in our experience, usually involves a tradeoff. Accepting audio evidence of a regurgitant lesion without hard-copy confirmation increases the sensitivity of the procedure but will also result in an increased number of false-positive diagnoses. Currently, we require hard-copy confirmation before we will report definite evidence of valvular regurgitation.

Second, it is important for the operator to take time to search for small regurgitant jets. When searching for insufficiency by pulsed wave with an instrument that has a variable sample volume size, one should not routinely begin the examination with a sample volume size that is as large as possible. Although this may seem desirable for locating small jets, the operator must remember that this process will frequently result in a loss of system sensitivity.

Third, the operator should expect regurgitant jets to exceed a velocity of 1.5 m/sec and result in aliasing when in pulsed wave mode. This is certainly true in most adults, since regurgitant lesions are located far enough away from the transducer to cause the Nyquist limit to be exceeded. Thus, in almost every instance, pulsed Doppler operators should expect aliasing of regurgitant lesion.

Fourth, Doppler operators, particularly beginners, should be prepared to switch back and forth between pulsed and continuous wave modes. This will help locate areas of turbulence more precisely and will also make it easier to recognize the typical spectral profiles of these lesions. The end result will be an enhanced ability to separate one abnormal lesion from another.

REFERENCES

1. Tunstall Pedoe DS: Blood velocity measurements in aortic regurgitation using heated thin film and ultrasonic techniques. Br. Heart J. 33:611, 1971
2. Kalmanson D, Veyrat C, Derai C, Chiche O: Diagnostic value of jugular venous flow velocity trace in right heart diseases. In Roberts C (ed): Blood Flow Measurement. Sector Publishing, London, 1972
3. Robertson JH, Krafchek J, Adams DB, Kisslo JA: Reassessment of Doppler ultrasound in minimal aortic and mitral regurgitation. Circulation, abstr., 70:suppl. 2, 387, 1984
4. Yock PG, Naasz C, Schnittger I, Popp RL: Doppler tricuspid and pulmonic regurgitation in normals: Is it real? Circulation, abstr, 70:suppl. 2, 40, 1984

5. Ward JM, Baker DW, Rubenstein SA, Johnson SL: Detection of aortic insufficiency by pulse Doppler echocardiography. J. Clin. Ultrasound. 5:5, 1977
6. Esper RJ: Detection of mild aortic regurgitation by range-gated pulsed Doppler echocardiography. Am. J. Cardiol. 50:1037, 1982
7. Diebold B, Peronneau P, Blanchard D, Colonna G, Guermonprez JL, Forman J, Sellier P, Maurice P: Non-invasive quantification of aortic regurgitation by Doppler echocardiography. Br. Heart J. 49:166, 1983
8. Saal AK, Gross BW, Franklin DW, Pearlman AS: Noninvasive detection of aortic insufficiency in patients with mitral stenosis by pulsed Doppler echocardiography. J. Am. Coll. Cardiol. 5:176, 1985
9. Handshoe R, Handshoe S, Kwan OL, Smith MD, DeMaria AN: Value and limitations of Doppler measurements in the estimation of left ventricular end diastolic pressure in patients with aortic regurgitation. Circulation, abstr., 70:suppl. 2, 117, 1984
10. Abbasi AS, Allen MW, DeCristofaro D, Ungar I: Detection and estimation of the degree of mitral regurgitation by range-gated pulsed Doppler echocardiography. Circulation 61:143, 1980
11. Quinones MA, Young JB, Waggoner AD, Ostojic MC, Ribeiro LGT, Miller RR: Assessment of pulsed Doppler echocardiography in detection and quantification of aortic and mitral regurgitation. Br. Heart J. 44:612, 1980
12. Blanchard D, Diebold B, Perronneau P, Foult JM, Nee M, Guermonprez JL, Maurice P: Non-invasive diagnosis of mitral regurgitation by Doppler echocardiography. Br. Heart J. 45:589, 1981
13. Patel AK, Rowe GG, Thompson JH, Dhanani SP, Kosolcharoen P, Lyle LEW: Detection and estimation of rheumatic mitral regurgitation in the presence of mitral stenosis by pused Doppler echocardiography. Am. J. Cardiol. 51:986, 1983
14. Wise NK, Myers S, Fraker TD, Stewart JA, Kisslo J: Contrast M-mode ultrasonography of the inferior vena cava. Circulation 63:1100, 1981
15. Yock PG, Popp RL: Noninvasive estimation of right ventricular systolic pressure by Doppler ultrasound in patients with tricuspid regurgitation. Circulation 70:657, 1984
16. Mark DB, Califf RM, Stack RS, Phillips HR: Cardiac cathteterization. In Sabiston DC (ed): The Davis-Christopher Textbook of Surgery. 13th Ed. W.B. Saunders, Philadelphia, in press
17. Nichol PM, Boughner DR, Persaud JA: Noninvasive assessment of mitral insufficiency by transcutaneous Doppler ultrasound. Circulation 54:656, 1976
18. Stewart WJ, Palacios I, Jiang L, Dinsmore RE, Weyman AE: Doppler measurement of regurgitant fraction in patients with mitral regurgitation: A new quantitative technique. Circulation, 68:suppl. 3, 111, 1983
19. Thompson PD, Mennel RG, MacVaughn H, Joyner CR: Evaluation of aortic insufficiency with a transcutaneous Doppler velocity probe. Ann. Intern. Med. 72:781, 1970
20. Boughner DR: Assessment of aortic insufficiency by transcutaneous Doppler ultrasound. Circulation 52:874, 1975
21. Sequeira RF, Watt I: Assessment of aortic regurgitation by transcutaneous aortovelography. Br. Heart J. 39:929, 1972

7 Doppler Evaluation of Valvular Stenosis

JOSEPH KISSLO
JACK KRAFCHEK
DAVID ADAMS
DANIEL B. MARK

One of the reasons why use of Doppler echocardiography is growing rapidly is because of its utility in detecting the presence of valvular stenosis and in estimating its severity. Detection of the presence of stenotic valvular heart disease using Doppler echocardiography was originally described over 10 years ago by Johnson et al.[1] Subsequently, Holen et al.[2] and Hatle et al.[3] demonstrated that Doppler blood velocity data could be used to estimate the severity of a stenotic lesion.

EFFECT OF STENOSIS ON BLOOD FLOW

The driving force for blood to move across any cardiac valve is the presence of a slight pressure difference normally found between the chambers (or chamber and great vessel) on either side of the valve. For example, systolic pressure builds within the left ventricle until it reaches a point at which the aortic valve is suddenly thrown open and blood is ejected into the aorta. In normal individuals, there is a very slight (1 or 2 mmHg) pressure difference between the left ventricle and aorta that helps drive the blood across the aortic valve.

Normal aortic valve blood flow is laminar (Fig. 7.1), and most of the red cells in the aortic root during systole are moving at approximately the same speed. Graphically, this translates into a narrow band of dark gray on the pulsed Doppler spectral recording (Fig. 7.1, arrow). Normal peak systolic velocity of blood flow across the aortic valve rarely exceeds 1.5 m/sec.

When the aortic valve is diseased, the leaflets become thickened and progressively lose their mobility. Eventually, the valve itself becomes narrowed to the point at which it begins to obstruct flow, and aortic stenosis is created.

124 BASIC DOPPLER ECHOCARDIOGRAPHY

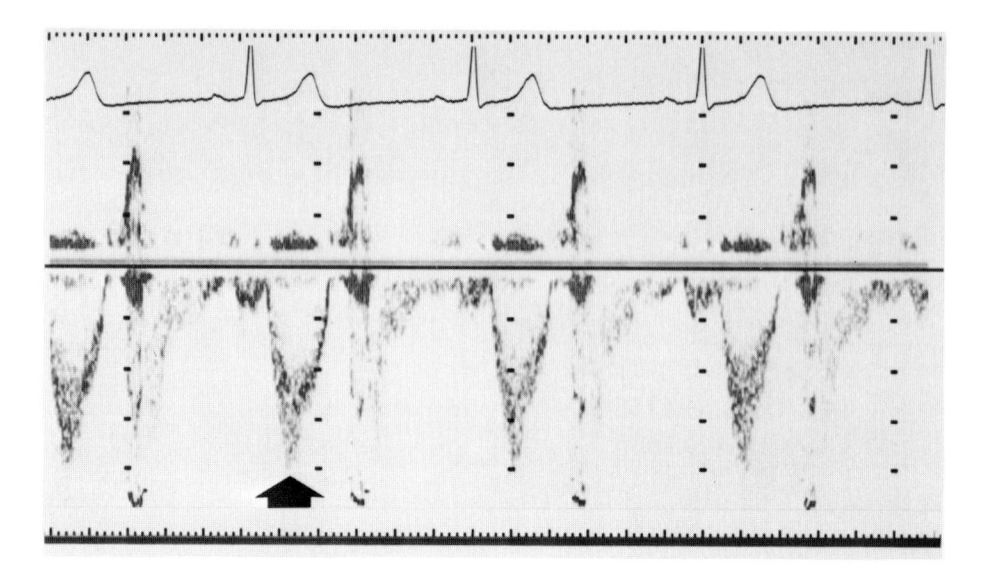

FIG. 7.1. Pulsed Doppler spectral recording of aortic root blood flow (arrow) taken from the apical window. Note the laminar appearance of normal flow. Scale marks are 20 cm/sec.

In the presence of aortic stenosis, systolic pressure in the ventricle must rise high enough to force the blood across the obstruction into the aorta. Thus, a pressure drop, or pressure gradient, is generated (Fig. 7.2). In fact, severe degrees of aortic stenosis may result in aortic valve gradients that exceed 100 mmHg in systole. As discussed in Chapter 2, the presence of such an obstruction results both in turbulent flow and an increase in velocity, two characteristics readily detected by Doppler echocardiography.

Doppler detection and evaluation of the presence or absence of aortic stenosis are based on recording turbulence and increased flow velocity in the ascending

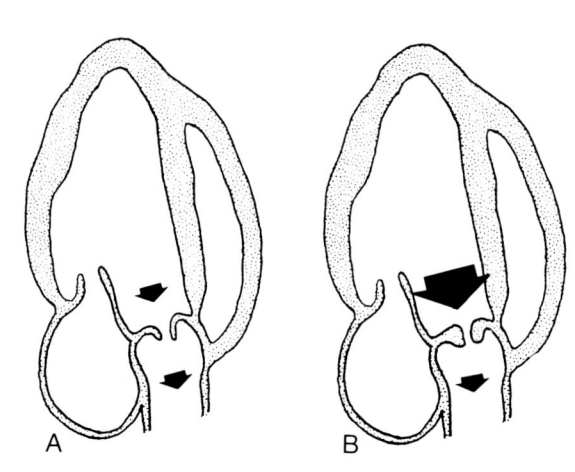

FIG. 7.2. (A) Without aortic valve obstruction, systolic pressures are almost the same in the ventricle and the aorta. (B) When significant aortic valve obstruction is present, left ventricular pressure rises much higher than aortic, and a systolic pressure gradient is present.

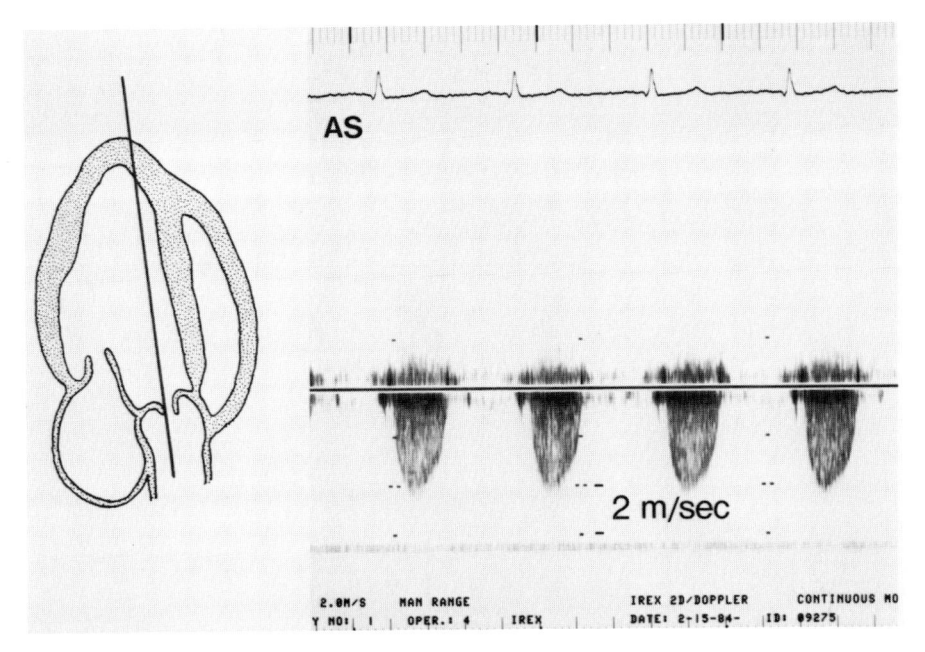

FIG. 7.3. CW spectral recording from the apex in a patient with aortic stenosis. The velocity spectrum is broadened, and systolic velocity is increased to 4 m/sec. Scale marks are 2 m/sec.

aorta. Figure 7.3 demonstrates these characteristics in a continuous wave spectral velocity recording of aortic systolic flow obtained from the apical window. Turbulent flow is represented by broadening of the velocity spectrum. There is also an increase in peak aortic velocity to 4 m/sec. The Doppler audio in this case had a harsh, higher-pitched quality during systole that was easily distinguished from the audio sound of laminar flow.

Similarly, the presence of these characteristics in the pulmonary artery during systole would indicate the presence of obstruction to right ventricular ejection. Figure 7.4 demonstrates a continuous wave Doppler spectral recording from the left parasternal window in a patient with mild pulmonic stenosis and insuffiency. Turbulent diastolic and systolic flows are noted with a slight increase in the peak systolic velocity to 1.4 m/sec (normal is less than 1 m/sec). Figure 7.5 shows a pulsed wave Doppler examination in the same patient and demonstrates the ability of pulsed wave to localize the level of the obstruction. With the cursor positioned on the ventricular side of the pulmonic valve (A), the turbulent diastolic spectral recording of pulmonic insufficiency is noted, although systolic flow is undisturbed (laminar) with a peak systolic velocity of just about 1 m/sec. When the sample volume is positioned distal to the diseased pulmonic valve (B), the systolic flow becomes turbulent, and the peak systolic velocity is elevated to 1.6 m/sec. The spectral recording of pulmonic insufficiency is lost because the sample volume is located distal to this lesion.

126 BASIC DOPPLER ECHOCARDIOGRAPHY

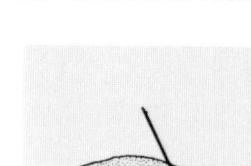

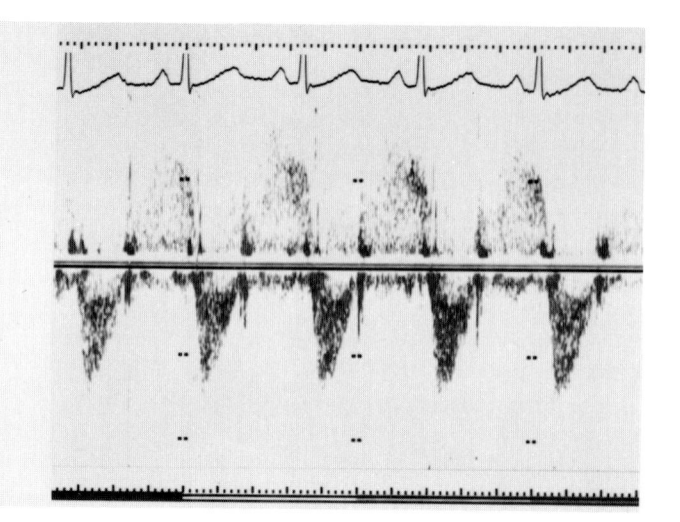

FIG. 7.4. CW spectral velocity recording of mild pulmonic stenosis and insufficiency. Flow away from the transducer reaches 1.4 m/sec in systole. The abnormal diastolic flow toward the transducer of pulmonic insufficiency is easily recognized. Scale marks are 1 m/sec.

Although pulsed Doppler is very useful for the localization of such obstructive lesions, it has limited value in establishing the severity of obstruction because most significant valvular obstructions result in velocities above 1.5 m/sec. As emphasized in Chapter 6, velocities above 1.5 m/sec will usually cause aliasing of the pulsed waved recording. This prevents the faithful recording of peak velocities necessary for calculation of valve gradients.

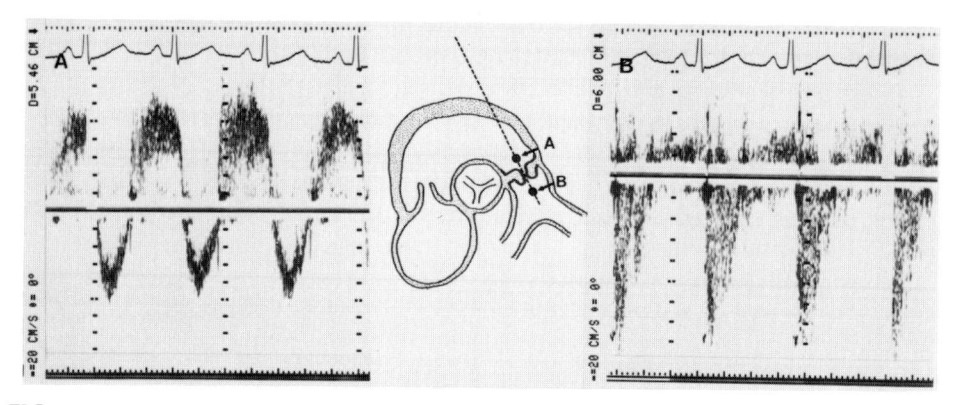

FIG. 7.5. Pulsed Doppler spectral recording from the same patient as Fig. 7.4. At position A, pulmonic insufficiency is noted, and systolic velocity is not yet elevated. At position B, on the distal side of the valve, the turbulence of pulmonic stenosis is encountered, and systolic velocity is elevated. Scale marks are 20 cm/sec.

ESTIMATION OF THE SEVERITY OF STENOSIS

Use of Doppler ultrasound to estimate the severity of a valve stenosis is based principally upon the fact that such obstructions result in an increase in the velocity of flow. In clinically significant mitral stenosis, the diastolic velocity of mitral flow usually exceeds 1.7 m/sec. Systolic velocity of aortic flow in clinically significant aortic stenosis may reach 5 or 6 m/sec (Fig. 7.6). Thus, continuous wave Doppler is required for detection of these increased velocities and for recording the full-spectral profiles.

We have already noted (Chapter 3) that there is a relationship between the pressure drop (or gradient) across a valve and the velocity of blood flow across that valve. For any given pressure gradient, there is a corresponding increase in velocity, as predicted by the simplified Bernoulli equation

$$p_1 - p_2 = 4V^2$$

where p_1 = pressure distal to obstruction, p_2 = pressure proximal to obstruction, and V = peak velocity of blood flow across the obstruction.

As the stenosis becomes more severe, the valve orifice area will become smaller, and the velocity of flow across the orifice will increase as a function of the increased pressure gradient. Thus, by measuring the peak velocity in a systolic aortic jet with Doppler echocardiography, it is possible to estimate the pressure gradient that produced it using the above simple algebraic expres-

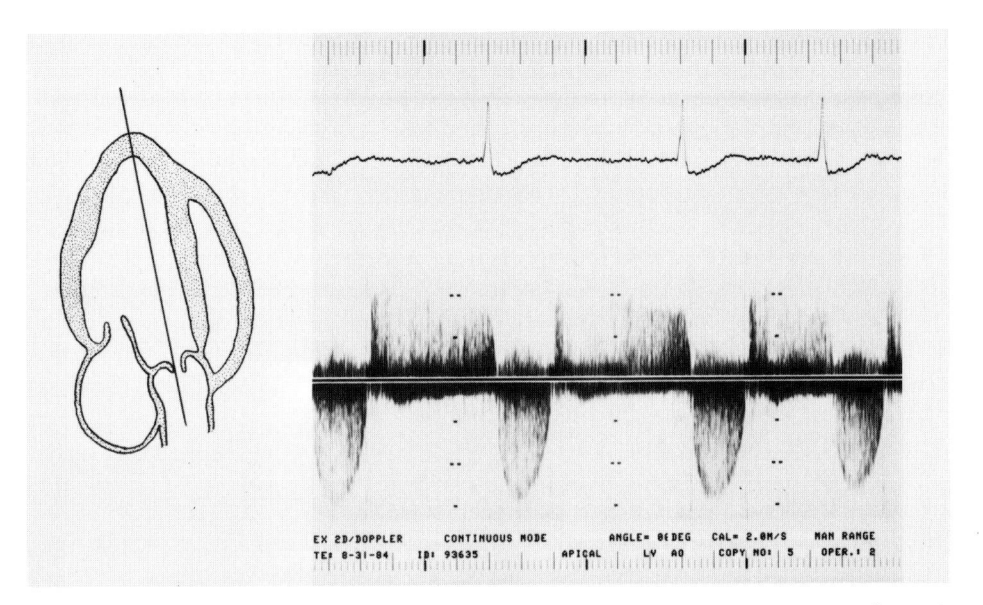

FIG. 7.6. Typical CW spectral velocity tracing from the apex in a patient with aortic stenosis and insufficiency. Peak systolic velocity is elevated to almost 6 m/sec, and peaking is delayed (compare with Fig. 7.1). Scale marks are 2 m/sec.

sion. The peak aortic velocity of the spectral recording in Fig. 7.6 is approximately 5.8 m/sec. Using the previous formula,

$$p_1 - p_2 = 4(5.8)^2$$

or pressure gradient = 135 mmHg.

There are, however, three major technical requirements that must be satisfied if Doppler is to be used for this purpose. First, an adequate window into the chest for ultrasound propagation and reception must be found so that well-formed Doppler profiles can be recorded. Second, as emphasized in Chapter 2, for the velocity measurements to be accurate, this window must allow orientation of the ultrasound beam so that it is as parallel to flow through the valve as possible (see Fig. 2.18). Third, the high velocities present in the disturbed jet often exceed the Nyquist limit of pulsed wave Doppler, so that continuous wave or high PRF Doppler must be used.

It should be recognized, however, that knowledge of the gradient across a stenotic valve does not provide all the information necessary to assess the severity of obstruction. The gradient will vary with flow across the stenotic valve orifice and will increase in high-flow situations and decrease in low-flow situations. Thus, a patient with a fixed valve area will have a higher gradient during exercise when cardiac output is increased than at rest, when cardiac output is lower. Valve orifice size is generally considered not to vary with the amount of flow across the valve and is, therefore, a preferred expression of the severity of a given stenosis. Unfortunately, there is, as yet, no generally accepted method of calculating aortic or pulmonic valve areas from Doppler flow-velocity measurement.

AORTIC STENOSIS

The most common windows utilized for recording peak aortic systolic velocity are the apical, suprasternal, and right parasternal. Although stenotic jets, like regurgitant jets, are often directed eccentrically, it is usually possible to find a fully formed aortic systolic profile from one of these windows. A comprehensive Doppler examination for aortic stenosis requires that the ascending aorta be examined from all possible windows in order to align the beam parallel to the jet. Figure 7.7 shows a continuous-wave examination of a patient with aortic stenosis from the suprasternal notch (Fig. 7.7A) and the apex (Fig. 7.7B). The spectral tracing from the apical window is superior as judged by the presence of a fully formed profile with a discrete ascent, peak, and descent.

Although we have found the apical window to be most productive, we always examine the aorta from every possible view. Occasionally, the suprasternal window will be perfectly aligned to flow and will present the typical spectral profile of aortic stenosis (Fig. 7.8). In severe aortic stenosis, there is marked spectral broadening, delayed systolic peaking, and a marked increase in velocity. In this patient, the peak systolic velocity is almost 5 m/sec (100 mmHg).

Considerable operator skill is required to obtain adequate spectral tracings for measurement of peak velocity. It is our experience that the Doppler exami-

DOPPLER EVALUATION OF VALVULAR STENOSIS   129

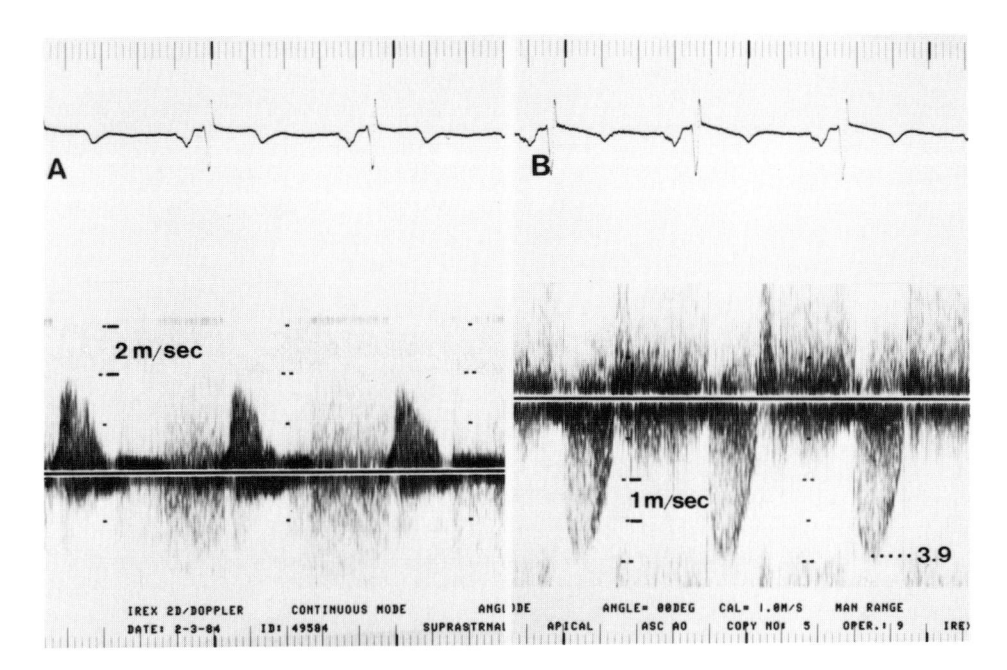

FIG. 7.7. CW Doppler spectral recordings of aortic outflow from the suprasternal notch with flow toward the transducer (A) and apex with flow away from the transducer (B). The spectral recording from the apex is better formed than the one from the suprasternal notch.

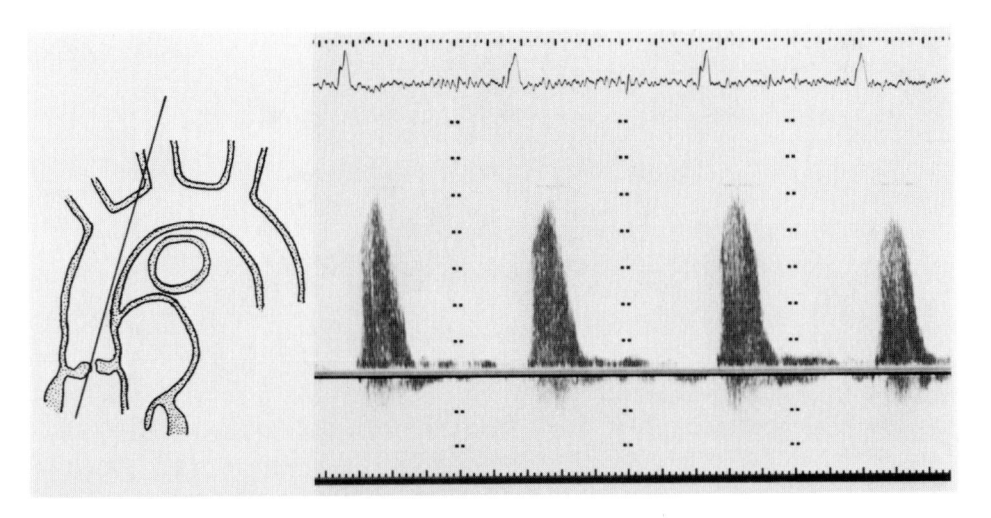

FIG. 7.8. Typical aortic systolic velocity recording from the suprasternal notch in a patient with aortic stenosis. Note that peak aortic velocity is almost 5 m/sec. As the gradient increases, so does peak systolic velocity. Scale marks are 1 m/sec.

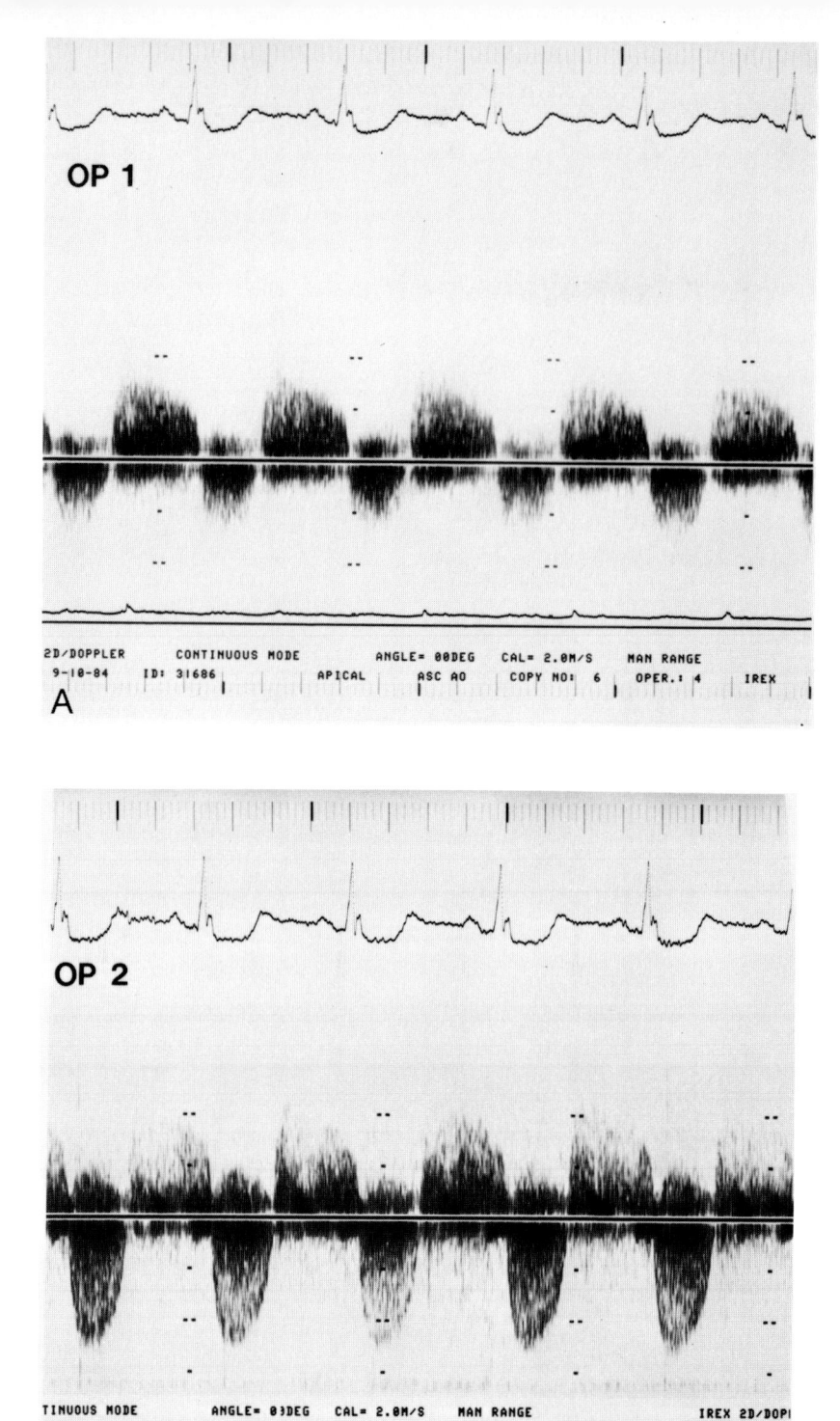

FIG. 7.9. Operator skill is very important in obtaining an adequate systolic aortic jet profile in aortic stenosis. (A) A recording done by less experienced operator (OP 1) is compared with one from (B) a more experienced operator (OP 2). OP 2 shows a more fully formed velocity profile away from the transducer, reaching 5 m/sec. Using the OP 1 tracing would result in severe underestimation of gradient.

nation for aortic stenosis will add an average of 15 to 30 minutes to the two-dimensional and routine Doppler echocardiographic examination, even with an experienced operator. Figure 7.9A shows a recording from the apical window obtained by an operator with only modest experience. Both aortic stenosis and aortic insufficiency are recorded, but the systolic flow away from the transducer fails to show a fully formed profile. The spectral recording in Fig. 7.9B was performed by a more experienced individual, and the fully formed systolic profile is seen. Had a measurement been made on Fig. A, peak systolic velocity would have been approximately 2.8 m/sec, whereas the true velocity shown in Fig. B is 5 m/sec. Use of the inadequate tracing would have severely underestimated the valve gradient.

Most experienced Doppler operators can obtain aortic systolic velocity profiles adequate for measurement of peak velocity in about 95 percent of patients (Fig. 7.10). Occasionally, only incompletely formed profiles are recorded. These should be considered inadequate and never used for estimation of gradient (Fig. 7.11). Another potential source for error is mistakenly interpreting the profile of mitral insufficiency for that of aortic stenosis. When recorded from the apical window, both occur in systole and are displayed as downward spectral velocity shifts (Fig. 7.12). These may be differentiated by remembering that the onset of ventricular systole and mitral regurgitation (arrow) occurs prior to aortic valve opening. Mitral regurgitation also is longer in duration (see Fig. 5.15).

Hatle, Berger, and colleagues were the first to use Doppler ultrasound to

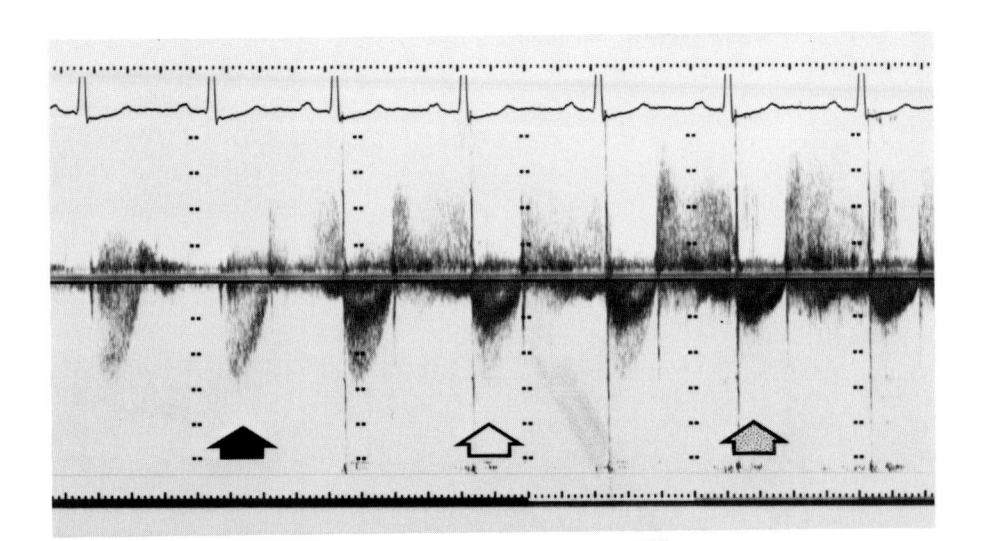

FIG. 7.10. The systolic jet of aortic stenosis and the diastolic jet of aortic insufficiency often cannot be recorded at the same time. As the transducer beam is angled from the stenotic jet (closed arrow) to intercept the aortic insufficiency, the left ventricular outflow tract velocity is encountered (stippled arrow). Both outflow tract velocities are superimposed during the beam sweep (open arrow). Scale marks are 1 m/sec.

132 BASIC DOPPLER ECHOCARDIOGRAPHY

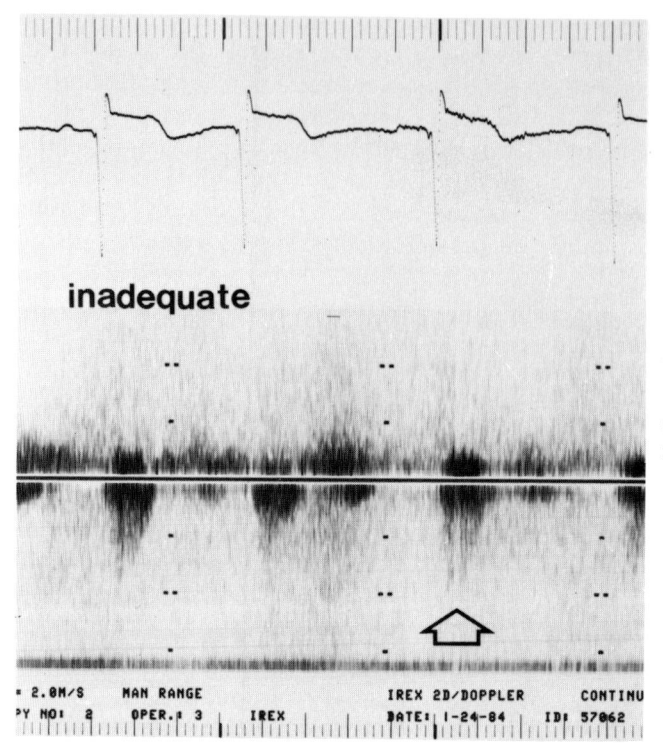

FIG. 7.11. Inadequate recordings of aortic systolic velocity do occur and should not be used for estimation of gradient. Scale marks are 2 m/sec.

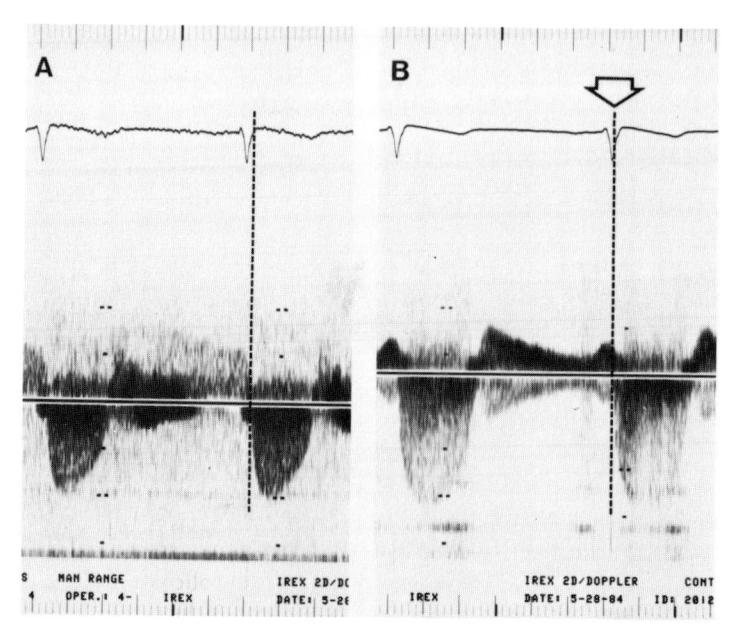

FIG. 7.12. Aortic stenosis (A) should not be mistaken for mitral insufficiency (B). Mitral systole begins before aortic (arrow) and is longer in duration. Scale marks are 2 m/sec.

FIG. 7.13. Schematic representation of simultaneous left ventricular (LV) and aortic (Ao) pressure recordings obtained at catheterization with representation of different gradient measurement methods.

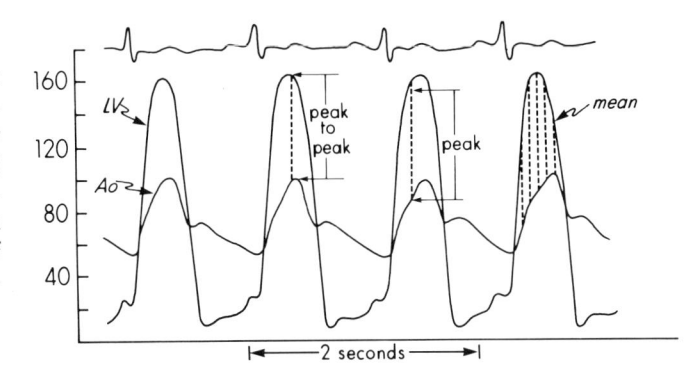

estimate the pressure gradient in patients with aortic stenosis.[4,5] Subsequently, others[6-8] have confirmed the accuracy of continuous wave Doppler echocardiography for assessing the severity of aortic valve gradients. In all of these studies, predicted Doppler gradients have been compared with those obtained at cardiac catheterization.

Figure 7.13 demonstrates three possible methods for calculating pressure gradients across the aortic valve, and all depend upon the recording of pressure from the left ventricle (LV) and aorta (Ao), or some peripheral artery. If a peripheral artery is used, it takes time for the systolic pulse to be conducted into the aorta, and there is usually a short delay in the upstroke of the aortic pulse when compared with that of the ventricle. This requires an individual measuring these pressures to trace the aortic pulse and move it slightly backward in time to adjust for the timing delay. A peak-to-peak gradient is measured from the peak of the left ventricular pressure recording to the peak of the aortic. Peak gradient is measured as the largest difference between the two and occurs somewhere on the ascending pressure tracings. Mean gradient is estimated by summing the gradients measured at sequential time intervals during systole and dividing by the number of measurements made.

Appreciation of three various invasive methods for calculation of the aortic valve gradient is very important for a critical interpretation of the Doppler literature on aortic stenosis. Almost all catheterization laboratories report peak-to-peak and mean gradients since both are readily performed. Accurate measurement of peak gradient, however, is somewhat more difficult and requires precise alignment of ventricular and aortic pressures in time and careful searching for the peak, or largest, instantaneous gradient. With the fluid-filled catheters commonly used, rapid changes in pressure, such as occur with ventricular ejection, occasionally create overshoot artifacts on the pressure recording.[9] Peak gradient is often not reported from catheterization data, in part because of these artifacts which can create large measurement errors. The peak gradient is usually higher than the peak-to-peak or mean gradients.

As Hatle and Angelsen[10] have pointed out, Doppler estimates of the aortic peak gradient calculated using the simplified Bernoulli formula generally overestimate severity when compared with catheterization peak-to-peak gradients.

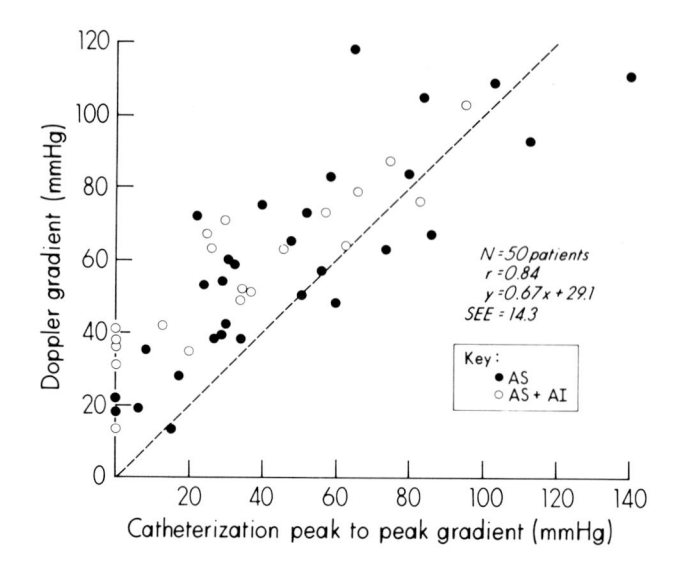

FIG. 7.14. Doppler-estimated peak aortic valve gradient compared with catheterization peak-to-peak gradient in a consecutive series of patients studied at Duke. There is sometimes marked overestimation of the gradient by Doppler.

N = 50 patients
r = 0.84
y = 0.67x + 29.1
SEE = 14.3

Key:
● AS
○ AS + AI

Accordingly, Doppler estimates of severity would be expected to correlate best with the peak gradient at catheterization.[6]

In an attempt to evaluate the use of Doppler echocardiography in clinical practice, we studied 60 consecutive patients who were referred to the catheterization laboratory with clinical findings suggestive of any possible aortic stenosis (aortic systolic murmur and peripheral pulse deficit).[11] All patients underwent cardiac catheterization at a time remote from the Doppler study (usually after 24 hours). The Doppler examination and interpretation were done without knowledge of the results of catheterization. Our patients were older than many of the groups reported from other centers (mean age 63 years), as one might anticipate in routine clinical practice, and 45 percent had 2+ or greater aortic insufficiency.

As can be seen in Fig. 7.14, Doppler overestimation of catheterization peak-to-peak gradient in our series was sometimes quite significant. Indeed, overestimations are evident over the entire spectrum of gradient values and vary in magnitude between 1 and 53 mmHg. In our view, this finding suggests that the clinician must be very careful in using catheterization laboratory criteria for the severity of an aortic gradient with Doppler peak aortic gradient values.

Doppler and catheterization estimates are more comparable when both laboratories report out the peak aortic valve gradient (Fig. 7.15). The scatter of our data is slightly greater than that of Hatle.[4] One reason for this difference may be that some of her Doppler data were collected at the time of catheterization whereas all of the patients in our series were studied at a time remote from catheterization (within 24 hours). Altered hemodynamic states with different volumes of blood flow across the aortic valve could easily account for the differences between catheterization and Doppler gradients seen in our data.

In routine clinical practice, Doppler estimates of severity of aortic stenosis

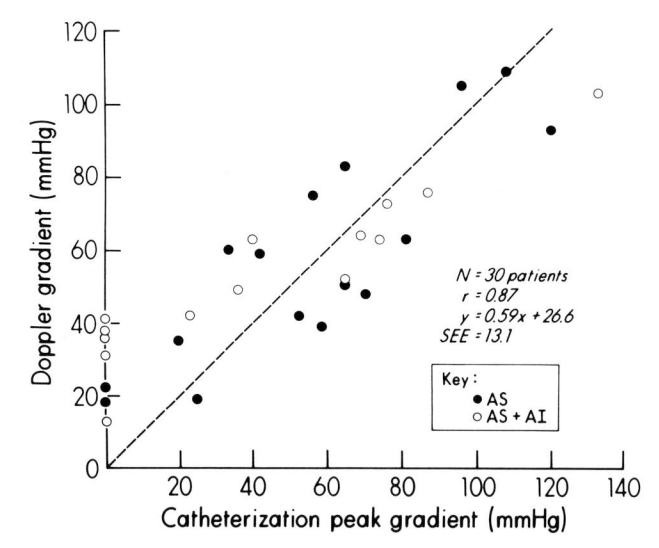

FIG. 7.15. Doppler peak gradient compared with catheterization peak gradient in the Duke series of patients.

[Scatter plot: Doppler gradient (mmHg) vs Catheterization peak gradient (mmHg). N = 30 patients, r = 0.87, y = 0.59x + 26.6, SEE = 13.1. Key: ● AS, ○ AS + AI]

are likely to be made at least 24 hours before the catheterization. These Doppler measurements may find a role in selecting patients for invasive study. Eventually, they may be used to refer some patients to surgery without prior catheterization.

What is encouraging is that even though comparative data were collected at different times in our study, peak gradients correlated favorably. In our experience, if heart rates are more than 20 beats different between the two studies, agreement between them will be reduced (due to differences in blood flow across the valve). Therefore, heart rate serves as one convenient index to assess the similarity of hemodynamic states, when Doppler and catheterization comparison studies are performed at remote times.

There are some limitations inherent in using Doppler peak-aortic gradient estimates. Few catheterization laboratories report peak-gradient data, and a suitable frame of reference to judge severity of stenosis, as exists for peak-to-peak gradients, is not available. Clinicians have commonly used peak-to-peak gradients in excess of 50 mmHg to identify severe aortic stenosis.[9] There is no corresponding figure for peak gradients in current use.

The comparison of mean Doppler gradient to mean catheterization gradient also shows good overall agreement (Fig. 7.16). Mean gradients may be less sensitive to individual measurement errors since they reflect an average of multiple measurement. The calculation of mean Doppler gradient also has the advantage that such gradients are available from most catheterization laboratories and are familiar to most clinicians.

Understanding the details of these various gradient comparisons is very important for the beginning user of Doppler echocardiography. We have seen significant credibility gaps develop between the echocardiography and catheterization laboratories when there is not a mutual understanding of the capabilities

136 BASIC DOPPLER ECHOCARDIOGRAPHY

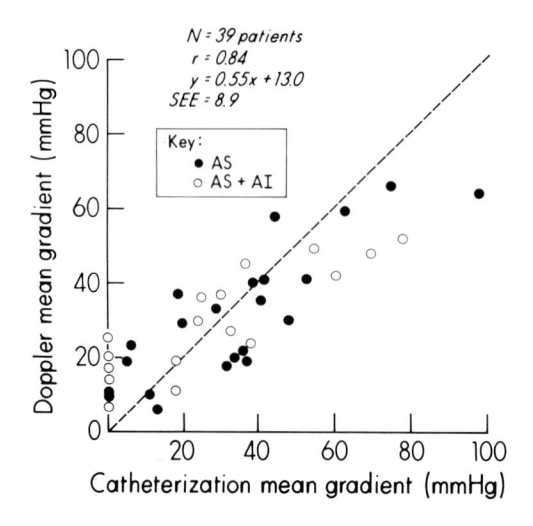

FIG. 7.16. Doppler mean gradient compared with catheterization mean gradient in the Duke series of patients.

and limitations of both techniques. Despite these cautions, we do believe that Doppler comparisons to catheterization data acquired with pressure transducer-tipped catheters should be most satisfactory when acquired simultaneously.

Seven of our patients had a gradient predicted by Doppler but did not have a gradient at catheterization (Figs. 7.14–7.16). In all seven of these patients,

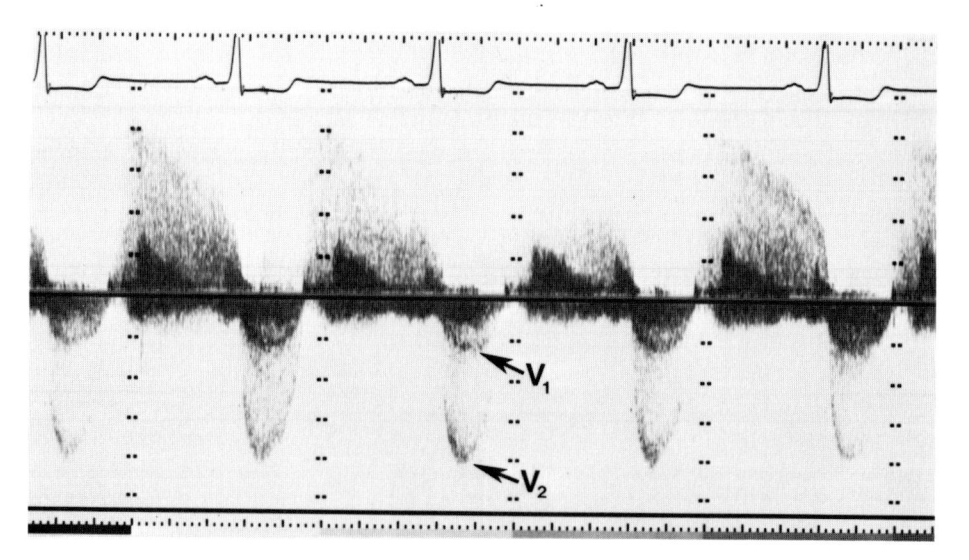

FIG. 7.17. Velocity below the valve (V_1) is not commonly recorded as often as velocity on the aortic side (V_2). V_1 is ignored in the simplified Bernoulli equation. Scale marks are 1 m/sec.

heart rates were nearly identical, making it unlikely that differences in hemodynamic status were responsible for the discrepancies. However, it is noteworthy that all seven patients had high cardiac outputs, and in five significant aortic regurgitation was present. It is possible that the use of the simplified Bernoulli equation in such patients may be at least partly responsible for the overestimates. The full Bernoulli equation takes into account blood velocity on both sides of the valve, whereas the simplified form only uses peak velocity after the valve is crossed (Fig. 7.17). Patients with hyperdynamic circulatory states, such as those with aortic regurgitation, may have a significant velocity component below the aortic valve. Failure to take this into account may lead the Doppler operator to attribute the elevated aortic velocity to an obstruction of the outflow tract, even in patients with pure aortic regurgitation. In our series, the effect of aortic insufficiency was most evident when there was minimal or no aortic valve gradient. It seemed to be less important in patients with combined stenosis and insufficiency.

Two observations may be helpful in recognizing such overestimated gradients. In all seven cases, early peaking of the aortic velocity profile suggested an insignificant gradient.[4] In addition, all patients whose aortic valve cusps opened to the periphery of the root on echocardiography had absent or small aortic gradients at catheterization.[12] Indeed, full mobility of the aortic valve cusps correctly classified one patient with a calculated Doppler gradient of 67 mmHg in whom catheterization revealed a gradient of only 25 mmHg.

It is well known that determining the severity of aortic stenosis by physical examination can be difficult, particularly in older patients.[13] One useful clinical role for Doppler echocardiography would be to serve as a supplement to the history and physical examination in the selection of patients for cardiac catheterization. Doppler studies of aortic valve gradients, including our own, have shown a good (but not perfect) correlation with catheterization aortic valve peak and mean gradients in older adult patients.

However, it is important for the beginner to appreciate that difficult patients do occur. When recordings of poor quality are seen, these should be disregarded since they will generally underestimate the severity of the gradient. Even when good-quality traces are obtained, it is possible to record falsely high gradients by Doppler, especially in the setting of aortic insufficiency. This may be suspected when there is an early peak in the Doppler profile, and retained aortic valve mobility is seen by echocardiography.

Hatle et al.[4] have proposed an additional method for judging the severity of aortic stenosis using the time to peak velocity in systole. The method is demonstrated in Fig. 7.18; Fig. A demonstrates a patient with lesser severity of stenosis and a shorter relative time to peak than in Fig. B. A value of 0.50 or greater has been found to correlate with moderate-to-severe obstruction.[10] The method is most accurate when clear evidence of aortic valve opening and closing is seen on the Doppler recording. If these are not evident, a phonocardiogram or Doppler signal amplitude tracing must be used to indicate the boundaries of the systolic ejection period.

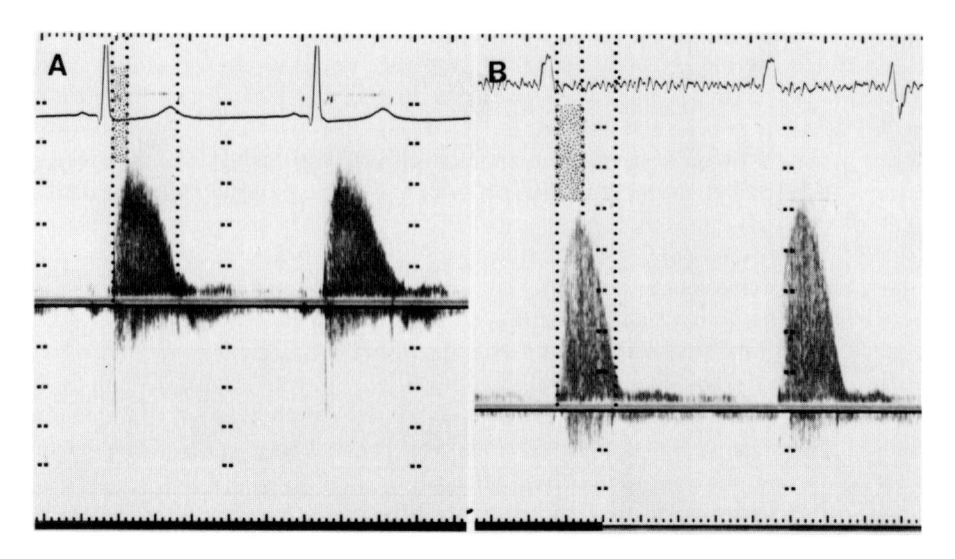

FIG. 7.18. The severity of aortic stenosis may also be judged by the relative proportion of total systolic time taken to reach peak velocity (stippled areas). Both are CW spectral recordings from the suprasternal notch. Both time-to-peak and peak velocity are lower in Fig. A than seen in Fig. B. Scale marks are 1 m/sec.

MITRAL STENOSIS

The best window for examination of mitral valve diastolic flow is invariably apical. With the transducer at the cardiac apex, the ultrasound beam should be directed posteriorly and a bit superiorly to intercept mitral valve flow. In normal individuals, pulsed Doppler is adequate for recording mitral valve diastolic flow. Mitral flow is typically laminar and biphasic (Fig. 7.19), peaking in early diastole (solid arrow) and rising again with atrial contraction in late diastole (open arrow).

The examination for mitral stenosis is usually much easier and more straightforward than that for aortic stenosis. The typical continuous wave spectral recording of mitral stenosis demonstrates spectral broadening in diastole, with peak flow in early diastole and a progressive but slowed diastolic descent (Fig. 7.20). The secondary increase in diastolic velocity due to atrial contraction is absent in patients with atrial fibrillation.

A mitral valve gradient is calculated using the modified Bernoulli equation, discussed previously. The spectral recording shown in Fig. 7.21 shows a peak diastolic velocity of 2 m/sec which is equivalent to a 16 mmHg peak transmitral gradient. Just as with aortic stenosis, the transmitral pressure gradient may be reported in several ways. Catheterization laboratories usually report the mean gradient. In order to compute a comparable mean gradient for Doppler data, one must measure multiple instantaneous peak gradients during diastole (such as 40- to 100-msec intervals) and average the values. At least 10 well-formed Doppler profiles should be averaged in this manner, if the patient is in atrial fibrillation.

DOPPLER EVALUATION OF VALVULAR STENOSIS   139

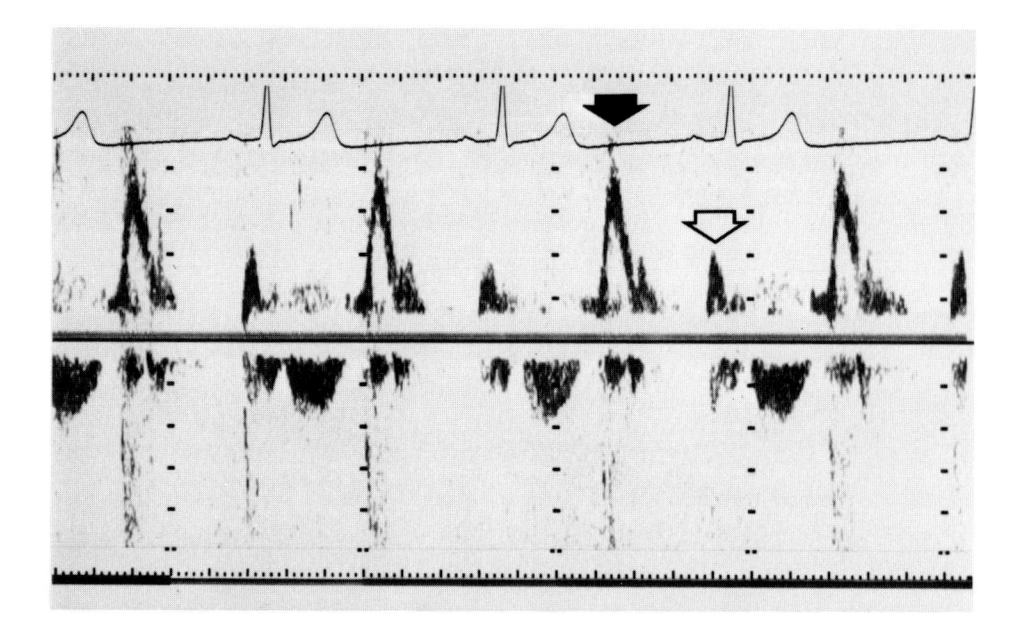

FIG. 7.19. Pulsed Doppler spectral recording from the mitral orifice taken by the apical window. Early diastolic flow is higher (closed arrow), followed by a rapid descent, and then peaks again after atrial contraction (open arrow). Use of the low-frequency filter has eliminated low velocities on either side of the baseline. Scale marks are 20 cm/sec.

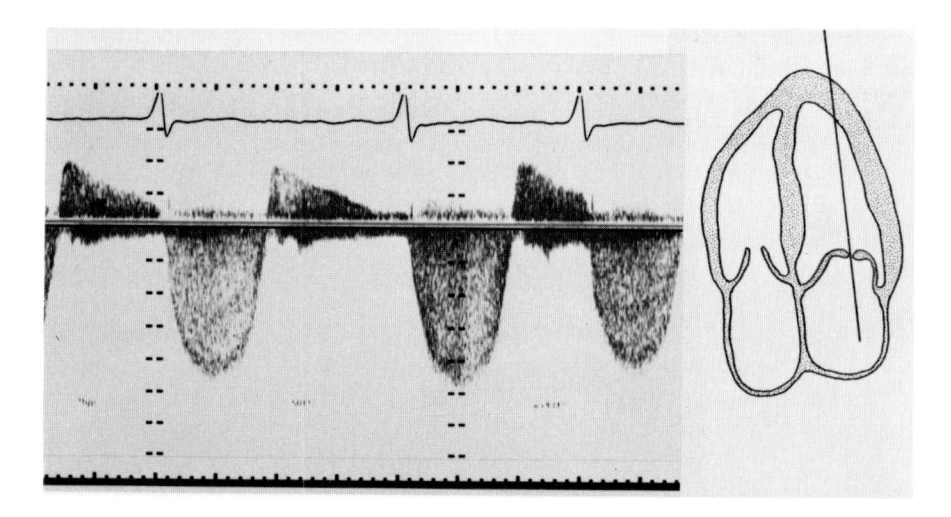

FIG. 7.20. Typical CW spectral velocity recording from a patient with mitral stenosis and insufficiency. From the apex, the diastolic flow of mitral stenosis is toward the transducer. There is a rise in velocity in early diastole followed by a slow diastolic descent. Note the spectral broadening. The patient is in atrial fibrillation, and the secondary rise in diastolic mitral flow seen in Fig. 7.19 is absent. Scale marks are 1 m/sec.

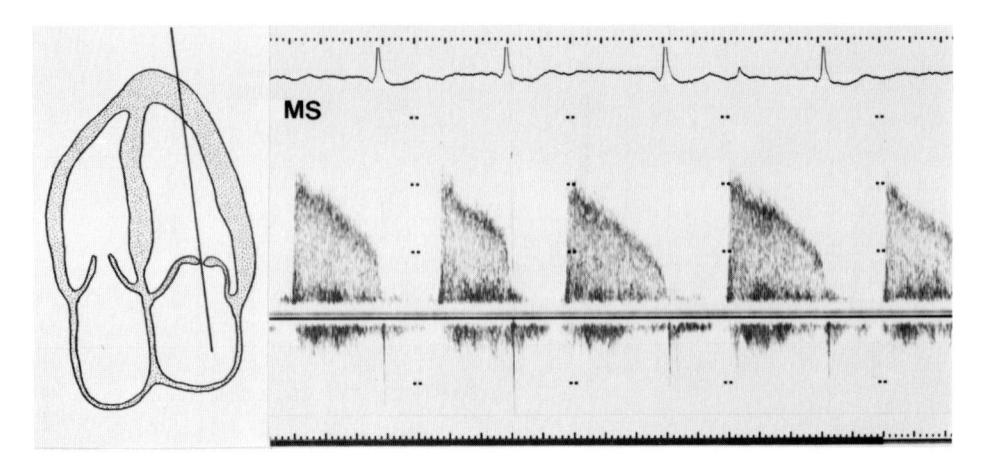

FIG. 7.21. Typical diastolic pattern of mitral stenosis using CW Doppler. Note early diastolic velocity rises to 2 m/sec. Mitral valve pressure gradients may be estimated using this technique. Scale marks are 1 m/sec. For details see text.

Results published to date have shown excellent agreement between CW Doppler estimates of the mitral valve pressure gradient using the simplified Bernoulli equation and simultaneous estimates derived from cardiac catheterization data.[2,3,10] However, when the two studies are done on separate days, the agreement between the two is reduced.[2,10] This apparent discrepancy derives, in part, from the labile nature of the mitral pressure gradient. The value of this parameter at any particular instant is determined not only by the extent of mitral valve obstruction present but also by the flow across the valve (i.e., cardiac output) and the length of the diastolic filling period, which is determined by the heart rate.[9] Therefore, if the heart rate during catheterization differs from the rate during the Doppler study, the pressure gradients estimated by these two techniques would be expected to differ. In this situation, the higher gradient would be recorded in the study done at the faster heart rate.

The sensitivity of the mitral pressure gradient to changes in heart rate clearly make it an incomplete descriptor of the severity of mitral stenosis. As stated previously, valve area is generally considered not to vary with changes in cardiac output and is the preferred method for expressing the severity of mitral stenosis. Mitral valve area may be calculated at catheterization or by two-dimensional echocardiography (Fig. 7.22). In our laboratory, catheterization-derived mitral valve area correlates well with that measured by two-dimensional echocardiography.[14] We find both two-dimensional echocardiography and Doppler to be useful for noninvasive assessment of the severity of mitral valve obstruction.

Hatle, Libanoff, and coworkers[10,15] have described a method for estimating mitral valve area from Doppler measurements. The method is based on the measurement of a parameter termed the atrioventricular (AV) pressure half-time. This quantity was originally proposed as an alternative to the Gorlin

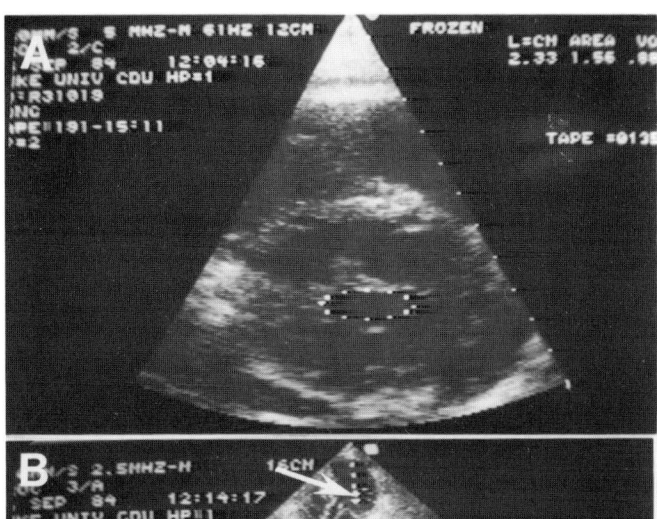

FIG. 7.22. Mitral valve orifice area may be measured by two-dimensional echocardiography (A). The peak mitral velocity and rate of diastolic descent (open arrow) of the Doppler tracing also contain information that allow for calculation of valve area by Doppler (B).

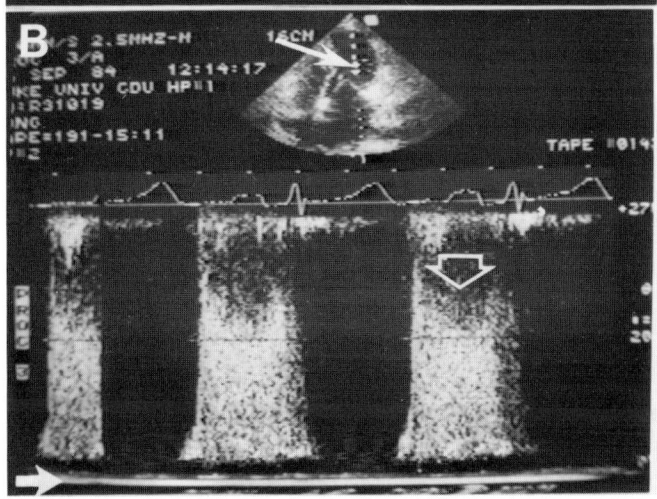

formula for estimating the severity of mitral stenosis from catheterization pressure data. It is defined as the time interval in milliseconds (msec) required for the diastolic pressure gradient across the mitral valve to fall to one-half of its initial value.

The original studies of AV pressure half-time done in the catheterization laboratory showed it to correlate well with effective mitral valve area and to be relatively insensitive to changes in heart rate or cardiac output.[15,16] In 40 normal subjects (20 adults and 20 children), Hatle et al. found pressure half-time values of 20 to 60 msec.[17] In 32 mitral stenosis patients, they found a strong correlation between the pressure half-time estimated from Doppler data and the mitral valve area calculated from catheterization data using the Gorlin formula. Pressure half-time was found to be relatively insensitive to the effects of exercise, atrial fibrillation, or coexisting mitral regurgitation. Patients with mitral stenosis had values from 100 to 400 msec, with the higher values seen in the subjects with smaller valve areas. Pressure half-times greater than 220

142   BASIC DOPPLER ECHOCARDIOGRAPHY

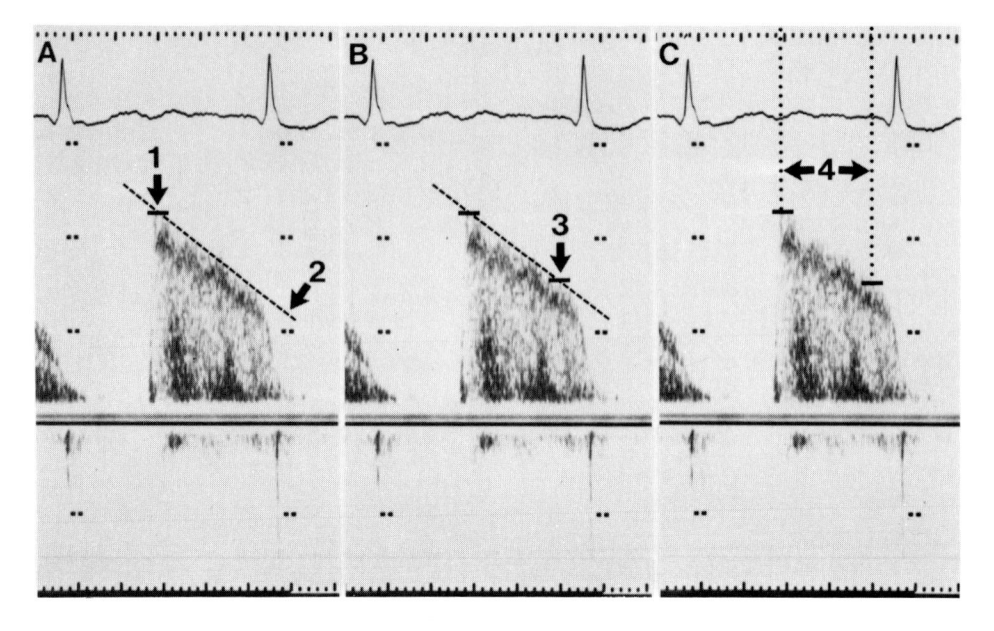

FIG. 7.23. Method for calculation of pressure half-time by Doppler. Scale marks are 1 m/sec. For details see text.

$$\text{MVA （cm}^2\text{)} = \frac{220}{\text{pressure half-time (ms)}}$$

FIG. 7.24. Formula for estimation of mitral valve area in centimeters squared (cm²) using the pressure half-time. The number 220 is an empiric constant.

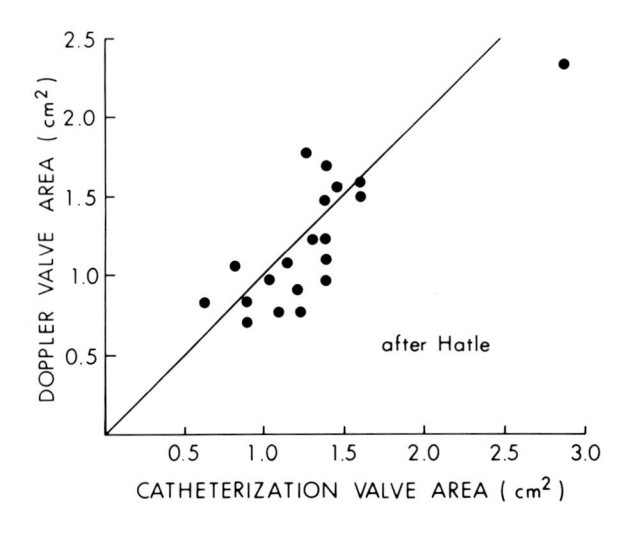

FIG. 7.25. Comparison of Doppler-estimated mitral valve area and catheterization valve area. (Redrawn after Hatle L, Angelsen B: Doppler Ultrasound in Cardiology. 2nd Ed. Lea and Febiger. Philadelphia, 1985.)

msec correlated well with a valve area less than 1.0 cm.² Patients with isolated mitral regurgitation had values ≤80 msec.

Figure 7.23 illustrates how the pressure half-time is measured. The starting point is the time of peak velocity (point 1), which in this case is 2.2 m/sec. This corresponds to a peak pressure gradient of 19 mmHg by the simplified Bernoulli equation. A line along the diastolic descent of the mitral valve velocity spectrum is drawn (step 2). A point is then found along this line where the pressure has dropped to one-half of its initial value (point 3). This point is rapidly determined by always dividing the initial velocity by the 1.4 (which is the square root of 2). In this case, 2.2/1.4 = 1.6 m/sec. Thus, when velocity falls to 1.6 m/sec, the pressure is at one half of its initial (point 1) value. The pressure half-time is simply the time interval between point 1 and point 3, in this case 250 msec (interval 4).

Subsequently, Hatle and Angelsen[10] found that pressure half-time could be used to estimate mitral valve area from an empirical formula shown in

FIG. 7.26. Pulsed Doppler recording of tricuspid stenosis (A, open arrow) with the sample volume placed at the tricuspid orifice using the apical four-chamber view. When the sample volume is moved into the right atrium (B), tricuspid insufficiency is noted (open arrow). Closed arrows at left show baseline location. Scale marks are 20 cm/sec.

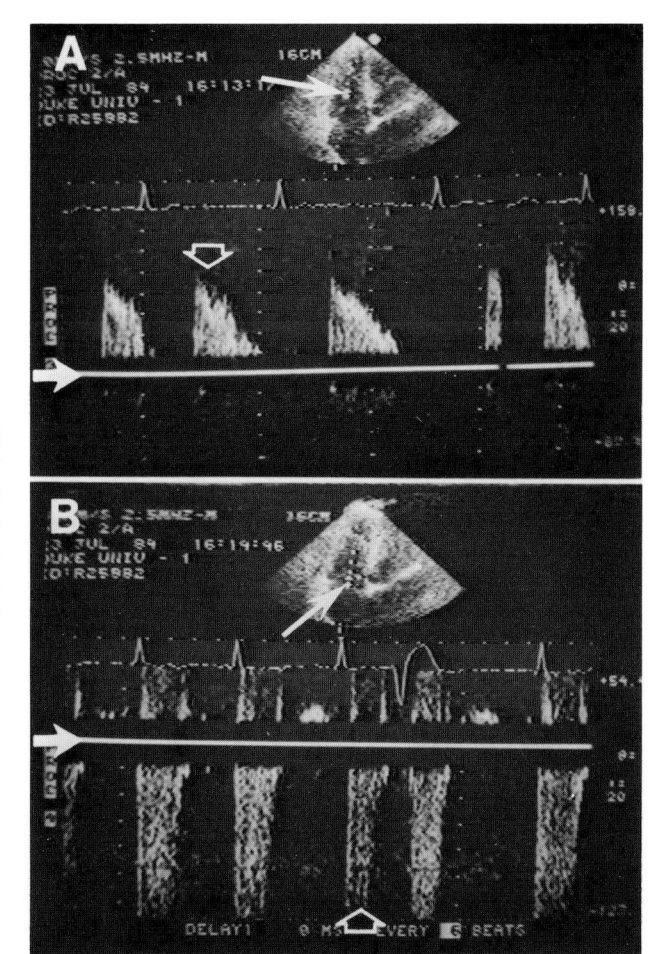

Fig. 7.24. In the case of the patient in Fig. 7.23, the predicted valve area would be 0.9 cm.[2] In a series of 20 patients, Hatle and colleagues found a strong correlation between this Doppler-derived estimate and catheterization-derived mitral valve area[10] (Fig. 7.25). These findings have been confirmed by other investigators.[8] However, more work will need to be done to define the accuracy of Doppler-generated mitral valve areas in routine clinical practice and validated in independent studies.[17]

Evaluation of triscuspid stenosis with Doppler poses problems similar to mitral stenosis but, since it is a rarer disease, the accumulated experience is less extensive. The presence of tricuspid stenois is readily determined with either pulsed or continuous wave Doppler by detecting turbulence and increased velocities in the right ventricle during diastole (Fig. 7.26). Since the pressure gradient across a stenotic tricuspid valve is fairly low, even with severe obstruction, peak Doppler velocities will be correspondingly reduced from those seen in severe mitral stenosis. Experience with both catheterization and Doppler-derived estimates of tricuspid valve areas is limited. Consequently, assessment of the severity of tricuspid obstruction in the noninvasive laboratory consists of a two-dimensional echocardiographic evaluation followed by Doppler measurement of the transvalvular mean pressure gradient.

REFERENCES

1. Johnson SL, Baker DW, Lute RA, Dodge HT: Doppler echocardiography: The localization of cardiac murmurs. Circulation 48:810, 1973
2. Holen J, Aaslind R, Lardmark K, Simonsen S: Determination of pressure gradient in mitral stenosis with a noninvasive ultrasound Doppler technique. Acta Med. Scand. 199:455, 1976
3. Hatle L, Grubakk A, Tromsdal A, Angelsen B: Noninvasive assessment of pressure drop in mitral stenosis by Doppler ultrasound. Br. Heart J. 40:131, 1978
4. Hatle, L: Noninvasive assessment and differentiation of left ventricular outflow obstruction with Doppler ultrasound. Circulation 64:381, 1981
5. Berger M, Berdoff RL, Gallerstein PE, Goldberg E: Evaluation of aortic stenosis by continuous wave Doppler ultrasound. JACC 3:150, 1984
7. Oliviera-Lima CO, Sahn DJ, Valdez-Cruz LM, Allen HD, Goldberg SJ, Grenadier E: Prediction of the severity of left ventricular outflow tract obstruction by quantitative two-dimensional echocardiographic Doppler studies. Circulation 63:348, 1983
8. Stamm RB, Martin RP: Quantification of pressure gradients across stenotic valves by Doppler ultrasound. JACC 2:707, 1983
9. Mark DB, Califf RM, Stack RS, Phillips HR: Cardiac catheterization. In Sabiston DC (ed): The Davis-Christopher Textbook of Surgery. (13th Ed.) W.B. Saunders, Philadelphia, in press
10. Hatle L, Angelsen G: Doppler Ultrasound in Cardiology. 2nd Ed. Lea and Febiger, Philadelphia, 1985
11. Krafchek J, Robertson JH, Radford M, Adams DB, Kisslo JA: A critical reappraisal of continuous wave Doppler in the assessment of severity of aortic stenosis. Circulation, abst., 70:suppl. 2, 115, 1984
12. DeMaria AN, Bommer W, Joye J, Lee G, Bouteller J, Mason DT: Value and limitations of cross-sectional echocardiography of the aortic valve in the diagnosis and quantification of valvular aortic stenosis. Circulation 62:304, 1980

13. Crawley IS, Morris DC, Silverman BD: Valvular heart disease. In Hurst JW (ed): The Heart. 4th Ed. McGraw-Hill, New York, 1978
14. Nichol PM, Gilbert BW, Kisslo JA: Two-dimensional echocardiographic assessment of mitral stenosis. Circulation 55:120, 1977
15. Libanoff AJ, Rodbard S: Evaluation of the severity of mitral stenosis and regurgitation. Circulation 33:218, 1966
16. Libanoff AJ, Rodbard S: Atrioventricular pressure half-time: Measurement of mitral valve orifice area. Circulation 38:144, 1968
17. Hatle L, Angelsen B, Tromsdal A: Noninvasive assessment of atrioventricular pressure half-time by Doppler ultrasound. Circulation 60:1096, 1979

8 Measurement of Ventricular Function Using Doppler Ultrasound

STEVE M. TEAGUE

As you see in the other chapters of this book, Doppler has wide application in the evaluation of valvular heart disease. However, the need to know ventricular function is a much more common reason for an echocardiographic evaluation. Interestingly, Doppler examinations can assess ventricular function from many perspectives. Description of ventricular function entails measurement of the timing, rate, and volume of ventricular filling and ejection. Doppler ultrasound examination reveals all of these aspects of ventricular function noninvasively, simply, and without great expense or radiation exposure.

DOPPLER VENTRICULAR FUNCTION EXAMINATION

Two Doppler echocardiographic windows are utilized in the determination of ventricular function: the suprasternal notch and the apex. As diagramed in Fig. 8.1, the suprasternal notch affords an excellent ultrasonic view of blood ejected from the left ventricle. With minimal training, the transducer can be placed in the suprasternal notch and rapidly positioned, obtaining maximal signal strength and velocity of ejection from the left ventricle. Either continuous or pulsed wave Doppler instrumentation may be employed. To assure measurements in the proximity of the aortic valve, the examiner should look for the clicks of aortic valve opening and closing that bracket the systolic velocity pulse. Signals that could contaminate this measurement originate from major systemic arteries: the innominate and the subclavians. If valve clicks are sought, these contaminations may be avoided.

The dynamics of left ventricular ejection may be studied from an apical

148 BASIC DOPPLER ECHOCARDIOGRAPHY

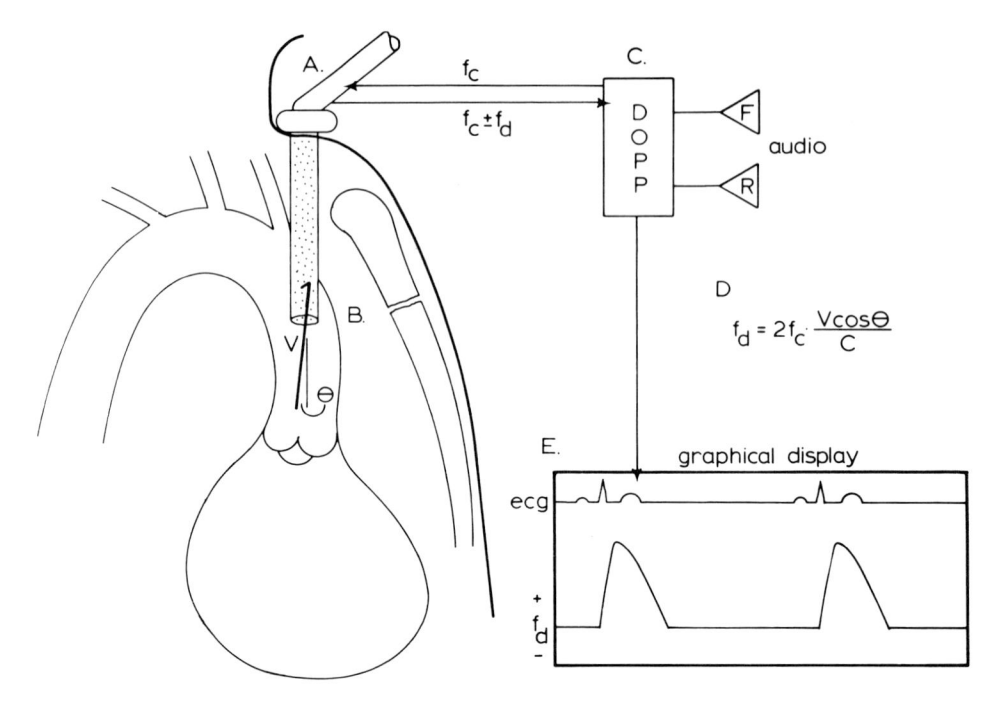

FIG. 8.1. A Doppler Transducer in the suprasternal notch (A) interrogates blood ejected from the left ventricle (B). The frequency of the reflected ultrasound is determined by the Doppler equation (D). The Doppler instrument (C) calculates the difference between transmitted and received signals, and displays this information as forward (F) or reverse (R) flow velocity in a video display or stereo speakers.

$$f_d = 2f_c \cdot \frac{V\cos\theta}{C}$$

window as well. From this position blood is accelerating out the left ventricular outflow tract and away from the transducer, so Doppler signals are recorded below the baseline. Again, this signal is easily found, and is often bracketed by aortic valve clicks. Chances of contaminating or confusing this signal would only occur in the case of aortic stenosis or hypertrophic cardiomyopathy. From the apical window, it is a simple matter to angle the transducer inferiorly and laterally, so as to interrogate blood flow toward the transducer during diastole across the mitral valve. From this velocity contour, information regarding diastolic function of the left ventricle may be ascertained.

From either window, Doppler information is processed and displayed acoustically and graphically. The acoustic output of the Doppler instrument is useful in properly aligning the beam for maximum signal strength and minimum noise. However, the acoustic output is of little use in quantitating ventricular function. For this information, we must turn to the visual display for accurate time and velocity measurements.

FIG. 8.2. The systolic velocity pulse, as observed in the aorta. Ap and Vp represent peak acceleration and velocity. Stroke volume is proportional to the area under the curve (SVI). Timing of the pulse in relation to the EKG is specified by the preejection period (PEP), left ventricular ejection time (LVET), and time to peak (TTP).

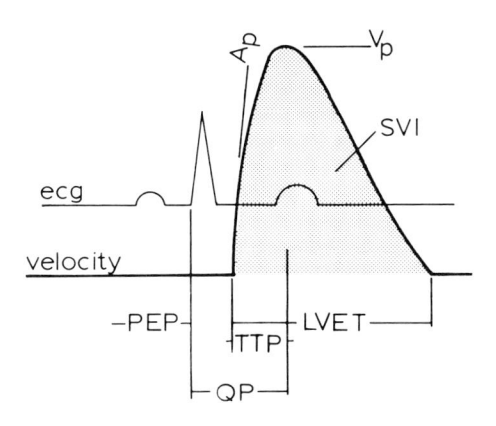

THE SYSTOLIC PULSE

From either apical or suprasternal windows, the systolic pulse similar to that diagramed in Fig. 8.2 may be obtained. If a simultaneous electrocardiogram is recorded, a wealth of information is available.

Regarding the timing of ventricular ejection, the classic systolic time intervals of preejection period (PEP) and left ventricular ejection time (LVET) can be measured between the occurence of the Q wave, the onset of Doppler ejection, and the termination of the velocity pulse. It is possible to obtain a host of other parameters, such as the time from the onset of ejection to attainment of peak ejection velocity, and the time from the Q wave to attainment of peak ejection velocity.

The rate of ventricular ejection is ascertained by analyzing peak ejection velocity and peak acceleration. Peak acceleration is simply the maximum upstroke slope of the velocity profile. Doppler instrumentation is available to measure both acceleration and peak velocity automatically.

The volume of left ventricular ejection is determined by finding the area bounded by the systolic velocity pulse, indicated in Fig. 8.2 by the systolic velocity integral (SVI). As we will soon see, the area under this curve is very important in the Doppler determination of stroke volume, which is the key element in the determination of cardiac output.

CARDIAC OUTPUT

Cardiac output is perhaps the most important descriptor of ventricular function in clinical use today. Doppler allows accurate assessment of cardiac output noninvasively. To determine cardiac output, we need two prime ingredients. The first is heart rate, and that may be determined by physical examination or automated EKG analysis. The second is stroke volume, and this can be determined by Doppler. Figure 8.3 shows the "cookbook" approach to cardiac output. To determine a stroke *volume*, one must know an area and a length.

"Stroke Volume"

AREA × LENGTH

A_o × [velocity/time curve SVI] × HEART RATE

CARDIAC OUTPUT

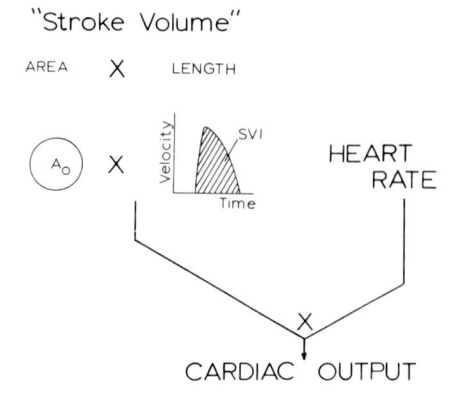

FIG. 8.3. Doppler determination of cardiac output (CO) requires measurement of heart rate (HR), cross-sectional aortic root area (Ao), and the area under the Doppler velocity curve (SVI). CO = HR × Ao × SVI.

Conceptually, the stroke volume that appears in the aortic root is a cylindrical plug with the base being the cross section of the aortic root (area) and the height being the distance that blood travels up the aortic root during a systolic ejection (length). The area of the aortic root is easily determined by M-mode or two-dimensional echocardiography. After determining the radius of the vessel, one needs only to square the result and multiply times π to determine the area.

The distance blood travels during a systolic ejection is determined by Doppler velocity information. Acceleration, velocity, and distance are all related. If one determines the area under an acceleration curve, velocity is measured, whereas the area under a velocity curve determines distance. By taking the area under the Doppler systolic velocity profile, we measure the distance blood travels up the aortic root during a single systolic ejection. By taking this distance and multiplying by the area of the root, one calculates the stroke volume, or the volume of the cylindrical plug that is ejected from the ventricle during systole. By measuring area and velocity, echocardiography allows determination of cardiac output at many other sites in the heart. Similar techniques using area and velocity allow determination of cardiac output in the pulmonary artery and at the mitral valve.

There are many possibilities for error in such calculations, and some problems exist with the technique. Debate continues regarding the correct place in the aorta to make the area measurement. From the suprasternal notch, we have found best results by taking the diameter of the aorta at the junction of the sinus of Valsalva and ascending aorta. From the apex, the most logical place is the narrowest diameter that blood must pass during systolic ejection: the aortic valve. Other observers found reliable assessments of cardiac output from the apex using this measurement. Since the calculation of cardiac output involves squaring the radius measurement, overall accuracy is highly influenced at this step. Great care and precision must be taken when these data are obtained.

Beyond the issue of the diameter determination, there are many assumptions that go into the calculation. One involves the consistency of aortic root diameter during systole. In fact, the aortic root probably expands slightly during systolic ejection. The other assumption concerns the existence of a flat velocity profile across the leading edge of the blood leaving the ventricle. Although we assumed the stroke volume to be a cylindrical plug, it more resembles a flattened bullet, with velocity peaking in the center of the vessel and falling off toward the walls. Despite this discrepancy, good correlations against clinical standards of cardiac output have been obtained.

CLINICAL APPLICATIONS

Cardiac Output

The accuracy of Doppler cardiac output determination has been verified in the animal laboratory and the clinical arena. Correlation studies have been performed against traditional forms of cardiac output determination; against thermodilution, Fick, and indicator dilution methods, and the electromagnetic blood flow probe. Studies have been performed in experimental animals, during routine cardiac catheterization, and in the intensive care unit. In all series, good correlation between Doppler and these standards have been found. In one such study, Huntsman et al. studied 45 patients undergoing Swan-Ganz catheterization in an intensive care unit. Patients with septic shock (high cardiac output), cardiogenic shock (low cardiac output), and patients with cardiac output between these extremes were represented. Despite a range of cardiac output between 2 and 14 L/min, Doppler simultaneous measurements correlated against thermodilution with an r value of .95 (a good correlation). Furthermore, the measurements were found to be repeatable from day to day, and tracked the clinical improvement or deterioration of these critically ill patients. Applications of Doppler cardiac output determinations have included the determination of treatment effects after diuretic therapy, inotropic drug administration, and volume replacement. The ability to measure cardiac output at multiple points in the heart has opened the possibility for noninvasive determination of intracardiac shunt volumes in ventricular and atrial septal defects, and regurgitant volume in valvular heart disease. With this information, it may be possible to screen patients for cardiac catheterization and help determine the need for surgical intervention. Doppler output determinations have been utilized to properly program multichamber and multimode pacemakers, optimizing cardiac output. In one such study, increments in cardiac output as high as 25 percent were seen after synchronizing atrial and ventricular pacing.

Rate of Ejection

A great deal of interest was directed at peak acceleration and peak velocity as descriptors of left ventricular function long before clinical Doppler ultrasound became available. Early investigators used electromagnetic blood flow probes on the tips of cardiac catheters positioned in the aortic root to study ejection dynamics. The universal finding in this work is that deterioration or impairment of ventricular function is reflected in lower values of acceleration and peak velocity. One such study utilized progressively increasing right atrial pacing rates during cardiac catheterization in patients with coronary artery disease. Left ventricular ejection velocity fell with pacing-induced angina in one such patient. After coronary bypass grafting and relief of myocardial ischemia, the patient experienced no angina and no fall in ejection velocity during a repeat study. In acute myocardial infarction, ventricular function as reflected in peak ejection acceleration and peak velocity appeared to correlate with survival and ejection fraction (Fig. 8.4). Another study utilized flowmeter-tipped catheters in the aortic root to show depression of ejection velocity and acceleration after the acute administration of propanolol, a depressant of contractility.

In general, relationships may be drawn between ejection velocity and acceleration and peak (dP/dt), velocity of circumferential fiber shortening, and ejection fraction. However, peak velocity and acceleration are not pure indices of ventricular contractility, as they are influenced by preload and afterload, as seen in animal models during exsanguination or cross-clamping of the ascending aorta. It does not appear that poor performance of these parameters at these unphysio-

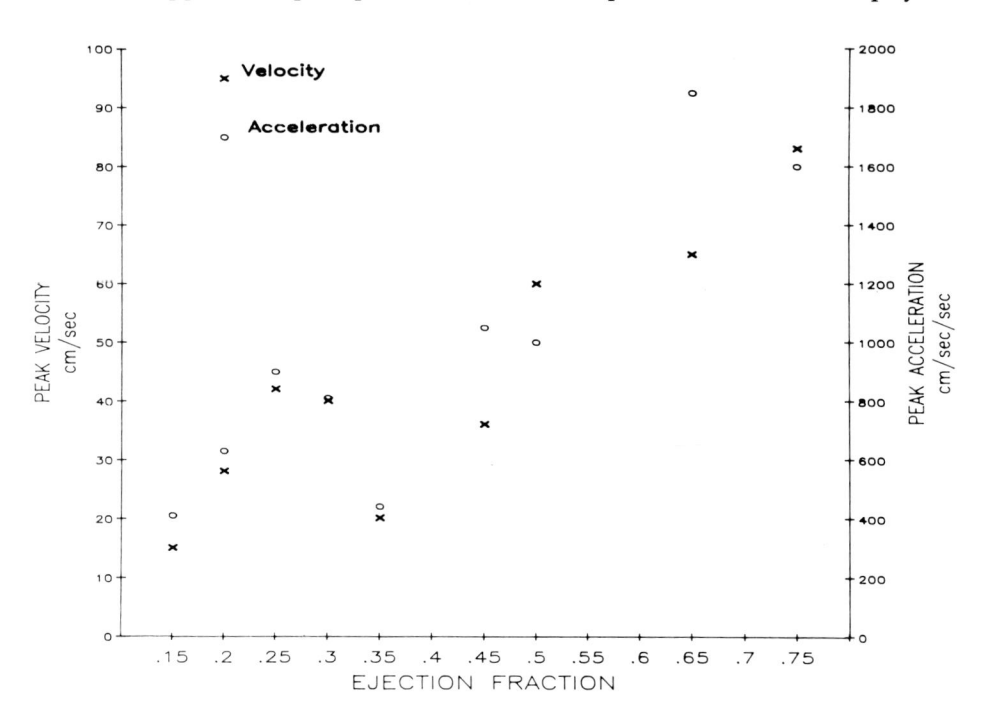

FIG. 8.4. Peak velocity and peak acceleration are correlated with one another and with ejection fraction in 14 coronary patients undergoing catheterization. (Modified from Bennett ED, Else W, Miller GAH, Sutton GC, Miller HC, Noble MIM: Maximum acceleration of blood from the left ventricle in patients with ischaemic heart disease. Clin Sci Mol Med 46:49, 1974.)

logical extremes would impair application of acceleration and velocity in the clinical domain.

Modern applications of Doppler ultrasound have shown results similar to those obtained with the invasive transducer-tipped catheter. In myocardial infarction, reduction in velocity and acceleration has been found. In vascular shock, Doppler showed reductions in peak velocity correlating with deteriorating clinical status, whereas clinical improvement was marked by increases in velocity.

We found it easy to employ continuous wave Doppler in subjects exercising on the treadmill for the diagnosis of coronary artery disease. The suprasternal notch provides an ideal location for stable placement of a hand-held transducer during exercise. By observing velocity profiles in subjects at rest and at peak exercise (Fig. 8.5), we found that patients with coronary disease have impaired ejection velocity responses. Patients with severe coronary disease and poor exercise tolerance actually have peak ejection velocity lower at peak exercise than at rest. Patients with moderate coronary disease and mild functional impairment have failure of ejection velocity to rise with increasing exertion, such that velocity at peak exertion is equal to that at rest. Patients with normal coronary arteries progressively increase ejection velocity under increasing exercise stress, often doubling velocity between rest and peak exertion.

From many studies and many perspectives it appears that ejection velocity and acceleration are strongly tied to the degree of systolic functional impairment brought on by coronary artery disease.

THE TIMING OF SYSTOLIC EJECTION

As already mentioned, the classic systolic time intervals, preejection period (PEP) and left ventricular ejection time (LVET), are easily determined by a Doppler assessment of the ejection pulse. The correlation between Doppler measurements and traditional measurements of systolic time intervals from the phonocardiogram and carotid pulse tracing has been validated. PEP/LVET is inversely related to ejection fraction in patients with coronary artery disease, and correlates with survival in acute myocardial infarction. Another interesting application of systolic timing has been found in the assessment of pulmonary hypertension. Normally, the ejection of blood from the right ventricle is much more gradual than the left ventricle. With the onset of pulmonary hypertension, the ejection from the right ventricle resembles the left ventricle; the time to the peak of ejection moves closer to the onset of ejection. By measuring this time interval (time to peak), a direct relationship to the degree of pulmonary hypertension has been established.

WHICH IS BEST?

As you can see, many measurements are possible from a single systolic velocity profile. The obvious questions are: Where should one focus attention when assessing ventricular function? Which is most sensitive to change? Is it cardiac

154 BASIC DOPPLER ECHOCARDIOGRAPHY

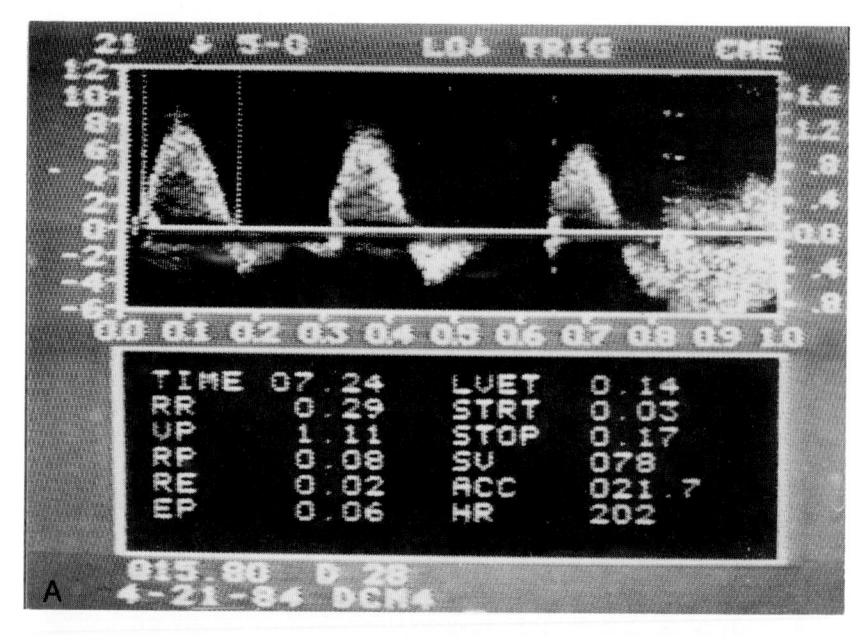

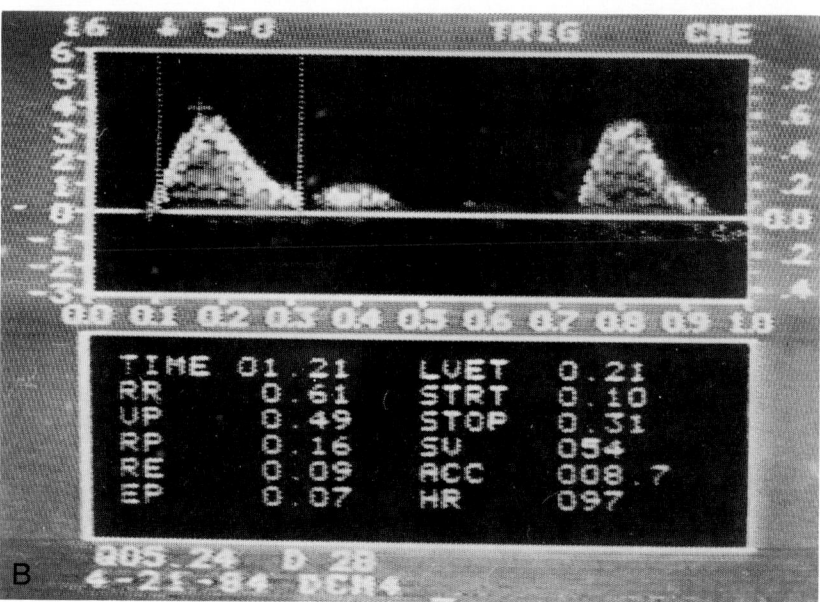

FIG. 8.5. Ascending aortic velocity profiles from a subject performing treadmill exercise at (A) Bruce stage 4 and (B) Bruce stage 1. The numeric readout documents time into study, peak velocity (VP), acceleration (ACC), stroke volume (SV), left ventricular ejection time (LVET), and heart rate (HR). As heart rate increased from 97 to 202, VP increased from 49 to 111 cm/sec, ACC rose from 8.7 to 21.7 meters/sec^2 (m/s^2) and SV increased from 54 to 78 cc. LVET shortened by 70 msec. (Courtesy of Carolina Medical Electronics, King, N.C.)

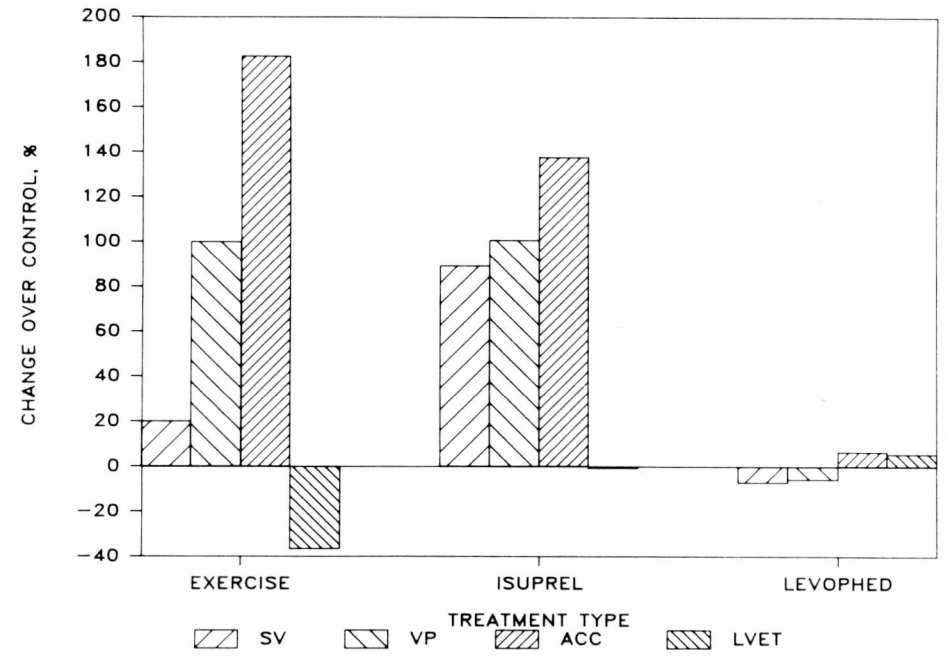

FIG. 8.6. Results of Doppler studies in 12 normal subjects undergoing submaximal bicycle exercise, Isuprel infusion, and Levophed infusion. Compared with control, acceleration is more sensitive than peak velocity, stroke volume, and left ventricular ejection time in the detection of changing inotropic state.

output? Rate of ejection? Or is it the timing of systolic ejection? To attempt to answer these questions, we studied normal subjects during exercise and during the infusion of Isuprel (to enhance contractility) and Levophed (to increase afterload). The results are seen in Fig. 8.6. Both exercise and Isuprel potently stimulated the Doppler ejection pulse, whereas a 20 percent elevation in mean artrial pressure after Levophed had little effect. Of stroke volume, acceleration, peak velocity, and left ventricular ejection time, acceleration was clearly the most sensitive indicator of changing ventricular performance. Ejection velocity superseded stroke volume, which in turn was more sensitive than LVET. It is anticipated that future Doppler work with acceleration and velocity will show a wide range of application in the assessment of ventricular function.

DIASTOLIC FUNCTION

Doppler evaluation of left ventricular diastolic function relies on diastolic velocity profiles across the mitral valve. This profile has a twin-peaked configuration similar to the M-shaped peaks of mitral valve opening on the M-mode echocardiogram. The first peak accompanies rapid ventricular filling whereas the second peak, which is normally lower than the first, is attributed to atrial contraction. States that alter left ventricular compliance, such as infarction, acute ischemia, and hypertrophy, appear to alter the relationship between these peaks. In the stiff ventricle, the velocity contribution from atrial systole is much higher than that of rapid filling. Drugs that increase left ventricular compliance, including calcium entry blockers and nitrates, can reverse this ratio, normalizing diastolic properties as reflected in mitral flow patterns. These are early results of research, and this area is yet to be fully explored.

SUMMARY

In summary, noninvasive Doppler ultrasound has a wide variety of applications in the determination of ventricular function. Included are the assessment of cardiac output, the ejection-phase indices of acceleration and velocity, and the timing of ventricular ejection. Of parameters that can be measured in single systolic Doppler pulses, acceleration appears to be most sensitive in detecting changes in ventricular systolic function. It appears possible to study diastolic properties of the ventricle utilizing Doppler ultrasound patterns of mitral valve flow. The noninvasive, accurate, and inexpensive nature of the technique makes Doppler ultrasound attractive for assessment of ventricular function in a wide range of applications and disease processes.

SUGGESTED READINGS

Velocity and Acceleration

Bennett ED, Barclay SA, Davis AL, Mannering D, Metha N: Ascending aortic blood velocity and acceleration using Doppler ultrasound in the assessment of left ventricular function. Cardiovasc Res 18:632, 1984

Bennett ED, Else W, Miller GAH, Sutton GC, Miller HC, Noble MIM: Maximum acceleration of blood from the left ventricle in patients with ischaemic heart disease. Clin Sci Mol Med 46:49, 1974

Buchtal A, Hanson GC, Peisach AR: Transcutaneous aortovelography: Potentially useful technique in management of critically ill patients. Br Heart J 38:451, 1976

Jewitt D, Gabe I, Mills C, Maurer B, Thomas M, Shillingford J: Aortic velocity and acceleration measurements in the assessment of coronary heart disease. Eur J Cardio 1:299, 1974

Kolettis M, Jenkins BS, Webb-peploe MM: Assessment of left ventricular function by indices derived from aortic flow velocity. Br Heart J 38:18, 1976

Kozlowski J, Gardin J, Dabestani A, Murphy M, Kusnick C, Allfie A, Russell D, Henry W: Changes in Doppler aortic flow velocity parameters during supine exercise. J Am Coll Cardiol 3:569, 1984

Noble MIM, Trechard D, Guz A: Left ventricular ejection in conscious dogs: Measurement and significance of the maximum acceleration of blood from the left ventricle. Circ Res 19:139, 1966

Rushmer RF, Watson N, Harding D, Baker D: Effects of acute coronary occlusion upon the performance of right and left ventricles in intact unanesthetized dogs. Am Heart J 66:522, 1963

Teague SM, Mark DB, Radford M, Robertson J, Albert D, Porter J, Waugh RA: Doppler velocity profiles reveal ischemic exercise responses. Circulation 70:II, 1984

Cardiac Output

Huntsman LL, Stewart DK, Barnes SR, Franklin BS, Colocousis JS, Hessel EA: Noninvasive Doppler determination of cardiac output in man. Clinical validation. Circulation 67:593, 1983

Nanna M, Chandraratna PAN, Nimalasuriya A, Kawanishi D, McKay C, Kotlewski A, Rahimtoola S: Noninvasive cardiac output monitoring during exercise stress test. Circulation 68:III, 1984

Sanders SP, Yeager S, Williams RG: Measurement of systemic and pulmonary blood flow and QP/QS ratio using Doppler and two-dimensional echocardiography. Am J Cardiol 51:952, 1983

Stewart WJ, Dicola VC, Harthorne JW, Gillam LD, Weyman AE: Doppler ultrasound measurement of cardiac output in patients with physiologic pacemakers. Am J Cardiol 54:308, 1984

Systolic Time Intervals

Hatle L: Noninvasive methods of measuring pulmonary artery pressure and flow velocity. In Cardiology, an International Perspective. Plenum Press, New York, 1984, p. 783

Lewis RP, Rittgers S, Forester WF, Boudoulas H: A critical review of the systolic time intervals. Circulation 56:146, 1977

Rothendler JA, Schick EC, Ryan TA: Systolic time intervals derived from Doppler measurement of temporal artery flow. Circulation 60:II, 1979

Diastolic Function

Iwase M, Yokota M, Takagi S, Kiode M, Ching HC, Kawai N, Hayashi H, Sotobata I: Effects of Diltiazem on left ventricular diastolic behavior in patients with hypertrophic cardiomyopathy: Evaluation with exercise pulse Doppler echocardiography. In Proceedings of the 2nd International Cardiac Doppler Symposium. Institute of Applied Physiology and Medicine, Seattle, Wash, 1983

Maron BJ, Arce J, Bonow RO, Wesley Y: Noninvasive assessment of left ventricular filling and relaxation by pulsed Doppler echocardiography in hypertrophic cardiomyopathy. Circulation 70:II, 1984

9 Doppler Echocardiography in Pediatric Cardiology

HUGH D. ALLEN
GERALD R. MARX

Congenital heart disease encompasses abnormalities in cardiac development which generally have in common either valve stenoses or connections between chambers or great vessels. Usually, abnormalities of intracardiac anatomy, and often, abnormalities of great vessel anatomy, can be unraveled by two-dimensional echocardiography. However, echocardiography offers little information regarding flow characteristics in the various congenital lesions. Addition of the Doppler principle, particularly when combined with the two-dimensional examination, can characterize the source of a flow disturbance, quantify gradients across a site of obstruction, and quantify flow volume across sites where flow is nonturbulent. These features make Doppler echocardiography unique for noninvasive accurate evaluation of children and adults with various forms of congenital heart disease.

In this report, we will discuss some of the present uses of Doppler echocardiography in congenital heart disease. Application of this technique requires greater understanding of certain physics principles than does routine echocardiography. These have been discussed elsewhere in this monograph, in texts, and in review articles.[1-3] The reader is encouraged to refer to these for specific details.

QUALITATIVE DOPPLER ECHOCARDIOGRAPHY

Localization of flow disturbances in various cardiac lesions comprised most of the beginning efforts in the use of Doppler echocardiography in patients with congenital heart disease, and remains an important aspect of the examination. For example, Is the source of the murmur at the base of the heart in

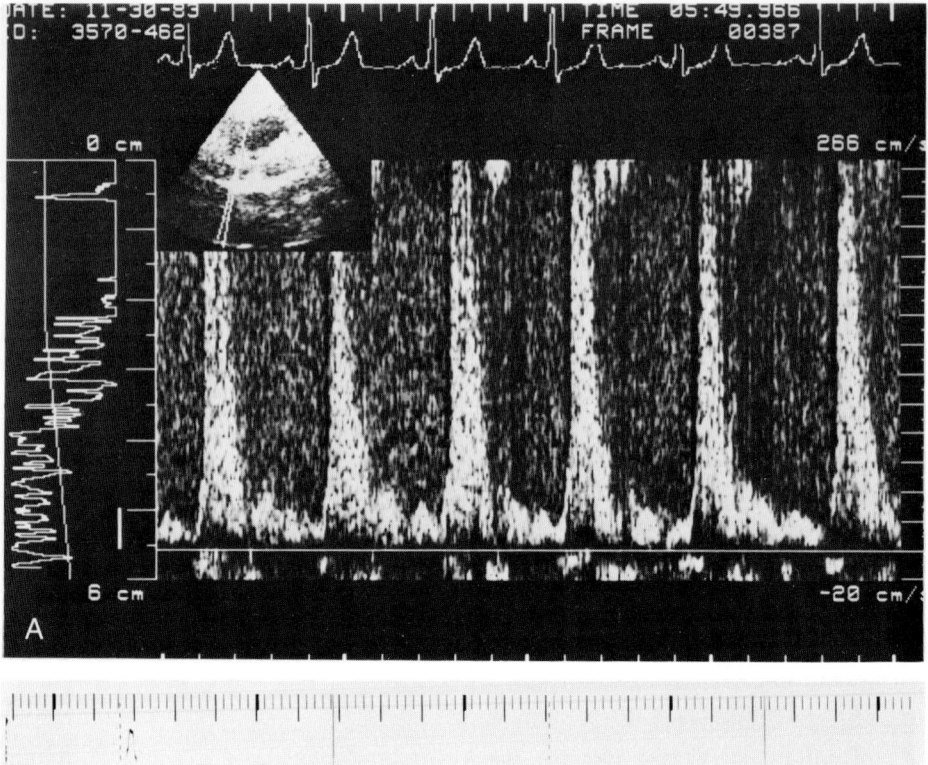

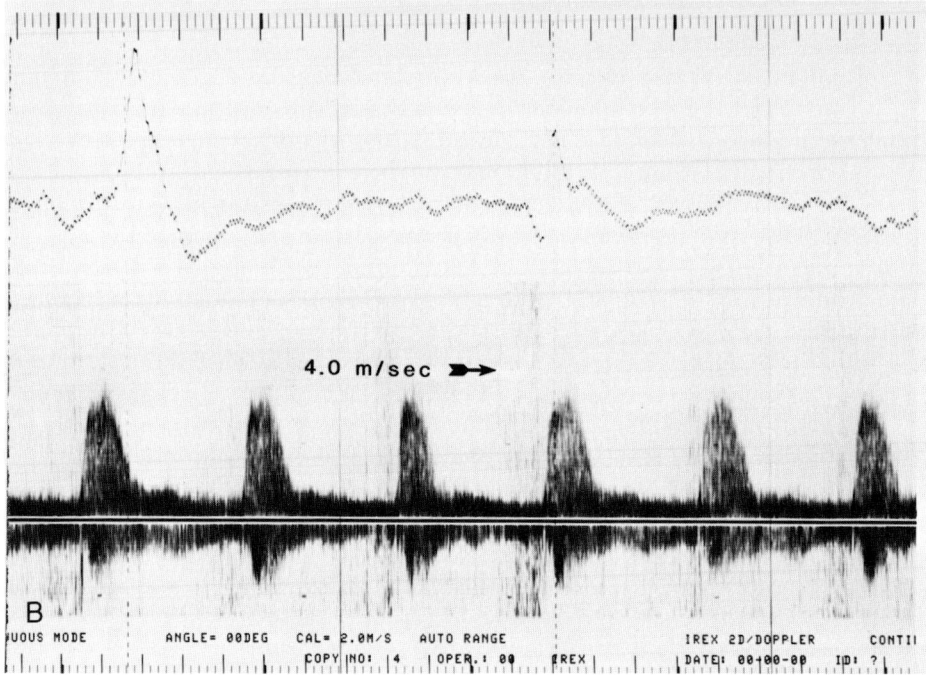

FIG. 9.1. Example of disturbed flow in a patient with aortic stenosis. Fig. A demonstrates aliasing of the Doppler signal because the Nyquist limit of the pulsed Doppler system has been exceeded. The insertion slows sample volume location in the dilated ascending aorta as viewed from the suprasternal notch. Fig. B shows a continuous wave Doppler evaluation of the same patient. A "blind" transducer was located in the suprasternal notch and moved until the maximal auditory and spectral signals were obtained. The arrow points to a 4 m/sec-calibration dot. This patient has mild-to-moderate aortic stenosis. (Goldberg SJ, Allen HD, Marx GR, and Flinn CJ: Doppler echocardiography, Lea and Febiger, Philadelphia, 1984.)

the patient with a suprasternal notch thrill and systolic ejection click a mildly stenotic aortic or pulmonary valve? The answer is important because aortic stenosis can progress whereas mild pulmonic stenosis is usually static. Thoracic roentgenography and electrocardiography are occasionally useful, but mild disease may not demonstrate the secondary findings often present in more significant disease. Furthermore, cardiac catheterization, although definitive, is invasive, costly, and carries some attendant risk. Since Doppler interrogation allows sampling of disturbed flow and two-dimensional echocardiography allows placement of the Doppler sample, accurate localization of a given flow disturbance is possible, and the diagnosis can be readily made (Fig. 9.1).

Other qualitative applications of Doppler echo in congenital heart disease include differentiation between ventricular septal defect and mitral regurgitation, mitral regurgitation and tricuspid regurgitation, and aortic versus pulmonary regurgitation. Doppler echocardiography also aids localization of atrial[4] and ventricular septal defects.[5] Other qualitative uses of Doppler echo include demonstration of the presence of left-to-right shunting through "silent" patent ductus arterioses in neonates[6-7] and patency of systemic artery to pulmonary artery shunts during the acute postoperative period when these shunts are not yet clinically apparent.[8]

QUANTITATIVE ASPECTS OF DOPPLER ECHOCARDIOGRAPHY IN PEDIATRIC CARDIOLOGY

Flow Measurement

One of the important questions in patients with congenital heart disease regards the magnitude of left-to-right shunting. This particularly applies to atrial and ventricular septal defects. Since Doppler echocardiography allows calculation of cardiac outputs from various sites [tricuspid valve,[9] pulmonary artery,[10] aorta,[11] and possibly the mitral valve[12-13]], the QP/QS ratio (ratio of pulmonary to systemic flow) can be determined.

With certain variations, all these sites have in common a flow orifice and a certain volume of blood passing through that orifice. Doppler velocities directly reflect blood flow. The orifice through which flow passes can be visualized by two-dimensional echocardiography and various mathematical approaches can be used to calculate orifice area. Aortic, pulmonary artery, and tricuspid orifices are generally circular and thus can be calculated by measuring orifice diameter; then area = $\pi(d/2)^2$. Caution should be exercised to measure the area at the site where flow is sampled. If not, invalid data can result in an inaccurate final flow calculation.

The mean velocity of blood flow is then determined by tracing several velocity curves over time. Mean velocity (cm/sec) × cm² (area) then yields cm³/sec (flow); this product times 60 (sec/m) gives flow in cc/min. We have found that the easiest method for computing mean velocity is by tracing the modal velocities of the flow curve with a light pen and digitizing pad. A dedicated software program (Biodata Co., Box 838, Davis, California, 95617) controls an Apple II computer for this purpose.

If Doppler velocities are not measured parallel to flow, correction for the beam-flow intercept angle (Θ) must be made. The two-dimensional echocardiogram allows alignment of the Doppler sample volume with flow in two planes, and correction for the third (nonvisualized) azimuthal plane is made during the examination by subtly moving the transducer while listening for the clearest auditory signal and obtaining the optimal time velocity profile which has minimal spectral dispersion. Once the Doppler sample is in the best plane of alignment, the angle Θ is measured, and its cosine is placed in the denominator of the above equation, allowing angle correction. All attempts should be made toward achieving an angle of <20° so that the cosine function is small. The formula is thus,

$$\frac{\text{Mean velocity in cm/s} \times \text{flow area in cm}^2 \times 60 \text{ sec/m}}{\text{Cosine of the angle } \Theta} = \text{flow in cc/min.}$$

VENTRICULAR SEPTAL DEFECTS

Goldberg et al.[10] and Sanders et al.[14] have demonstrated that the QP/QS ratio can be accurately calculated in pediatric patients with ventricular septal defects. Systemic flow is calculated from the ascending aorta, and pulmonary flow is calculated from the main pulmonary artery. Occasionally pulmonary flow in ventricular septal defects is too disturbed to allow accurate sampling by pulsed Doppler, and in those cases transmitral flow should be measured, unless an atrial septal defect coexists. The mitral orifice is more elliptical than the tricuspid orifice, and thus the above-mentioned formula may not apply. Several centers are evaluating the best mathematical model for mitral flow measurement in humans.

ATRIAL SEPTAL DEFECTS

Since shunting in atrial septal defects occurs at the atrial level, pulmonary flow can be sampled from the tricuspid orifice or, more often, in the main pulmonary artery. Systemic flow is sampled in the ascending aorta.

Marx et al.[15] have demonstrated that measurement of transatrial septal velocities not only confirms the presence of an atrial septal defect but that the measurement correlates well with QP/QS ratios determined at cardiac catheterization by radioisotope techniques or by Doppler echocardiography. We have found this technique quite useful, especially when detection of the presence of an atrial septal defect is equivocal by two-dimensional echocardiography (Fig. 9.2).

ECHOCARDIOGRAPHY IN PEDIATRIC CARDIOLOGY   163

FIG. 9.2. Transatrial septal velocities in a patient with a secundum atrial septal defect. (A) The atrial septal defect location as viewed in a subcostal view. The sample volume is positioned in the right atrium as near to the perpendicular as possible. (B) The Doppler velocities which were obtained. The dotted line shows where the outer edge of the velocities were digitized from EKG R wave to R wave or successive beats. The mean value was 32.1 cm/sec. (C) Comparison of transatrial septal velocities in ASD patients compared with QP/QS obtained by Doppler. The value of 32.1 in this patient suggests a QP/QS ratio of 1.9:1, which was confirmed by cardiac catheterization at 2:1. Abbreviations: RA = right atrium; LA = left atrium; ASD = atrial septal defect; QP/QS = ratio of pulmonary flow to systemic flow; TASV = transatrial septal velocities. (Goldberg SJ, Allen HD, Marx GR, and Flinn CJ: Doppler echocardiography, Lea and Febiger, Philadelphia, 1984.)

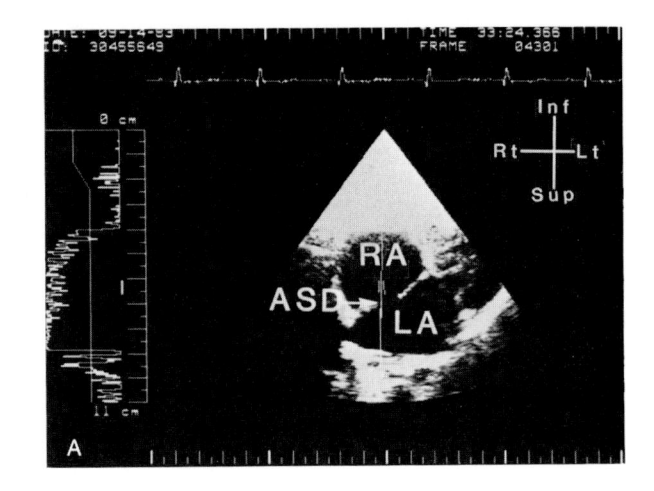

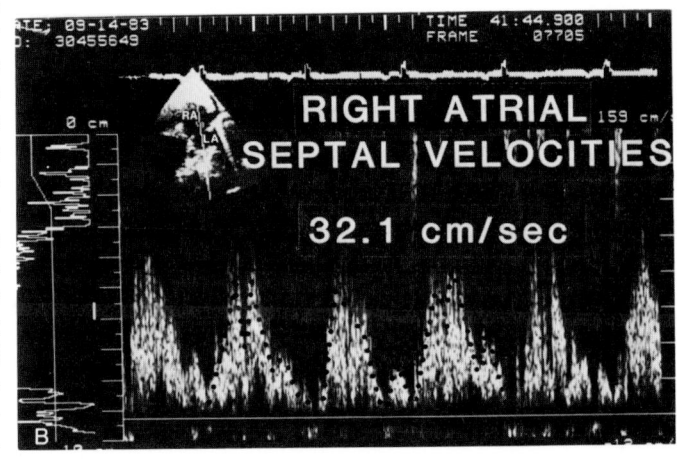

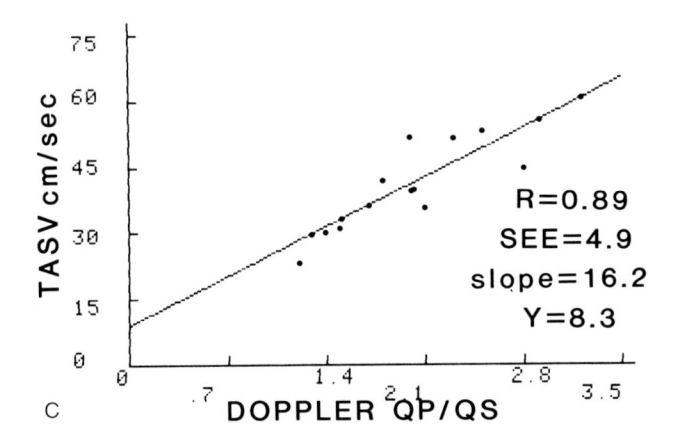

PATENT DUCTUS ARTERIOSUS

No published reports exist regarding measurement of the QP/QS ratio in patent ductus arteriosus. However, we think that the following concepts are true: Since the Doppler pulmonary flow signal is so disturbed, pulmonary flow must be sampled at other sites, including transmitral or ascending aorta. Systemic flow, in the absence of an atrial septal defect, can be sampled across the tricuspid valve. Studies evaluating this concept are presently underway in our institution.

FLOW MEASUREMENT IN CLINICAL SITUATIONS

Drug Management

We routinely use the Doppler echocardiogram for assessment of the postoperative patient who is in a low-output state. Effects of preloading, inotropic agents, and afterload-reducing agents can be serially monitored at the bedside in the intensive care unit. This is especially useful in infants in whom indwelling thermodilution catheters are not practical, such as those who have had arterial switch operations for transposition of the great vessels. Clinical decisions about optimal therapies can be made as frequently as necessary in this setting.

Valvar Insufficiency

Goldberg and Allen[16] have demonstrated that the degree of regurgitation can be quantitated by Doppler echocardiography in patients with aortic or pulmonary valvar insufficiency. The concept behind quantification is that the regurgitant flow can be digitized as described above for regular wave forms. In this case the diastolic wave form is digitized separately. Then the systolic wave form is digitized. The systolic wave form represents total forward flow, and the diastolic wave form represents regurgitant flow. The regurgitant fraction is then

$$RFr = \frac{\text{regurgitant flow}}{\text{total forward flow}} \times 100$$

A cross-check on the accuracy of this calculation is to subtract the regurgitant flow from the total forward flow and to compare this forward output figure with forward flow measured from a separate site (Fig. 9.3).

The quantitative values correlate with clinically mild regurgitation (~30 percent regurgitant fraction). When values are in the 50 to 70 percent range, overlay exists between moderate and severe insufficiency as judged by clinical standards. More studies correlating the regurgitant fraction and clinical states are necessary.

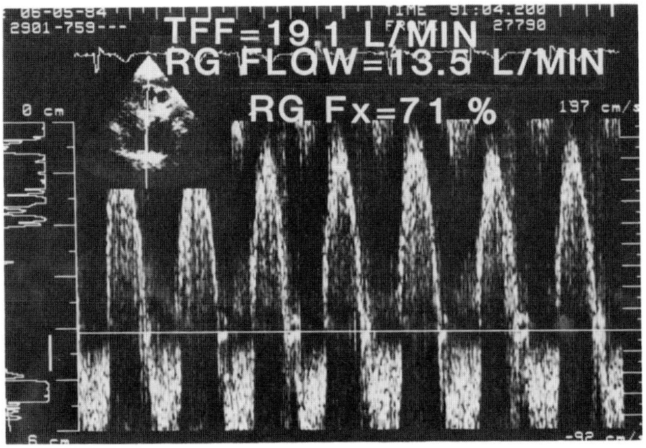

FIG. 9.3. Aortic Doppler velocities from a 3-year-old with a severe aortic regurgitation after aortic valvotomy. The sample volume is located in the ascending aorta from the suprasternal notch (insert). Total forward flow obtained from the aortic tracing was 19.1 1/min. Forward flow across the tricuspid valve was 5.6 1/min. The regurgitant fraction was thus: 19.1 − 5.6/19.1 = 71 percent. Abbreviations: TFF = total forward flow; RG flow = regurgitant flow; RG FX = regurgitant fraction.

PRESSURE GRADIENT ESTIMATION IN STENOSIS

When Doppler flows are disturbed and signal aliasing exists, either high pulse repetition frequency or continuous wave Doppler techniques are employed to allow measurement of the flow-velocity curves. The flow-velocity curve is proportional to the pressure drop across a narrowed orifice.

The energy balance equation was used by Hatle and Angelsen[2] and later by several investigators to show that pressure gradients calculated from Doppler tracings by a modification of the Bernoulli equation correlated quite well with pressure gradients measured at cardiac catheterization. The equation, although complex, considers three major factors: conductive acceleration, flow acceleration, and viscous friction. Generally, flow acceleration and viscous friction effects are negligible when stenosis is discrete. Therefore, the equation is shortened to

$$P_1 - P_2 = 4(V_2^2 - V_1^2)$$

where $P_1 - P_2$ = pressure drop, V_2 = velocity beyond obstruction, and V_1 = velocity proximal to obstruction. The second term V_1 is usually less than 1.5 m/sec and, unless proximal velocities are higher, this term can generally be ignored.

Pulmonary Stenosis

Various studies[17,18] have shown that pulmonary stenosis can be not only detected by echocardiography but that the severity of the transvalve gradient can be accurately predicted. The pulmonary artery is sampled from both the

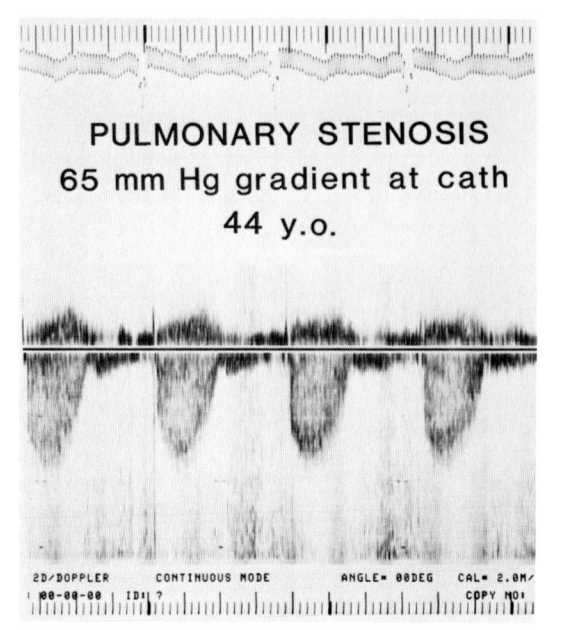

PULMONARY STENOSIS
65 mm Hg gradient at cath
44 y.o.

FIG. 9.4. Pulmonary stenosis in a 44-year-old female. Continuous wave Doppler tracing was obtained from the precordial location with the patient in a very exaggerated lateral position. Peak gradient calculated from the Bernoulli equation is 64 mmHg (4 m/sec squared × 4 = 64). Gradient measured at catheterization ranged from 60 to 70 mmHg. (Goldberg SJ, Allen HD, Marx GR, and Flinn CJ: Doppler echocardiography, Lea and Febiger, Philadelphia, 1984.)

short axis and subcostal positions. The suprasternal notch plane can occasionally be used if the transducer is directed anteriorly and somewhat leftward. Whichever plane is used, the highest velocities are used in the calculation (Fig. 9.4). The above-mentioned studies in patients with valvar pulmonary stenosis have shown close correlation between the Doppler-calculated gradients and gradients measured at cardiac catheterization.

Aortic Stenosis

The principles for gradient quantification in valvar aortic stenosis are the same as were used for pulmonary stenosis. The Doppler sample is generally best obtained from either the suprasternal notch or right upper sternal border positions. Other planes can include the apex long-axis plane, five-chamber plane, or subcostal planes. The examiner should take care to measure velocities proximal to the stenotic aortic valve to assure that velocities in this area are not excessive. If they are, they should be included in the equation as V_1^2 to obviate overestimation of the valve gradient. Further, if a long area of subaortic stenosis exists, frictional losses may come into play. This requires further study.

Coarctation of the Aorta

Although pressure drop across coarctation of the aorta is usually readily assessed by appropriate measurement of upper and lower extremity blood pressures, occasionally previous catheterizations, surgeries, or incorporation of a vessel into the anatomy of the coarctation itself prevent accurate measurement. Accordingly, we have evaluated Doppler results of transcoarctation pressure drop with cardiac catheterization pressure gradient measurements, and have found a close correlation (Fig. 9.5). In evaluation of coarctation of the aorta, the gradient is measured from the suprasternal notch by either high pulse repetition frequency or continuous wave Doppler. The examiner should measure precoarctation velocities and include them in the equation as V_1, since these velocities are generally high. We have used this technique to serially assess patients after balloon angioplasty and have found it quite useful.

Ventricular Septal Defect

Since ventricular septal defects vary in size, a pressure drop between the left and right ventricle may or may not exist. Further, the flow across a ventricular septal defect will be governed by the balance between the systemic and the right ventricular outflow resistances. Right ventricular outflow resistance can occur in the form of muscle bundles, infundibular stenosis, pulmonary valve stenosis, or a pulmonary artery band. Branch or peripheral pulmonary artery stenosis or pulmonary vascular obstructive disease can modify flow across a ventricular septal defect.

Careful examination with either high-pulse repetition frequency Doppler incorporated with direct visualization of a defect or by continuous wave Doppler by methodically searching the left precordium (in most cases) allows evaluation of the peak systolic velocities which exist across a ventricular septal defect. One hint for obtaining peak transseptal velocities is to palpate for a left sternal border thrill. This is generally the area in which the jet is maximal. If the ventricular septal defect is restrictive, its velocities will be high. Magnitude of the pressure drop across the ventricular septal defect can then be calculated. When an upper extremity blood pressure is measured in the absence of aortic stenosis, left ventricular systolic pressure can be inferred. Subtracting the pressure drop across the ventricular septal defect from this value allows estimation of right ventricular pressure. Further, pulmonary artery pressures can be estimated by the same technique. If pulmonary valve stenosis coexists, the degree of pressure drop across the pulmonary valve must be subtracted from the estimated right ventricular pressure to predict the pulmonary pressure. Figure 9.6 shows an example of this deductive approach to prediction of pulmonary artery pressure in a patient with an interventricular communication.

Valve Area Calculation in Aortic or Pulmonary Valve Stenosis

Calculation of pulmonary or aortic valve stenosis at cardiac catheterization is accomplished by use of the Gorlin and Gorlin equation where valve area equals systolic cardiac output divided by 44.5 × square root of the mean gradient. Using a separate mathematical analysis, Kosturakis et al.[19] showed that a direct

168 BASIC DOPPLER ECHOCARDIOGRAPHY

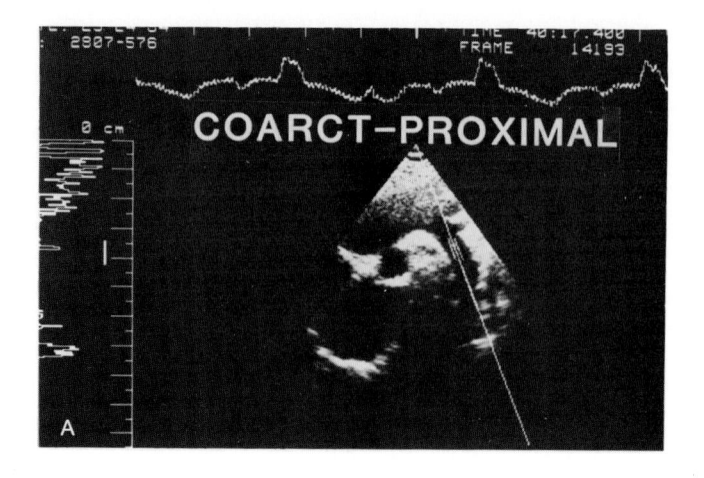

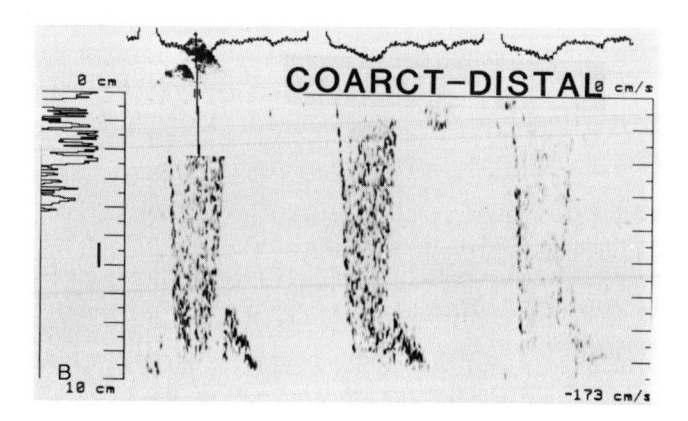

FIG. 9.5. Aortic velocities in a patient who had surgically repaired coarctation of the aorta. (A) Sample volume location in the descending aorta proximal to the repair. Velocities here were 2.2 m/sec. (B) Distal to the repair the signal aliased as shown. (C) Continuous wave Doppler velocities of 2.6 m/sec are shown. If the distal velocities were used alone in the equation, a pressure drop of 27 mmHg would be predicted. However, when V_1 is taken into account, the gradient is negligible.

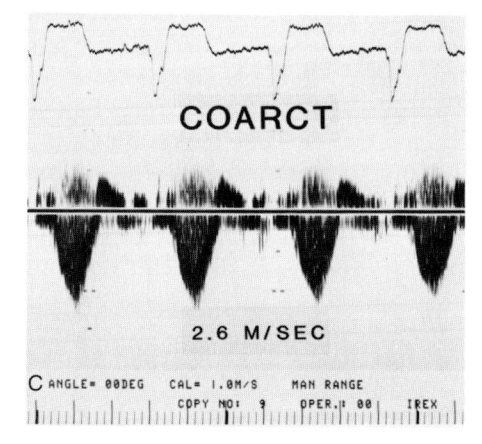

Gradient = $4(V_2^2 - V_1^2) = 4(6.76 - 4.84) = 8$ mmHg

This was confirmed at cardiac catheterization which was performed to evaluate other intracardiac abnormalities.

ECHOCARDIOGRAPHY IN PEDIATRIC CARDIOLOGY   169

FIG. 9.6. Noninvasive prediction of pulmonary artery pressure in a patient with ventricular septal defect. Arm blood pressure was 90 mmHg. No aortic stenosis was evident with aortic velocities of 90 cm/sec. Fig. A shows location of the sample volume in the right ventricle across the ventricular septal defect. Fig. B shows trans-VSD velocities at 3 m/sec measured by high pulsed repetition frequency Doppler which was confirmed by continuous wave Doppler. Therefore, trans-VSD gradient = 36 mmHg. Thus, AOP = LVP = 90 mmHg. RVP = LVP − ΔP = 90 − 36 = 54 mmHg. Fig. C shows pulmonary velocities measured by high-pulsed repetition frequency Doppler at 1.8 m/sec. Note that the time to peak velocity is accelerated at 90 m/sec, consistent with mild pulmonary hypertension. Therefore, ΔP = 14 mmHg, PAP = RVP − ΔP = 54 − 14 = 40 mmHg, at cath PAP = 45 mmHg at the same aortic pressure. Abbreviations: VSD = ventricular septal defect; HPRF = high pulsed repetition frequency Doppler; PA = pulmonary artery; TPV = time to peak velocity = acceleration time.

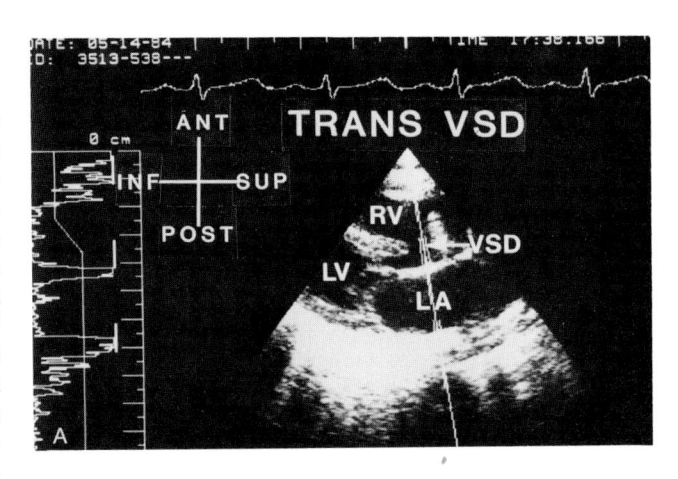

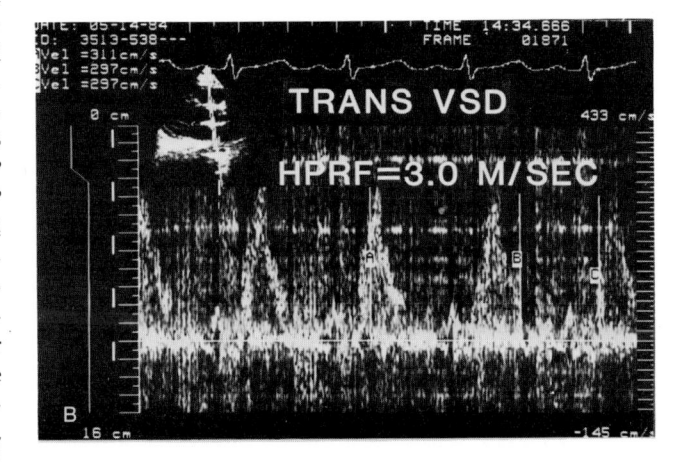

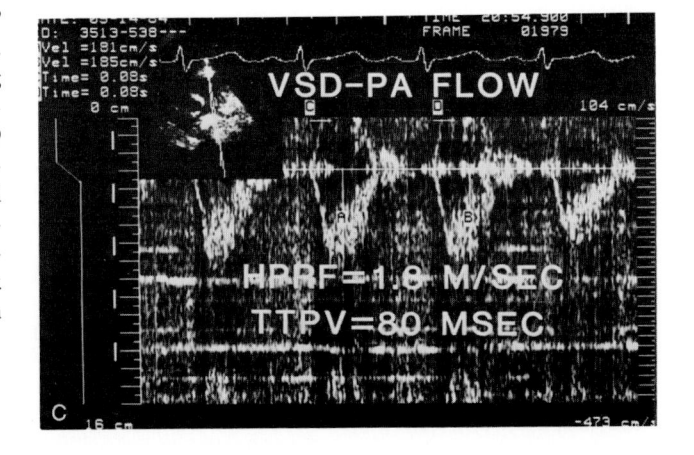

relationship existed between the peak velocity across a stenotic valve and valve area. The formula, which was mathematically derived, is valve area equals stroke volume in cubic centimeters divided by $0.88 \times V_2 \times VET$, where ventricular ejection time (VET) is measured from the velocity curve in seconds, V_2 is peak Doppler velocities in centimeters per second, and 0.88 is a constant for the aortic and pulmonary valves which takes into account fluid column height, gravity acceleration, and blood viscosity.

Cardiac output can be derived either from invasive techniques, such as thermodilution cardiac output measured in the intensive care unit, or it can be measured by Doppler echocardiography as described above. Assuming that no shunts exist, a site separate from the area of involvement must be used.

When Kosturakis et al. compared valve areas obtained from Doppler-derived data and catheterization-derived data in patients with aortic and pulmonic valve stenosis, a close correlation was determined. Subsequently, we have found that the prediction of valve area by this technique continues to be valid.

SUMMARY

Doppler echocardiography is an integral part of the pediatric cardiologist's armamentarium. It has advantages of being noninvasive, safe, and can be used serially. Qualitative assessment of the origin of organic murmurs is possible. Blood flow can be measured, allowing calculation of cardiac output, pulmonary artery-to-systemic artery flow ratios, and regurgitant fractions. Pressures can be estimated either directly or inferentially, and stenotic pulmonary or aortic valve areas can be predicted. Doppler echocardiography is a complement to the entire evaluation of a patient with congenital heart disease and should not be approached in isolation. When the test is performed carefully, data are valid and in some cases may replace cardiac catheterization. Future applications of quantitative Doppler should be of great value for the care of patients with congenital heart disease.

REFERENCES

1. Goldberg SJ, Allen HD, Marx GR, Flinn CJ: Doppler echocardiography. Philadelphia, Lea and Febiger, 1984
2. Hatle L, Angelsen B: Doppler Ultrasound in Cardiology. Physical Principles and Clinical Applications. Lea & Febiger, Philadelphia, 1982
3. Goldberg SJ: A review of pediatric Doppler echocardiography. Am J Dis Child, 138:1003, 1984
4. Stevenson JG, Kawabori I: Sequential 2D Echo/Doppler: Improved noninvasive diagnosis of atrial septal defect. Circulation, abstr., 68(3):110, 1983
5. Stevenson JG, Kawabori I, Dooley T, Guntheroth WG: Diagnosis of ventricular septal defect by pulsed Doppler echocardiography. Sensitivity, specificity, and limitations. Circulation 58:322, 1978
6. Allen HD, Goldberg SJ, Valdes-Cruz LM, Sahn DJ: Use of echocardiography in newborns with patent ductus arteriosus: A review. Pediatr Cardiol 3:65, 1982

7. Stevenson JG, Kawabori I, Guntheroth WG: Pulsed Doppler echocardiographic evaluation of the cyanotic newborn: Identification of the pulmonary artery in transposition of the great vessels. Am J Cardiol 46:849, 1980
8. Allen HD, Sahn DJ, Lange L, Goldberg SJ: Noninvasive assessment of surgical systemic-to-pulmonary artery shunts by range-gated pulsed Doppler echocardiography. J Pediatr 94:395, 1979
9. Meijboom E, Valdes-Cruz LM, Sahn DJ, Horowitz S, Scagnelli S, Larson D, Allen HD: Echo Doppler method for calculating volume flow across the tricuspid valve: Validation in an open chest canine model and initial clinical studies. Circulation abstr., 68(2):232, 1982
10. Goldberg SJ, Sahn DJ, Allen HD, Valdes-Cruz LM, Hoenecke H, Carnahan Y: Evaluation of pulmonary and systemic blood flow by two-dimensional Doppler echocardiography using fast Fourier transform spectral analysis. Am J Cardiol 50:1394, 1982
11. Magnin PA, Stewart JA, Myers S, von Ramm O, Kisslo JA: Combined Doppler and phased array echocardiographic estimation of cardiac output. Circulation 63:388, 1981
12. Fisher DC, Sahn DJ, Friedman MJ, Larson D, Valdes-Cruz LM, Horowitz S, Goldberg SJ, Allen HD: The mitral valve orifice method for noninvasive two-dimensional echo Doppler determination of cardiac output. Circulation 67:872, 1983
13. Loeber CP, Goldberg SJ, Allen HD: Doppler echocardiographic comparison of flows distal to the four cardiac valves. J Am Coll Cardiol 4:268, 1984
14. Sanders SP, Yeager S, Williams RG: Measurement of systemic and pulmonary blood flow and QP:QS ratio using Doppler and two-dimensional echocardiography. Am J Cardiol 51:952, 1983
15. Marx GR, Allen HD, Goldberg SJ, Flinn CJ: Transatrial septal velocity measurement by Doppler echocardiography in atrial septal defect: Correlation with QP: QS ratio. Am J Cardiol 55:1162, 1985
16. Goldberg SJ, Allen HD: Quantitative measurement of semilunar insufficiency by Doppler echo with an internal accuracy check. Circulation abstr., 68(3):260, 1983
17. Lima CO, Sahn DJ, Valdes-Cruz LM, Goldberg SJ, Barron JV, Allen HD, Grenadier E: Noninvasive prediction of transvalvular pressure gradient in patients with pulmonary stenosis by quantitative two-dimensional echocardiographic Doppler studies. Circulation 67:866, 1983
18. Johnson GL, Kwan OL, Handshoe S, Noonan JA, DeMaria AN: Accuracy of combined two-dimensional echocardiography and continuous wave Doppler recordings in the estimation of pressure gradient in right ventricular outlet obstruction. J Am Coll Cardiol 3:1013, 1984
19. Kosturakis D, Allen HD, Goldberg SJ, Sahn DJ, Valdes-Cruz LM: Noninvasive quantification of pulmonary arterial hypertension in congenital heart disease. Am J Cardiol 53:1110, 1984

10 Pulsed Doppler Analysis of Human Fetal Blood Flow

CHARLES S. KLEINMAN
ELLEN M. WEINSTEIN
JOSHUA A. COPEL

Echocardiographic imaging techniques have been applied successfully for the diagnosis of structural heart disease in the second- and third-trimester human fetus.[1-3] These studies have also provided structural information that has increased our understanding of normal fetal cardiac development, and have furthered our concepts of the pathophysiology of congenital heart disease.

The application of pulsed Doppler technology for examination of the fetal cardiovascular system offers the promise of increasing our understanding of fetal cardiovascular development, by providing information concerning directional blood flow, as well as estimates of volume flow within the fetus.

It is the purpose of this report to review the experience that has been amassed in the application of pulsed Doppler technology for the analysis of blood flow within the human fetus.

QUANTITATIVE ANALYSIS OF FETAL BLOOD FLOW

Several workers have reported their experience with the application of the pulsed Doppler modality for quantitation of flow within the umbilical circulation.[4-8] Eik-Nes et al.[4,5] have utilized a linear-array imaging system with an off-line pulsed Doppler transducer that ensures accurate measurement of the angle of incidence between the ultrasound beam and the vector of blood flow within the fetal umbilical vessels. The linear-array device may thus be used to image the blood vessel at a right angle, allowing the vessel to be measured using the axial resolution of the imaging system, whereas the Doppler incident angle is fixed below 60°, keeping error inherent in inaccurate measurement of angle of insonation at a minimum. Using this equipment, these workers have reported reproducible measurements of volume flow in the umbilical vein and artery within the physiological range, predicted on the basis of previous reports of fetal lamb blood flow studies and the relatively sparse data available from studies of human abortuses. This linear-array equipment has been useful for estimation of descending aortic and umbilical arterial and venous blood flow, but is unwieldy when applied to measurement of volume flow within the central circulation. Using mechanical scanning devices with in-line pulsed Doppler transducers, it is possible to accurately locate the Doppler sample volume within the central circulation; however, the Doppler beam is then parallel to the imaging beam making it necessary to choose between ideal imaging angle (90°) and an ideal angle for Doppler insonation (less than 60°). Sahn[9] has documented preliminary evidence, derived from studies with mechanical duplex scanning devices, that suggests that transtricuspid valve flow exceeds transmitral valve flow, with a right ventricular/left ventricular flow ratio of 55:45.[9] These findings suggest, as predicted on the basis of fetal lamb flow studies, that the fetal right ventricle is relatively volume-loaded in utero, but that the disparity between the two ventricles in the human fetus is less marked than that in the fetal lamb (where it approximates 2:1). This is due, in large part, to the proportionately larger cerebral blood flow in the human fetus. The substantial error that may be introduced by small errors in measurement of flow orifice and/or insonation angle may account for a large variation in flow calculation, making such measurements only rough estimates of regional blood flow.

QUALITATIVE ANALYSIS OF BLOOD FLOW

We have focused our attention on the qualitative analysis of blood flow within the central circulation.

Normal Blood Flow Patterns

Using pulsed Doppler assessment of directional blood flow, we have been able to characterize normal flow patterns within the fetal cardiovascular system, and to analyze directional flow within the shunt pathways that are unique to fetal cardiovascular physiology.

Venous flow profiles, obtained within the fetal venae cavae and pulmonary veins, show characteristic unidirectional flow toward the fetal atria (Fig. 10.1). Alterations in flow velocity, attending atrial and ventricular contraction as well as rapid ventricular filling periods, are reflected.

Transatrioventricular valve flow profiles are easily obtained within the ventricular inflow tracts, on either side of the mitral or tricuspid valve mechanism. Biphasic flow profiles are obtained. Normally the biphasic flow suggests dominance of the secondary peak (Fig. 10.2). This pattern suggests that active ventricular filling, associated with atrial contraction, makes the major contribution to ventricular filling—a pattern seen postnatally in ventricular hypertrophy,[10] suggesting decreased ventricular compliance. Romero et al.[11] have previously

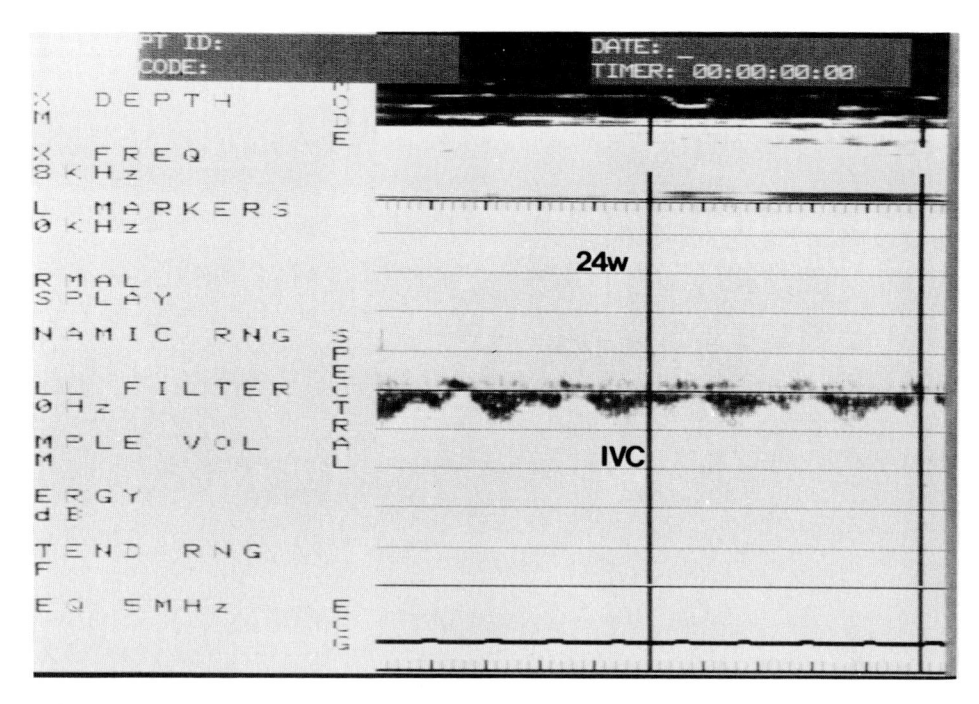

FIG. 10.1. Doppler wave form generated with the sample volume located in the inferior vena cava of a 24-week fetus. Phasic flow in the great veins reflects changes in velocity and direction of flow accompanying atrial and ventricular contraction. Flow is unidirectional, toward the fetal right atrium (in this case below the baseline, away from the source of ultrasound).

FIG. 10.2. Doppler wave form generated with the sample volume in the right ventricular (RV) inflow tract of a midtrimester fetus. Transatrioventricular valve flow is biphasic. The secondary (*a*) peak dominates in utero. This suggests that active ventricular filling, associated with atrial contraction, makes the major contribution to ventricular filling. This pattern is seen postnatally when there is decreased ventricular compliance. (RA = right atrium)

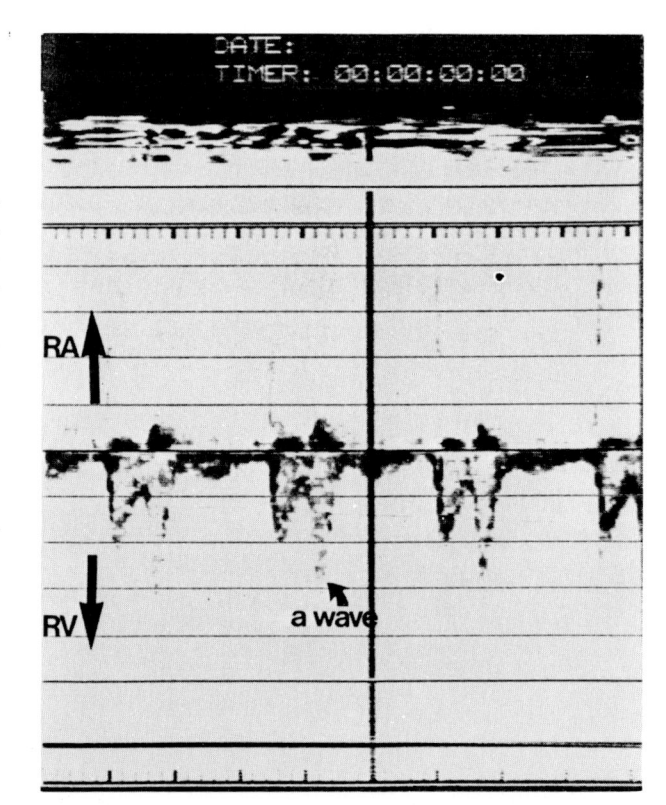

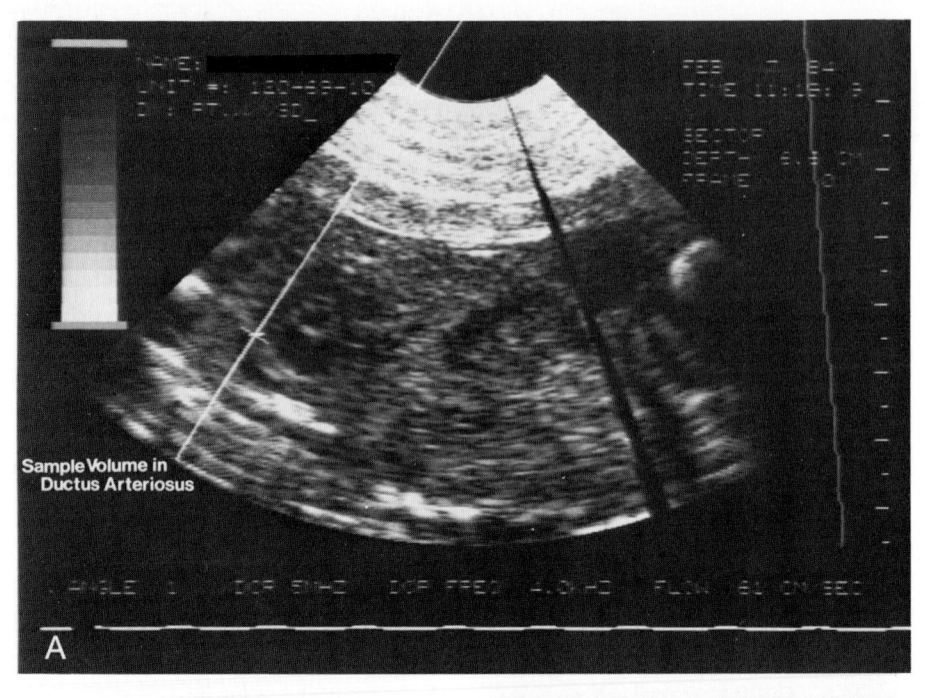

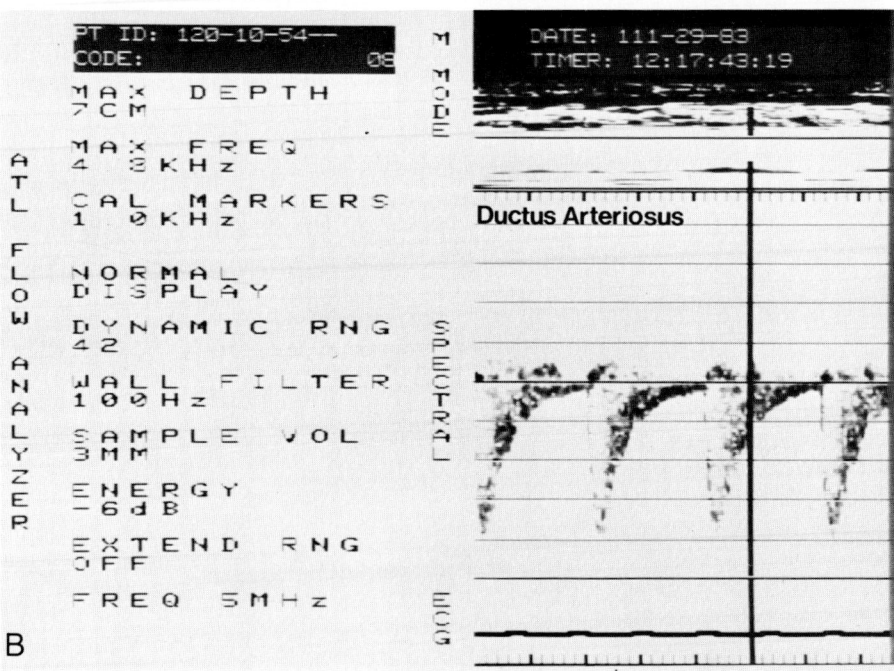

FIG. 10.3. (A) Two-dimensional scan showing sample volume within the fetal ductus arteriosus. The ductus arteriosus is continuous with the fetal descending aorta. (B) Doppler wave form generated in the fetal ductus arteriosus. Fetal ductal flow is from the main pulmonary artery into the descending aorta.

shown that fetal myocardium is less compliant than neonatal and adult myocardium, due to a relative abundance of fibrous tissue between fetal myocytes. The Doppler flow-velocity profile of ventricular filling in the human fetus therefore fits the pattern that would have been predicted based on these studies in the lamb.

Flow profiles in the supravalvar region of the ventricular inflow tracts normally fail to demonstrate evidence of atrioventricular regurgitation. The biphasic pattern of ventricular filling is seen again, with the secondary peak predominating.

Ventricular outflow tract flow is similar to that seen postnatally, with no evidence of semilunar valve regurgitation during diastole.

Arterial flow patterns in the fetus are unique, due to the presence of the ductal shunt. Laminar systolic flow is detected both in the main pulmonary trunk and in the ascending aorta. The ductus arteriosus is easily visualized, and flow is from the main pulmonary trunk into the descending aorta (Fig. 10.3). Both ductus arteriosus and descending aorta demonstrate continuous antegrade diastolic flow into the low-impedance descending aortic-placental vascular bed. This antegrade diastolic flow becomes more prominent as the sample volume is placed further distally into the descending aorta and umbilical arterial system, where Doppler wave forms suggest parabolic flow profiles (Fig. 10.4).

Within the fetal atrial cavities continuous flow from right to left atrium, across the foramen ovale, is seen. When the sample volume is in the left atrium, a high-frequency clicking sound secondary to the phasic motion of the flap-valve mechanism of the foramen ovale may be heard.

Abnormal Flow Patterns

Rudolph[12] has described the pathophysiological impact of a variety of different congenital cardiac abnormalities upon fetal cardiovascular flow pathways. Using pulsed Doppler flow analysis, a number of laboratories have been successful in detecting abnormalities of fetal blood flow which, when added to two-dimensional imaging studies and interpreted in light of Rudolph's concepts of cardiovascular development, have increased the diagnostic accuracy of these techniques and have increased our understanding of the pathogenesis of congenital heart disease.

Using pulsed Doppler analysis we have detected atrioventricular valve regurgitation in a fetus with Ebstein's malformation of the tricuspid valve, whose two-dimensional scan had suggested right atrial enlargement and only a minimal amount of apical displacement of the tricuspid valve apparatus (Fig. 10.5).

Doppler analysis allowed us to detect antegrade pulmonary blood flow into the main pulmonary artery in a fetus in whom a diagnosis of atrial isomerism with obstructed pulmonary outflow was noted (Fig. 10.6). Two-dimensional scan had, incorrectly, suggested the diagnosis of pulmonary atresia.

Bierman et al.[13] have described the use of pulsed Doppler technique for the detection of retrograde flow within the fetal descending aorta in a fetus

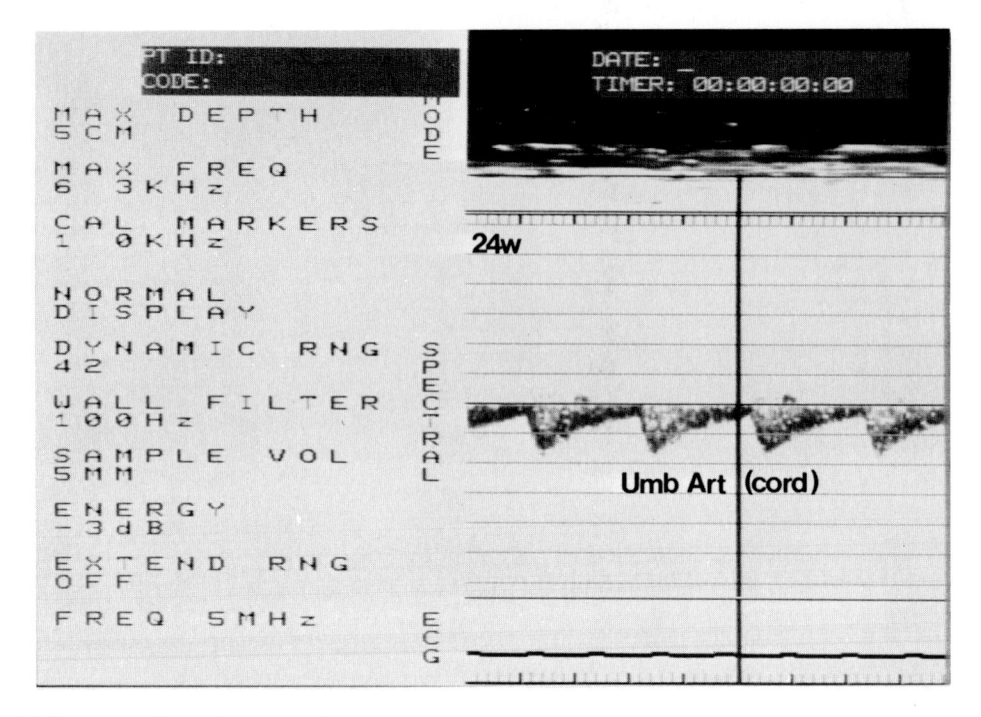

FIG. 10.4. Doppler wave form generated from the fetal umbilical artery within the umbilical cord of a 24-week fetus. The spectral pattern in the umbilical artery suggests that the wavefront of blood flow within the umbilical artery is parabolic. Flow is away from the source of ultrasound. There is continuous antegrade diastolic flood flow, suggesting low impedance to flow within the placenta.

subsequently diagnosed to have severe aortic regurgitation secondary to an absent aortic valve mechanism.

Silverman et al.[14] have reported the use of range-gated pulsed Doppler flow analysis for the evaluation of flow into the hypoplastic ascending aorta of a patient with mitral-aortic atresia and hypoplastic left heart syndrome.

Redel and Hansmann[15] have described a fetus with upper body edema in whom pulsed Doppler study documented premature closure of the foramen ovale.

As pulsed Doppler flow studies are applied with greater frequency, it is likely that abnormal flow patterns will be described in a wide variety of congenital heart diseases.

Nonimmune Hydrops Fetalis

Our observations of fetal cardiac anatomy have led us to consider nonimmune hydrops fetalis to be a manifestation of end-stage fetal heart failure,[16] with systemic venous hypertension the "common denominator." In some cases, we speculated that atrioventricular valve regurgitation could have resulted in ve-

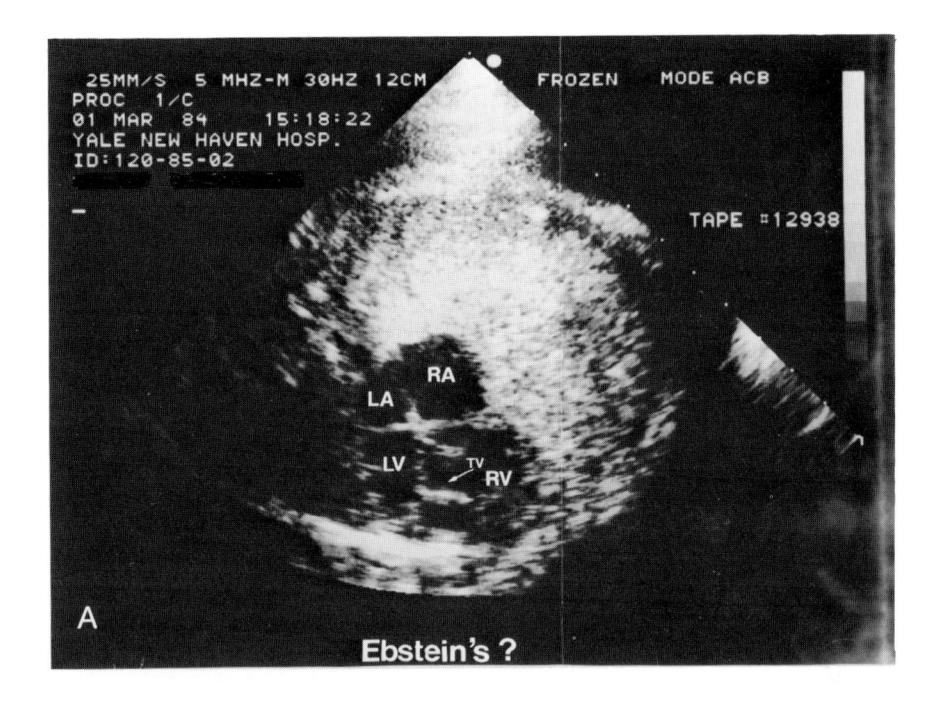

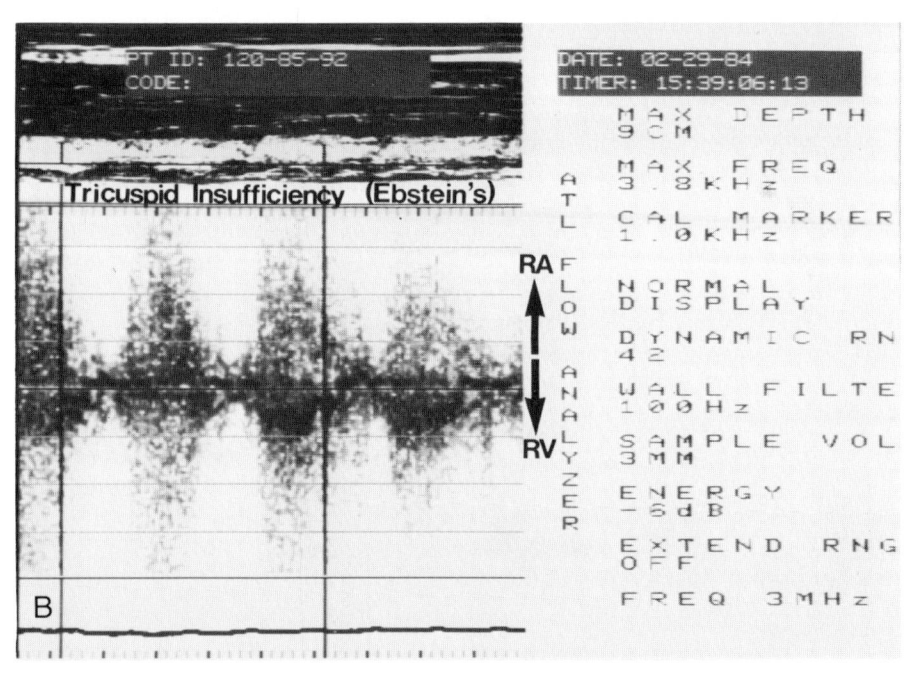

FIG. 10.5. (A) Two-dimensional four-chamber view of the heart of a 34-week fetus of a mother who ingested lithium salts throughout pregnancy. Right atrial enlargement and moderate apical displacement of the tricuspid valve apparatus suggested Ebstein's malformation (LA = left atrium; LV = left ventricle; RA = right atrium; RV = right ventricle). (B) Doppler wave form recorded in the same fetus, with the sample volume within the right atrium. Holosystolic tricuspid regurgitation is detected.

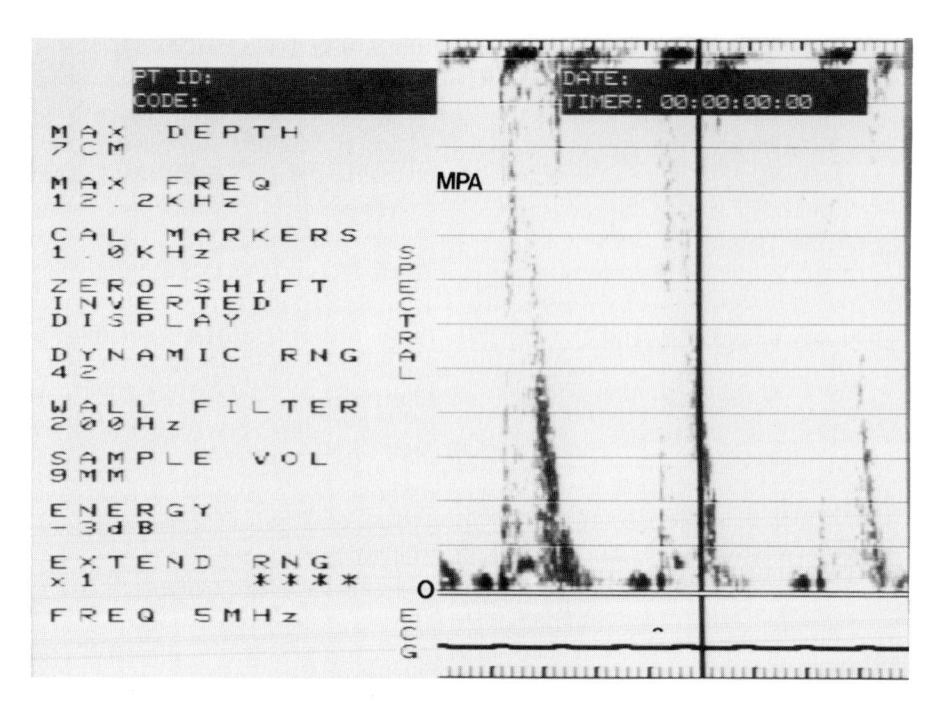

FIG. 10.6. Doppler wave form recorded with the sample volume in the main pulmonary artery of a 34-week fetus with atrial isomerism and pulmonary outflow tract obstruction. Antegrade pulmonary arterial flow (above the 0 baseline) is detected, ruling out the possibility of pulmonary atresia.

nous hypertension. We have recently encountered two cases in whom pulsed Doppler study was invaluable. A 31-week hydropic fetus with complete atrioventricular septal defect was noted to have mitral regurgitation into the right atrium, and a 34-week hydropic fetus with endocardial fibroelastosis was noted to have mitral regurgitation into the left atrium in utero.

We have been impressed that many of the hydropic fetuses that we have encountered with primary cardiovascular explanations for fetal edema (e.g., fetuses with sustained tachyarrhythmias) have vigorously contracting ventricles that do not appear to manifest systolic pump failure. We believe that these fetuses have abnormalities of diastolic filling of the noncompliant fetal ventricles, resulting in systemic venous hypertension. Pulsed Doppler analysis of ventricular filling has increased our insight into the diastolic events in the fetal heart.

PULSED DOPPLER ANALYSIS OF FETAL CARDIAC ARRHYTHMIAS

During the past several years an increasing amount of attention has been paid to the analysis of disturbances of fetal cardiac rhythm.[17] In the absence of a reliable means of recording the fetal electrocardiographic signal, most investigators have relied upon two-dimensional and M-mode echocardiography to relate cardiac motion against time to the underlying electromechanical events. The application of this information for the development of rational treatment protocols for sustained arrhythmias has increased the need for accuracy in the assessment of fetal cardiac rhythm disturbances. Using the pulsed Doppler technique, we have analyzed transatrioventricular valve flow. Atrial extrasystoles result in extra peaks of transvalve flow into the fetal ventricle (Fig. 10.7). The effects of fetal arrhythmias on arterial blood flow may also be analyzed using pulsed Doppler examination. Isolated extrasystoles may be associated with diminished arterial stroke volume, as reflected in decreased peak flow velocity and decreased area under the flow-velocity curve. Similarly, the first postextrasystolic beat can be demonstrated, using similar criteria, to be potentiated (Fig. 10.8).

With the Doppler sample volume located in the left ventricle at the junction of the inflow and outflow tracts, it is possible to time systolic and diastolic flow phenomena within the fetal heart. This technique has been especially helpful in analyzing rhythm disturbances associated with various degrees of atrioventricular block. The effects of sustained arrhythmias, such as supraventricular tachycardia, on arterial blood flow (decreased stroke volume), ventricular filling characteristics, and venous flow (retrograde inferior vena caval blood flow) (Fig. 10.9) may be analyzed using pulsed Doppler flow analysis. The effects of in utero treatment on heart rate as well as on vascular flow characteristics may be monitored using these techniques.

INTRAUTERINE GROWTH RETARDATION

Griffin et al.[18] have recently reported their observations of altered fetoplacental flow characteristics in pregnancies with growth-retarded fetuses. Normal arterial blood flow wave forms within the fetal descending aortic and umbilical arterial beds characteristically show marked forward flow throughout diastole, implying a continuous arterial "runoff" into the relatively low-impedance placental bed. Similarly, vigorous atrioventricular (AV) fistulalike continuous antegrade blood flow may be detected within the normal maternal uterine-arcuate arterial bed. In cases of intrauterine growth retardation, associated with placental insufficiency, decreased diastolic runoff into the placental circulation suggestive of elevated placental vascular resistance may be detected using pulsed Doppler flow analysis. Griffin et al. have been quite successful in characterizing normal fetoplacental blood flow patterns and have used these techniques to identify fetuses at risk due to critically decreased uterine blood flow. We have found similarly altered fetoplacental flow patterns in growth-retarded fetuses and have recently encountered a severely growth-retarded fetus, with a calcific placenta, in whom retrograde diastolic flow within the umbilical artery and descending aorta were noted (Fig. 10.10). This fetus was found to have retrograde diastolic flow in both the ascending aorta and the main pulmonary artery, and was found to have semilunar valve regurgitation. These data have furthered our understanding of the profound effect that increased placental vascular resistance has upon fetal cardiovascular function, and offer the promise of providing diagnostically important information which may be used to identify the fetus who requires emergent delivery.

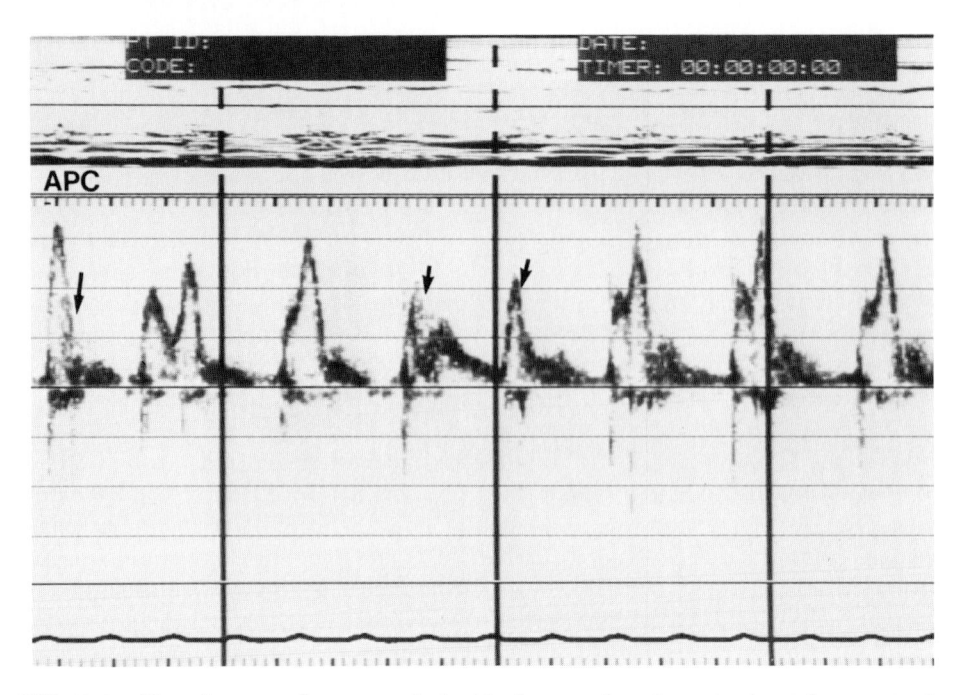

FIG. 10.7. Doppler wave form recorded with the sample volume in the right ventricular inflow tract. Transtricuspid flow into the right ventricle is detected as a deflection above the baseline. Atrial extrasystoles result in the early appearance of transvalvar flow (arrows) peaks on the wave form.

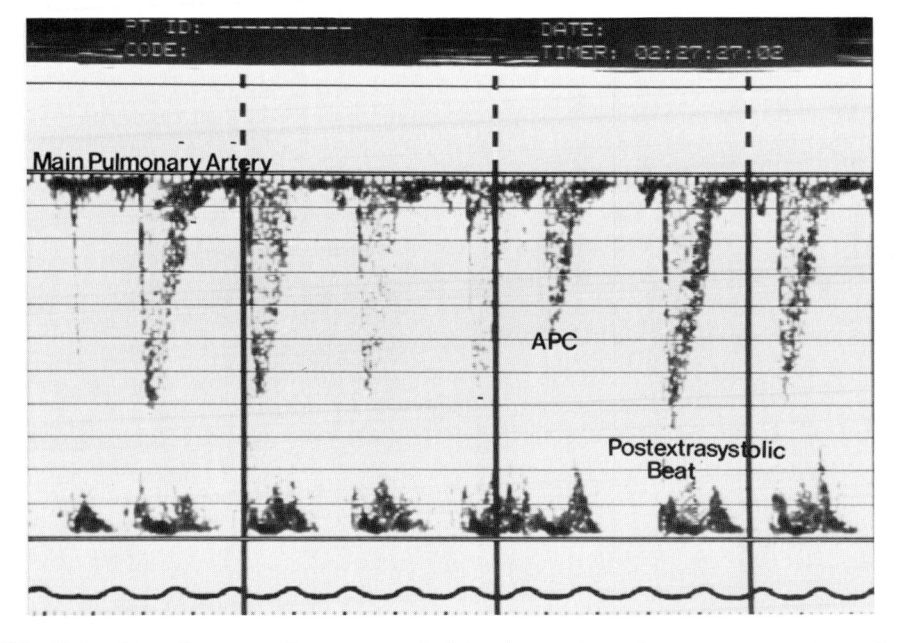

FIG. 10.8. Doppler wave forms recorded in the main pulmonary artery in a fetus having occasional spontaneous atrial extrasystoles (APC). Flow is away from the source of ultrasound. The wave form of the first postextrasystolic beat suggests potentiation, as reflected by increased flow velocity (amplitude) and flow volume (proportional to the area subtended by the wave form).

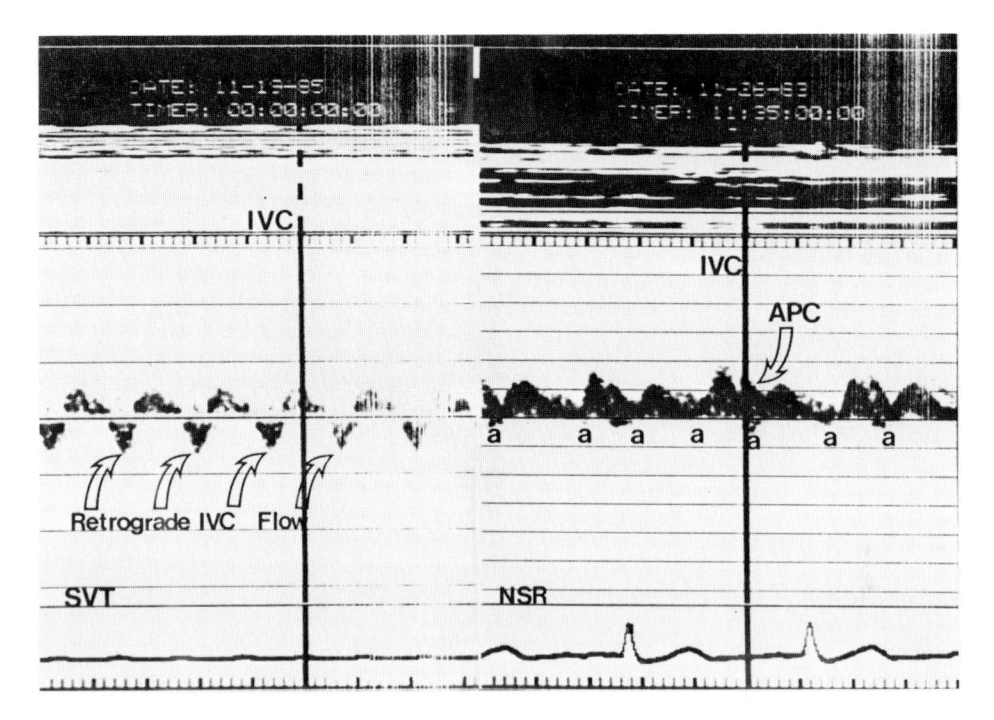

FIG. 10.9. Doppler wave forms recorded with sample volume within the fetal inferior vena cava (IVC). In the left-hand panel the fetus was in supraventricular tachycardia (SVT). Retrograde flow down the vena cava is seen (arrows). Immediately after conversion to normal sinus rhythm (NSR) (right-hand panel) unidirectional flow, toward the right atrium, is seen. An atrial extrasystole (APC) causes an alteration in phasic flow within the vena cava (ECG is the maternal signal).

SUMMARY

In summary, pulsed Doppler flow analysis of fetoplacental circulation may provide important insights into normal fetal cardiovascular development. Qualitative analysis of directional blood flow may provide an increased understanding of normal fetal shunt pathways, as well as an enhanced appreciation of the alterations in fetal blood flow that may be associated with structural or rhythm abnormalities of the fetal heart. The Doppler wave form may also provide information of use in evaluating arterial impedance and ventricular filling characteristics, and may be used to assess the effects of various environmental factors, including transplacentally administered medications on the fetal cardiovascular system. The combined use of two-dimensional imaging techniques and quantitative evaluation of the Doppler flow-velocity wave form offers the promise of providing a means of analyzing regional blood flow distribution within the fetus. These quantitative data may ultimately prove to be a most valuable means of assessing the integrity of the fetal circulation, as well as the fetal response to in utero therapy.

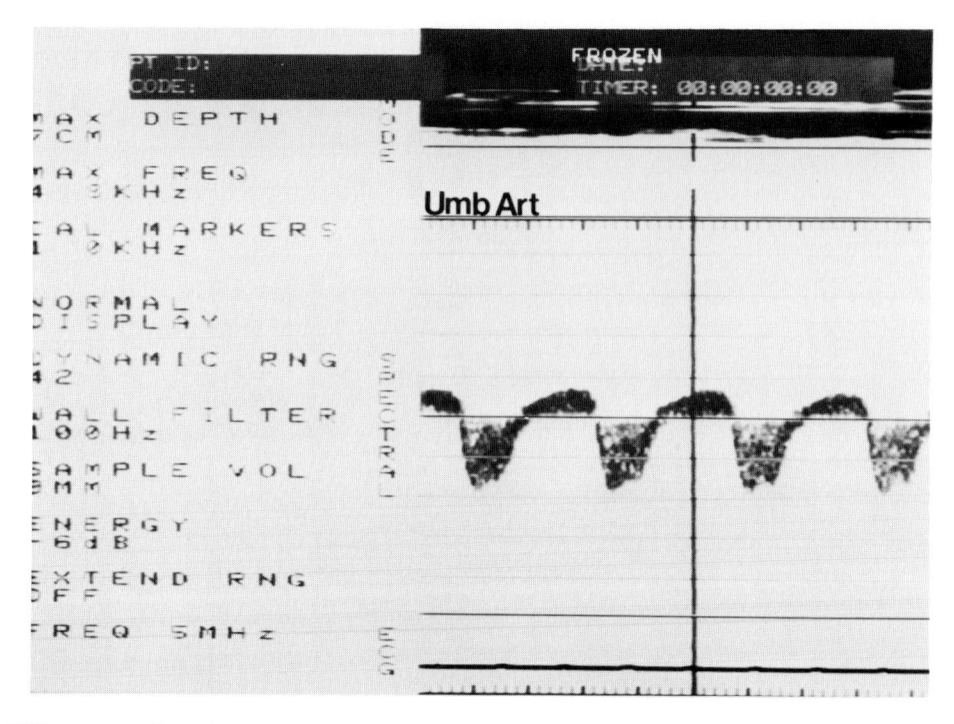

FIG. 10.10. Doppler wave form within the umbilical artery of a severely growth-retarded 37-week fetus. Retrograde diastolic flow (above the baseline) was recognized. This fetus had retrograde flow within the descending aorta and had both aortic and pulmonary valve insufficiency. The placenta was severely fibrotic and calcified.

ACKNOWLEDGMENT

This work supported by Clinical Research grant 6-225 from the March of Dimes Birth Defects Foundation, White Plains, New York.

REFERENCES

1. Kleinman CS, Santulli TV Jr: Ultrasonic evaluation of the fetal human heart. Sem Perinatol 7:90, 1983
2. Allan LD, Tynan M, Campbell S, Anderson RH: Identification of congenital cardiac malformations by echocardiography in midtrimester fetus. Br Heart J 46:358, 1981
3. Sahn DJ, Lange LW, Allen HD, Goldberg SJ, Anderson C, Giles H, Haber K: Quantitative real-time cross-sectional echocardiography in the developing normal human fetus and newborn. Circulation 62:588, 1980
4. Eik-Nes SH, Brubakk HO, Ulstein MK: Measurement of human fetal blood flow. Lancet 1:283, 1980
5. Eik-Nes, SH, Marsal K, Brubakk HO, Kristofferson K, Ulstein M: Ultrasound measurement of human fetal blood flow. J Biomed Eng 4:28, 1982

6. Gill RW, Trudinger BJ, Garrett WJ, Kossoff G, Warren PS: Fetal umbilical venous blood flow measured in utero by pulsed Doppler and B-mode ultrasound. Am J Obstet Gynecol 139:720, 1981
7. Fitzgerald DE, Drumm JE: Non-invasive measurement of the fetal circulation using ultrasound: A new method. Br Med J 2:1450, 1977
8. Campbell S, Diaz-Ricasens J, Griffin DR, Cohen-Overbeck TE, Pearce JM, Willson K, Teague MJ: New Doppler technique for assessing uteroplacental blood flow. Lancet 1:675, 1983
9. Sahn DJ: Personal communication. November 1984
10. Hatle L, Angelsen B: Doppler Ultrasound in Cardiology. Lea and Febiger, Philadelphia, 1982
11. Romero T, Covell J, Friedman WF: A comparison of the pressure-volume relations of the fetal, newborn, and adult heart. Am J Physiol 222:1285, 1972
12. Rudolph AM: Congenital Diseases of the Heart. Yearbook, Chicago, 1974
13. Bierman FZ, Yeh M-N, Swersky S, Martin E, Wigger JH, Fox H: Absence of the aortic valve: Antenatal and postnatal two-dimensional and Doppler echocardiographic features. J Am Coll Cardiol 3:833, 1984
14. Silverman, NH, Enderlein MA, Golbus MS: Ultrasonic recognition of aortic valve atresia in utero. Am J Cardiol 53:391, 1984
15. Redel DA, Hansmann M: Fetal obstruction of the foramen ovale detected by two-dimensional Doppler echocardiography. In Rijsterborgh H (ed): Echocardiology. Martinus Nijhoff, The Hague, 1981
16. Kleinman CS, Donnerstein RL, DeVore GR, Jaffe CC, Lynch DC, Berkowitz RL, Talner NS, Hobbins JC: Fetal echocardiography for evaluation of in utero congestive heart failure: A technique for study of nonimmune fetal hydrops. N Engl J Med 306:568, 1982
17. Kleinman CS, Donnerstein RL, Jaffe CC, DeVore GR, Weinstein EM, Lynch DC, Talner NS, Berkowitz RL, Hobbins JC: Fetal echocardiography, A tool for evaluation of in utero cardiac arrhythmias and monitoring of in utero therapy: Analysis of 71 patients. Am J Cardiol 51:237, 1983
18. Griffin D, Cohen-Overbeek T, Campbell S.: Fetal and utero-placental blood flow. Clin Obst Gynecol 10:565, 1983

11 Patient-Exposure Data for Doppler Ultrasound

HAROLD F. STEWART
PETER X. SILVIS
STEPHEN W. SMITH

In recent years ultrasound imaging and Doppler blood flow measurements have become important tools for use in diagnostic medicine. Commercial pulse-echo imaging equipment was first introduced into commerce in 1963.[1] The first commercial continuous wave Doppler unit was introduced to the marketplace in 1966. As equipment improved and applications developed, the industry experienced rapid growth in the 1970s. One of the more recent growth areas in the application of diagnostic ultrasound has been the use of pulsed Doppler equipment for cardiac applications. Prior to 1976, some continuous wave Doppler ultrasound was used for cardiovascular diagnosis. However, only a single manufacturer marketed a pulsed Doppler clinical instrument for cardiac or peripheral vascular diagnosis. Currently, many continuous wave and pulsed Doppler instruments are commercially available for both peripheral vascular and cardiac diagnosis.

This chapter will (1) briefly review current safety guidelines, regulations, and recommendations for diagnostic ultrasound; (2) discuss the patient-exposure intensities associated with Doppler ultrasound medical equipment and compare these levels of exposure with intensities from other medical ultrasound devices; and (3) consider some of the current information as it relates to the safety of diagnostic ultrasound.

EXISTING GUIDES, REGULATIONS, AND RECOMMENDATIONS

The need for information concerning patient-exposure levels associated with diagnostic ultrasound is widely recognized. For example, groups reviewing available ultrasound biological effects data such as the World Health

Organization[2] and the National Council on Radiation Protection and Measurements[3] have recently recognized and addressed this need. A joint effort by the American Institute of Ultrasound in Medicine (AIUM) and the National Electrical Manufacturers Association (NEMA) resulted in the development of a voluntary safety standard[4] for ultrasound equipment which provides definitions and measurement techniques for specifying the output from diagnostic ultrasound equipment. The Canadian government has published *Guidelines For the Safe Use of Ultrasound*,[5] which recommends that ultrasound exposure levels be made available to purchasers of equipment by labeling every ultrasound device. The desirability of making exposure levels generally available to users has also been recognized and encouraged by the AIUM Commendation Panel.[6]

In February of 1984, a consensus panel[7] cosponsored by the National Institutes of Health (NIH) and the Food and Drug Administration (FDA) reviewed the safety and efficacy of ultrasound imaging as it applies to obstetrical applications, and recommended that patient-exposure levels from the equipment be measured and reported to the user and that exposure information for imaging equipment and Doppler devices be recorded for each clinical examination.

Because of the fundamental importance of the knowledge of patient exposure levels in the evaluation of any potential risk of diagnostic ultrasound, manufacturers of medical ultrasound equipment are required to provide such information to the Food and Drug Administration. This is required by two different federal laws. The first is the Radiation Control for Health and Safety Act of 1968.[8] Under this legislation, diagnostic ultrasound manufacturers are required to provide ultrasound intensities and other equipment performance data to the FDA in their reports on new ultrasound products. In addition, under authority of the Medical Device Amendments[9] of 1976 to the Food, Drug, and Cosmetic Act, diagnostic ultrasound manufacturers are required to file information concerning exposure and other performance data in their premarket notifications of intent to market these devices. To aid manufacturers in providing this information, the FDA's Center for Devices and Radiological Health (CDRH) developed and published a diagnostic ultrasound reporting guide.[10] The guide was specifically written to aid manufacturers in the preparation of their submissions of diagnostic ultrasound equipment output intensities and other performance-related information to the FDA. It was prepared to be consistent, where possible, with the definitions used in the AIUM/NEMA *Safety Standard for Diagnostic Ultrasound Equipment.*[4]

EXPOSURE LEVELS FROM DOPPLER EQUIPMENT

This chapter reports patient-exposure data from commercial continuous wave and pulsed Doppler equipment. The data were submitted to the FDA by manufacturers between 1981 and 1984 for currently marketed equipment. Each manufacturer obtained the data by determining the ultrasound output intensities of his or her Doppler instrument in combination with each Doppler ultrasound transducer marketed for that particular model.

The capability of various manufacturers to provide these exposure data varies considerably. Therefore, the testing section of the FDA guide[10] requires that the procedures used in determining the ultrasonic output parameters submitted to the FDA be specified. This is of particular importance in that it provides a means of evaluating the reliability of the information provided. Experience has shown that only measured data rather than calculated values can be considered accurate. The accuracy of the information provided by each manufacturer is not known. However, data used for selection of transducers with output values within specified limits indicate that such data should be sufficiently reliable for a general comparison of the output levels from different equipment. For example, in measured output data for several hundred transducers of the same model coming off the production line, the 95 percent confidence interval was within about ±50 percent of the mean output value. This was prior to rejection of those transducers with output levels outside certain acceptable limits set by the manufacturer.

Exposure intensities reported by the manufacturers to the FDA include the spatial peak temporal average intensity (SPTA) for both continuous wave Doppler and pulsed Doppler equipment, and the spatial peak pulse average intensity (SPPA) for pulsed Doppler equipment. Fig. 11.1 and 11.2 illustrate the concept of these intensities. Figure 11.1 shows a focused Doppler ultrasound transducer which can emit a continuous wave ultrasound beam or a pulsed Doppler burst. The ultrasound spatial intensity distribution is sketched in the focal region of the transducer, and the spatial peak (SP) intensity is noted. Figure 11.2A is a graph of ultrasound intensity versus time for a continuous wave Doppler instrument. The time average exposure intensity is noted. Figure 11.2B is a graph of ultrasound intensity versus time for a pulsed Doppler burst, four cycles in length. The level of the ultrasound intensity time averaged (TA) over the interval between Doppler bursts (the pulse repetition period) is noted. The ultrasound intensity averaged over the burst length (pulse average, PA) is also noted.

The SPTA intensity is thus the maximum ultrasound intensity value in space averaged over time. This intensity is important in biological effects investigations, and it is the exposure parameter which characterizes ultrasound effects due to thermal mechanisms (i.e., heating). The SPPA intensity is the maximum ultrasound intensity in space averaged only while the Doppler burst is on. The SPPA intensity is often approximately 1,000 times higher than the SPTA intensity during its brief on time. This SPPA exposure parameter may be associated with biological effects arising from nonthermal mechanisms.

Patient-exposure levels reported to the FDA by manufacturers representing currently marketed continuous wave and pulsed Doppler equipment for peripheral vascular and cardiac diagnosis are summarized in Fig. 11.3–11.5. Figure 11.3 is a histogram of the manufacturers' reported values of SPTA exposure intensities for 20 different continuous wave (CW) Doppler devices in combination with the 37 transducers marketed with these instruments for cardiovascular application. Peripheral vascular (PV) transducers are noted by the clear areas. Cardiac or combination cardiac/PV units are denoted by cross-hatched areas in the histogram. The CW SPTA patient exposures range from less than 50

190 BASIC DOPPLER ECHOCARDIOGRAPHY

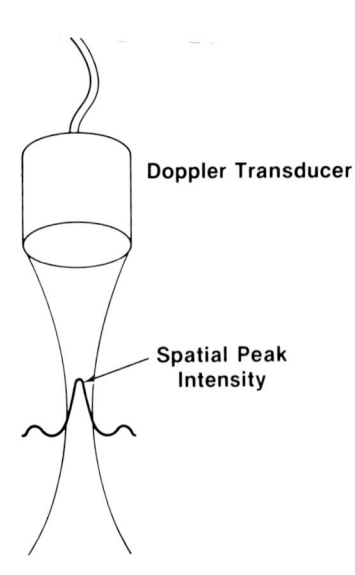

FIG. 11.1. Schematic of focused beam from Doppler transducer indicating location of spatial peak intensity.

mW/cm² to greater than 1,000 mW/cm². The median SPTA exposure is 160 mW/cm², and the mean is 255 mW/cm². As a reference point, the 100-mW/cm² level is noted in the figure. This is the level in the AIUM bioeffects statement discussed in this chapter under the section entitled "Safety Considerations." Note that many of the continuous wave Doppler instruments exceed the AIUM level.

Figure 11.4 is a histogram of the values of SPTA exposure intensities reported

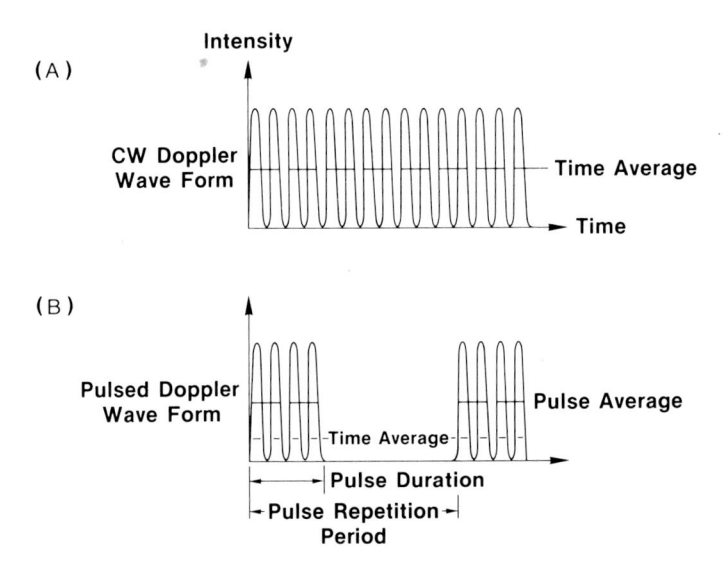

FIG. 11.2. Graph of intensity versus time for (A) CW Doppler and (B) pulsed Doppler indicating levels of time averaged intensity and pulse average intensity.

PATIENT-EXPOSURE DATA FOR ULTRASOUND   191

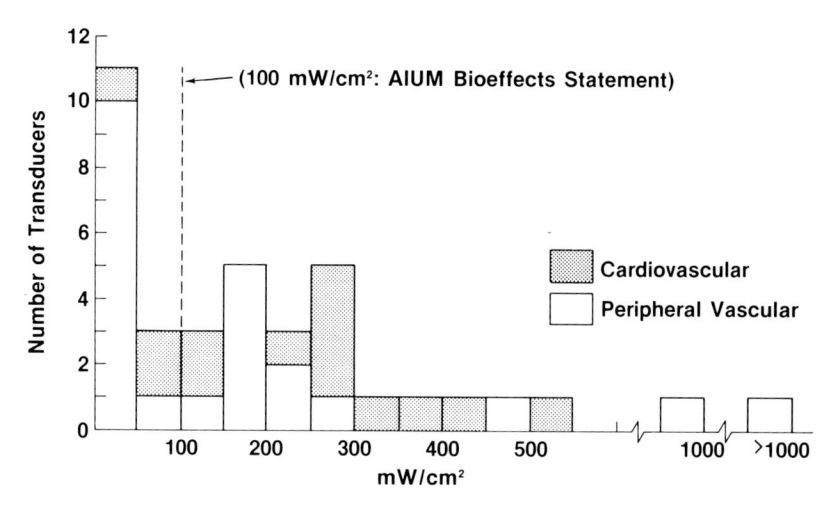

FIG. 11.3. Histogram of distribution of measured spatial peak temporal average intensities reported by manufacturers to the FDA for continuous wave Doppler devices.

by manufacturers to the FDA for 59 transducers used in 28 *pulsed* Doppler devices for cardiovascular applications. Again PV transducers are noted by the clear areas in the histogram. Cardiac or combination cardiac/PV units are denoted by cross-hatched areas. The pulsed Doppler SPTA patient exposures range from less than 100 mW/cm² to about 2,000 mW/cm². The median value of the histogram is 293 mW/cm², and the mean value is 553 mW/cm². For both the CW histogram and the pulsed Doppler histogram, the patient exposure varies over an order of magnitude from devices designed to perform the same function. Again the 100-mW/cm² value from the AIUM bioeffects statement

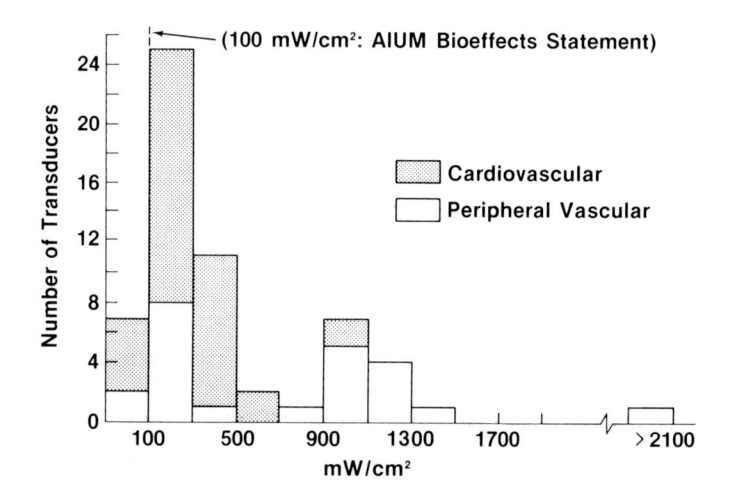

FIG. 11.4. Histogram of distribution of measured spatial peak temporal average intensities reported by manufacturers to the FDA for pulsed Doppler devices.

192 BASIC DOPPLER ECHOCARDIOGRAPHY

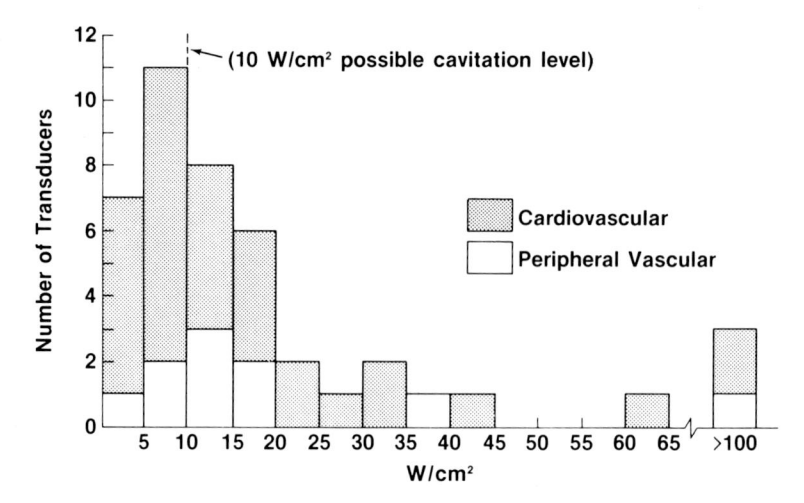

FIG. 11.5. Histogram of distribution of measured spatial peak pulse average intensities reported by manufacturers to FDA for pulsed Doppler devices.

is noted as a reference, and again a substantial fraction of the Doppler units exceed this level.

It should be noted that the majority of the Doppler SPTA intensities are less than 600 mW/cm², therefore it seems reasonable to question the need for systems which operate above 600 mW/cm², since the majority of manufacturers can achieve diagnostic quality Doppler information below 600 mW/cm². It is also important to note that these values of Doppler SPTA intensity are significantly higher than analogous levels for pulse-echo imaging equipment. We previously described[11] patient exposure intensities for pulse-echo equipment including 20 different echocardiographic devices. Specifically, the SPTA intensities reported for 96 pulse-echo transducers ranged from less than 10 mW/cm² to 180 mW/cm². The median pulse-echo SPTA intensity was 15 mW/cm², and the mean SPTA intensity was 38 mW/cm². Finally, one notes that some Doppler instruments emit SPTA intensities which approximate patient exposures typical of ultrasound physical therapy intended for deep tissue heating. In physical therapy practice, exposure levels range from about 100 mW/cm² to 3 W/cm,² with typical exposures in the range of 1.5 to 2 W/cm.²

Figure 11.5 shows the reported (SPPA) intensities from 26 pulsed Doppler devices marketed with 43 different transducers. These values range from less than 5 W/cm² to about 100 W/cm², with the majority having SPPA intensities less than 15 W/cm.² The median value is 12 W/cm², and the mean value is 29 W/cm². These values are comparable with those reported from pulse-echo imaging equipment.[11] The 10 W/cm² level which is discussed in the section "Safety Considerations" is noted as a reference. Many pulsed Doppler instruments exceed this level.

SAFETY CONSIDERATIONS

Doppler ultrasound is being shown to be of significant value in cardiovascular diagnosis, and to date there have been no confirmed reports of adverse effects associated with the clinical use of diagnostic ultrasound including Doppler. However, there are several recent reviews[7,12,13] of published biological effects in animals and in vitro studies using ultrasound at intensity levels representative of current diagnostic ultrasound applications. These include effects in human blood in vitro, reduced animal fetal weight, reduction in immune response, cell death, changes in cell membrane function, and free radical formation.[14] One may argue that many of the studies do not represent the exact exposure conditions of the clinical situations, or that the dosimetry is imperfect, or that the data have not been verified by other investigators. However, not all such studies can be dismissed as irrelevant, particularly because some of the studies involved the use of clinical devices.[15]

One widely referenced analysis of biological effects data was prepared by Nyborg.[16] The curve Nyborg developed was expressed in terms of spatial peak temporal average (SPTA) values and was an important step in the recognition that biological effects from diagnostic equipment may be related to spatial peak intensities. Nyborg's analysis was partially based on a thermal model estimating the intensity required for a temperature rise of 2.4°C in tissue. This value came from published data by Lele[17] indicating that a temperature of 2.4°C (above 37°C) represents a threshold for teratological effects to be produced, especially when maintained over an extended time period. Out of the analysis by Nyborg came the SPTA intensity of 100 mW/cm^2, suggesting a lower limit where thermal effects may be important.

Nyborg's analysis, along with other data, served as a basis for the American Institute of Ultrasound in Medicine's statement[18] made in August 1976, revised in October 1978 and reaffirmed in 1982, which reads, "In the low MHz frequency range there have been (as of this date) *no independently* [emphasis added] confirmed significant biological effects on mammalian tissues exposed to intensities (SPTA) below 100 mW/cm.^{2} Furthermore, for ultrasonic exposure times less than 500 seconds and greater than 1 second, such effects have not been demonstrated even at higher intensities, when the product of intensity and exposure time is less than 50 J/cm^2." The 100-mW/cm^2 level is identified in Figs. 11.3 and 11.4 which show the reported SPTA intensities from continuous-wave and pulsed Doppler equipment. Many of the patient exposures from Doppler equipment significantly exceed the 100-mW/cm^2 SPTA level.

A recent extensive review has identified a number of reported effects particularly with pulsed diagnostic exposures with temporal average intensities below 100 mW/cm^2 where one would not expect a thermal mechanism to be of predominant importance.[14] This would suggest that the mechanisms of importance for some of the effects reported in the literature using pulsed sources with low temporal average intensities may be nonthermal. There is growing recognition of the potential importance of the temporal peak intensity rather than the temporal average intensity in relation to some nonthermal mechanisms.[19-21]

Theoretical work indicating that transient cavitation under certain conditions can be produced by a single microsecond pulse suggests the need to report the exposures in terms of temporal peak intensities in addition to other pulse parameters and temporal average values.[19,20] Experiments in aqueous media detecting free radicals associated with ultrasound exposure are also suggestive that transient cavitation can be produced by pulsed ultrasound.[21] Ten W/cm^2 is the temporal maximum intensity above which the possibility of transient cavitation has been suggested.[22,23] The 10-W/cm^2 temporal maximum intensity can be approximated by the 10-W/cm^2 pulse average intensity. This level is identified as a reference in Fig. 10.5 which shows the reported SPPA intensities from pulsed Doppler equipment. Again, many of the patient exposures from pulsed Doppler equipment significantly exceeds the 10-W/cm^2 pulse average intensity at this level.

In view of these existing data, more extensive research into potential biological effects of diagnostic ultrasound is clearly necessary. Furthermore, in light of our uncertainty concerning the risk or safety of diagnostic ultrasound, it seems only prudent that an individual's exposure to ultrasound energy be kept as low and as brief as possible consistent with obtaining clinically useful diagnostic information. The physician certainly should request from the manufacturer the patient-exposure intensities for his or her Doppler instrument. The length of time the patient is exposed to ultrasound is also important and should be noted by the physician. Furthermore, ultrasound exposure for purposes of commercial demonstrations or for final quality testing by the equipment manufacturers' employees is unwarranted. These precautions are particularly important in the use of Doppler equipment with the associated high SPTA exposures. Finally, because of the increased sensitivity of fetal and neonatal tissues, it would seem particularly important to exercise prudence in the use of Doppler ultrasound in obstetrical and neonatal applications.

REFERENCES

1. The Ultrasonic Medical Market: Frost and Sullivan, New York, 1975
2. World Health Organization. Environmental Health Criteria for Ultrasound. World Health Organization, Geneva, 1982
3. National Council on Radiation Protection and Measurements. Biological Effects of Ultrasound. Report of NCRP SC-66. Bethesda, Md., NCRP Report No. 74, 1983
4. AIUM/NEMA: Safety Standard for Diagnostic Ultrasound Equipment. AIUM/NEMA Standards Publication No. UL1-1981. National Electrical Manufacturers Association, Washington, D.C., 1981
5. Department of National Health and Welfare, Ottawa, Canada: Safety Code-23. Guidelines for the Safe Use of Ultrasound. Part 1. Medical and Paramedical Applications. Minister of National Health and Welfare. 80 EHD-59, 1980
6. AIUM Manufacturers Commendation Panel: AIUM awards first commendation. Reflections 5(2):79, 1979

7. National Institute of Child Health and Human Development (NICHD) of the National Institutes of Health (NIH)/Center for Devices and Radiological Health (CHRD) of the Food and Drug Administration (FDA): Consensus conference on use of diagnostic ultrasound imaging in pregnancy, February 6-8, 1984. U.S. Government Printing Office, Washington, D.C., 1984

8. Radiation Control for Health and Safety Act of 1968, Title 42, Code of Federal Regulations, Section 263b-263n: Electronic Product Radiation Control. U.S. Government Printing Office, Washington, D.C., 1968

9. Food, Drug and Cosmetic Act, Medical Device Amendments of 1976: Code of Federal Regulations 21, Parts 800 to 1000:5. U.S. Government Printing Office, Washington, D.C., April 1983

10. Center for Devices and Radiological Health: Diagnostic Ultrasound Reporting Guide (21 CFR 1002.10). HHS Publication (FDA) 81-8145. U.S. Government Printing Office, Washington, D.C., November 1980

11. Stewart HF: Output levels from commercial diagnostic ultrasound equipment. Ultrasound Med, suppl., 2(10):39, 1983

12. Stewart HF, Moore RM: Development of health risk evaluation data for diagnostic ultrasound. J Clin Ultrasound, 12:493-500, 1984

13. Stewart HF, Stratmeyer ME: An Overview of Ultrasound: Theory, Measurement, Medical Applications, and Biological Effects. USHHS Publication (FDA) 82-8190, CDRH/AB/DBE. U.S. Government Printing Office, Washington, D.C., 1982

14. Stewart HD, Stewart HF, Moore RM, Garry J: Compilation of reported biological effects data and ultrasound exposure levels. J Clin Ultrasound, 13:167-168, 1985

15. Department of Health, Education, and Welfare, Food and Drug Administration: Diagnostic ultrasound equipment, notice of intent to propose rules and develop recommendations. Fed Register 44:9542, 1979

16. Nyborg WL: Physical mechanisms for biological effects of ultrasound. HEW Publication (FDA) 78-8062. U.S. Government Printing Office Washington, D.C., May 1978

17. Lele PP: Ultrasonic teratology in mouse and man. p. 22. In Proceedings of Second European Congress of Ultrasonics in Medicine. Excepta Medica, Amsterdam, 1975

18. American Institute of Ultrasound in Medicine: Report of the AIUM Bioeffects Committee. Reflections 4:330, 1978

19. Flynn J: Generation of transient cavities in liquids by microsecond pulses of ultrasound. J Acost Soc Am 72(6):1926, 1982

20. Carstensen EL, Flynn HG: The potential for transient cavitation in pulsed ultrasound. J Ultrasound Med, suppl., 1(7):140, 1982

21. Carmichael AJ, Mosoba MM, Riesz P, Christman CL: Detection of transient cavitation in aqueous solutions exposed to microsecond pulses of ultrasound. Proc Radiat Res Soc, 23rd annual meeting, Orlando, Florida, March 25-29, 1984

22. Carstensen EL, Berg RB, Child SZ: Pulse average versus maximum intensity. Ultrasound Med Biol 9:L451, 1983

23. Carstensen EL, Allen HG: The effects of pulsed ultrasound on the fetus. J Ultrasound Med 3:145, 1984

12 Recommendations for Terminology and Display for Doppler Echocardiography

THE DOPPLER STANDARDS AND NOMENCLATURE COMMITTEE OF THE AMERICAN SOCIETY OF ECHOCARDIOGRAPHY*

PREAMBLE

Doppler echocardiography has recently emerged as a major noninvasive technique with many applications in cardiology. To a large extent, this has been based upon a combination of clinical and engineering advances which now make possible the use of quantitative Doppler echocardiography in combination with two-dimensional imaging for measurement of volume flows, transvalve gradients, and other physiologic flow parameters which reflect cardiac function. It was the purpose of this Committee to provide a glossary of terms which could be used in standard fashion for papers and discussions related to Doppler echocardiography. As part of its task, the Committee also undertook an attempt to recommend a standard for display of Doppler information which would be useful, both for manufacturers and for clinicians. The document, therefore, includes: Section I, the Committee's recommendations for Doppler display. Section II, the glossary of Doppler terms, related to engineering and to clinical applications.

* By permission of the American Society of Echocardiography. Recommendations for Terminology and Display for Doppler Echocardiography. The Doppler Standards and Nomenclature Committee, August, 1984. Chairman: David J. Sahn, M.D. Members: Donald W. Baker; Anthony DeMaria, M.D.; Jim Gessert; Stanley J. Goldberg, M.D.; Howard Gutgesell, M.D.; Walter Henry, M.D.; Richard Popp, M.D.; Normal Silverman, M.D.; Rebecca Snider, M.D.; Geoffrey Stevenson, M.D.

SECTION I

This Committee makes the following recommendations for page print outputs of Doppler information related to studies in the cardiovascular system:

Doppler records should contain information related to the area which was interrogated and the type of interrogation performed. This could be an inserted, freeze-frame image, as a spatial locater showing the position of the sample volume and the direction of sampling, or an alphanumeric display designating the structure, the area of the cardiovascular system sampled and the echocardiographic view used, suprasternal notch, apex, etc. The display should denote the depth and the type of sampling whether single pulsed-gate, high pulse repetition frequency, multi-gate or continuous wave Doppler. In addition, to this spatial localization, this Committee suggests that the angle of incidence estimated for the Doppler interrogation be shown either by a cursor or alphanumerically with a statement included "angle corrected" or "uncorrected" to denote whether the calibrations of the Doppler record shown have or have not already been corrected for the angle of interrogation.

With regards to the Doppler content of the record, the Committee recommends that Doppler waveform should be calibrated in centimeters or in meters per second. We believed this to be preferable to kilohertz calibrations since it provides a more physiologic means for communication of Doppler information as a velocity within the circulatory system. The Doppler record should be displayed with flow towards the transducer, shown as positive in direction and upward on the record and flow away from the transducer as negative and downward, regardless of the direction of the beam or area of interrogation. As stated, Doppler records should specify the frequency of interrogation and the type of Doppler interrogation (pulsed, high PRF, or continuous). If a pulsed or high PRF record, the record should show the pulse repetition frequency being used and the Nyquist limit for that pulse repetition frequency, denoted in centimeters per second. The inclusion of this information as to spatial localization and Doppler interrogation parameters, should allow records to be passed between laboratories, and provide a complete documentation of the data obtained during a Doppler examination.

SECTION II

GLOSSARY

The following suggestions are made regarding a standardized Doppler nomenclature for use by physicians, clinicians and engineers. The nomenclature is subdivided into general Doppler terms, Doppler instrumentation and engineering parameters, Doppler display outputs, and hydrodynamic terms relevant to pulsatile blood flow within the circulatory system.

General Doppler Terminology

Doppler Echocardiography:

Analysis of intracardiac or intravascular flow by ultrasonic techniques involving the Doppler effect with or without a spatial reference by A-mode, M-mode, two-dimensional imaging, or auditory signals for the localization of the site being sampled.

Doppler Effect:

A shift in frequency and wave length caused by relative motion between transducers and scatterers, such as from motion of targets within the blood stream, when there is a component of relative motion parallel to the direction of ultrasound interrogation.

Doppler Frequency Shift:

The difference in frequencies of transmitted and received sound energy. This difference is directly proportional to the velocity of relative motion between the transducer and reflectors and the interrogation frequency. It is inversely proportional to the velocity of sound in the intervening medium.

$$\Delta F = \frac{V \times 2F_0 \times \cos\theta}{\text{velocity of sound}}$$

$$V = \frac{\Delta F \times \text{velocity of sound}}{2F_0 \times \cos\theta}$$

Where V = velocity ΔF = frequency shift

F_0 = frequency of interrogation (mHz)

θ = Angle of incidence between the direction of motion of the scatterers and the direction of interrogation

Doppler Instrumentation and Engineering Terms

Aliasing:

Ambiguous plotting of velocities which are too high to be determined with certainty due to PRF (Nyquist) sampling limitation in pulsed or range gated Doppler. For example, the very high velocity may wrap around and be displayed as negative velocity, or i.e., two different velocities may be displayed as the same velocity.

200   BASIC DOPPLER ECHOCARDIOGRAPHY

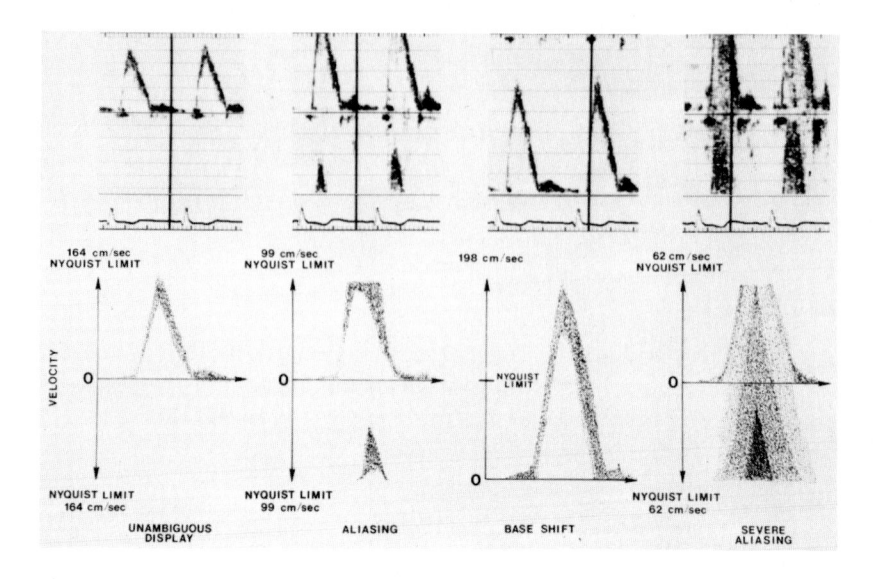

FIG. 12.1. Diagrammatic and spectral illustration of normal and aliased Doppler displays. The third panel shows a baseline shift to allow flow to be shown above the Nyquist limit, and the fourth panel, severe aliasing with more than one "wrap around."

Continuous Wave Doppler:

A wave of almost constant amplitude which persists for a large number of cycles and is used for sampling Doppler shifts regardless of distance from the transducer. There is no sampling limitation or inherent limitation on peak detected velocity, as there is for range gated Doppler. This technique can be achieved along a known line of interrogation from within a two-dimensional image. It always uses one transducer or transducer elements for sending and another or others for receiving the back-scattered ultrasound.

Doppler Interrogation Frequency:

The frequency of the transmitted acoustic energy relative to which a Doppler frequency shift is measured. This frequency is usually, but not necessarily, the nominal transducer frequency.

2D Doppler (Duplex) Scanner:

A real-time two-dimensional ultrasonic imaging device which is capable of simultaneous or sequential Doppler sampling from an area within the planar image.

Pulsed Doppler (Range Gated Doppler):

Doppler interrogation using a pulsed mode of transmission wherein establishment of a temporal gate allows determination of Doppler shift from within a specific axial area or areas at a known distance from the transducer. This area is known as the sample volume and it has axial and lateral dimensions which should be defined.

High PRF Doppler:

A method of achieving high sampling rates: multiple pulses, and their return signals from within the heart are present at any one point in time and Doppler shifts along the beam are summed along sample volume depths which are multiples of the initial sample volume depth to give a single output.

Nyquist Frequency:

One-half the pulse repetition frequency in pulsed/range gated Doppler. Frequency shifts exceeding this limit cannot be unambiguously displayed unless other information such as the time history of a narrow band flow spectrum is available.

Multigate Doppler:

A pulsed/range gated Doppler interrogation approach in which multiple range gates sample Doppler shift information from multiple, closely spaced depths along the untrasound beam. As opposed to high PRF Doppler, multigate Doppler is implemented to sample and display separately the information from the individual gates.

Power Output in Doppler Mode:

Manufacturers should be prepared to make available to the user, information relevant to the power output for their instrumentation in its various modes of Doppler interrogation. Power output in Doppler mode, as defined in the AIUM NEMA Standards* may be defined as a spatial peak intensity averaged over time.

Pulse Repetition Frequency:

The rate at which pulses of acoustic energy are transmitted in a pulsed or range gated Doppler system. This is usually a function of the depth of the

---

* American Institute of Ultrasound in Medicine and National Electrical Manufacturers Association Safety Standard for Diagnostic Ultrasound Equipment, Draft V, January 27, 1981. Copies available from the NEMA Executive Office, 2101 L Street NW, Washington, DC 20037, and from the AIUM Executive Office, 4405 East-West Highway, Suite 504, Bethesda, MD 20814.

202 BASIC DOPPLER ECHOCARDIOGRAPHY

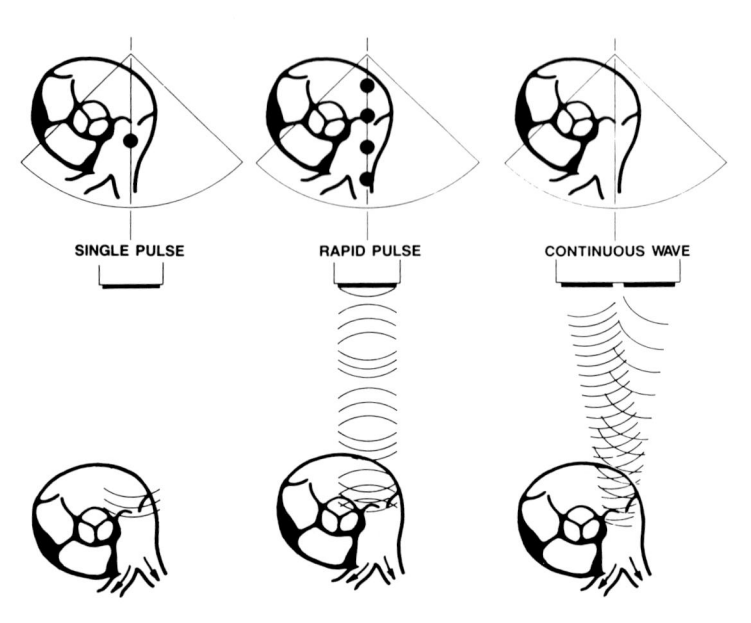

FIG. 12.2. (A) Modes of Doppler interrogation. In single pulsed Doppler, a single range, or time gate, is established distal to the pulmonary valve, as shown here, and ultrasound information from that gate shown as the wavelets in the diagram below is processed for the Doppler shift. On the right hand panel for continuous Doppler, one transducer is sending and the other is receiving ultrasound from all along the line of site. Velocities from along the complete line of the right ventricular outflow tract area, therefore, summed into the resultant display. In the center panel, a rapid pulse, or high pulse repetition frequency Doppler, has been implemented. Individual sample volumes are shown with Doppler information being processed from gates with depths which are multiples of the depth of the first gate. This is illustrated by the position of four sample volumes in the upper panel and by the fact that ultrasound information is coming and going at the same time from within the tissue. The multiple sampling depths in the lower panel are also illustrated by the individual wavelet packets. Information may be coming back to the transducer from depths of either two, three, or four times the initial sample volume depth, returning from previous pulse bursts and having traveled and arrived back at the transducer at the same instant in time as the information from the first range gate from the pulse just sent. This allows implementation of rapid pulse repetition frequencies, since the device is not listening for the required period of time necessary to receive information from the fourth gate, but receives it back within the specified time gate period while functioning at four times the pulse repetition frequency (Figure continues).

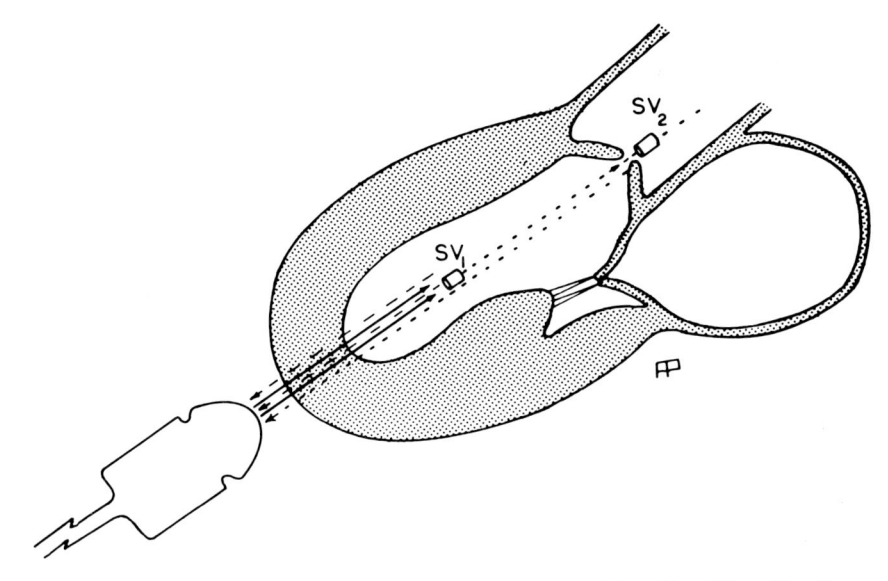

FIG. 12.2 (Continued). (B) This figure, kindly supplied by Dr. Allen Pearlman and reproduced from "Assessment of Valvular Heart Disease by Doppler Echocardiography" in Clinical Cardiology 6:573–587, 1983 by permission, clarifies the concept of multiple sample volumes in high pulsed repetition rate Doppler. Despite placement of a sample volume at position shown as SV$_1$, half the distance to the aorta in this apex view, the diagram shows how information can be derived about flow in sample volume 2, since sound energy from the previous pulse will have gone out to sample volume 2 and returned to the transducer at the same time as sound energy will be returning from sample volume 1 in the reception phase from the most recent pulse. Hence, information can be obtained from sample volume 2 by setting up the scanner with a range gate at sample volume 1, achieving the desired aortic flow while doubling the pulse repetition frequency. (Reprinted by permission of Clinical Cardiology Publishing Company, Inc.)

(first) sample volume and determines peak velocity limit which can be unambiguously detected by range gated or pulsed Doppler systems.

Sampling Angle:

The angle of incidence (see Doppler frequency shift) between the direction of flow and the direction of sampling within the imaged plane. This angle may be estimated during the Doppler examination.

Sample Volume:

The region in space from which Doppler data is collected for analysis in pulsed/range gated Doppler systems. The size of the sample volume is axially determined by the length of the transmitted acoustic pulse and the length of the range gate. The width is determined by the lateral width of the ultrasound beam.

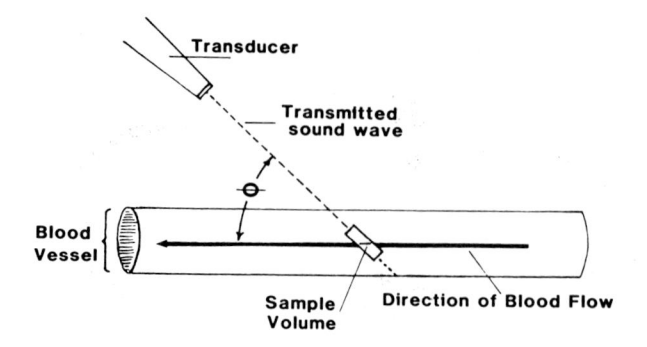

FIG. 12.3. Relationship of sampling direction to the direction of flow is shown and the designation of the angle θ illustrated in this figure.

Wall (Thump) Filter:

A filter in a Doppler system which rejects echo information from low velocity reflectors such as stationary or slow moving tissue. This filtering is needed to keep high amplitude tissue echos from saturating the Doppler receiver, masking very low amplitude echoes from flowing blood.

Section III

Doppler Signal Processing and Displays

Chirp Z Transform:

An algorithm which may be used to generate the discrete Fourier transform for spectral analysis. It is commonly used to implement spectrum analysis utilizing primarily analog electronics.

Doppler Image (D)-Mode Flow Map (Color Flow Map) (Flow Image):

A display method in which only areas containing moving targets are displayed. It is a Doppler imaging technique in which the flow information can be shown as an overlay on the image to denote areas with flow. A spatial plot of Doppler flow may be superimposed upon the two-dimensional image with the direction and spectral content of flow shown either by color coding or gray scale overlay and the area of flow denoted by specific overlay on the image itself.

At an early stage in this technology, the Committee feels strongly that color flow map color schemes should, in fact, be standardized. Historically, the first published color flow mapping by Brandestini used orange to yellow colors as flow towards the transducer and blue as flow away from the transducer. With this historical perspective, the Committee believes this general color scheme is visually and informationally acceptable and that spectral broadening and disturbances can be shown as variance and mixtures of these colors with an additional hue, probably green.

Discrete Fourier Transform:

Sampled data representation of the Fourier transform which converts a waveform from the time to the frequency domain.

Fast Fourier Transform FFT:

An algorithm for efficient rapid computation of the discrete Fourier transform. The FFT is commonly used to implement spectral analysis.

Modal Velocity (Frequency Mode):

The mode in the frequency analysis of a signal is the frequency component which contains the most energy. In display of the Doppler frequency spectrum, the mode corresponds to the brightest (or darkest) display points of the individual spectra and represents the velocity component which is most commonly encountered among the various moving reflectors.

M-Mode Velocity (MQ) Display:

Doppler shift information along with the M-mode echocardiogram, usually derived along the line of sampling and displayed as a function of time, usually with an accompanying EKG.

Maximal Velocity:

The highest velocity found with significant amplitude within the sampled area usually for use in Bernouli type gradient estimations.

Mean Spectral Velocity of Blood Flow:

A mathematical mean of the spectral shifts in velocity within a given sample volume.

Mean Velocity/Time:

(Mean temporal velocity) (Mean velocity as a function of time as in mean systolic velocity, mean diastolic velocity, or mean velocity for the cardiac cycle). Velocity time integral divided by the time period over which the integral was determined.

Spectral Analysis:

A method of analyzing waveforms derived from Doppler shift information by separating the waveform into its frequency velocity components.
   Multiple frequency components may be derived from a single waveform. A common technique for spectral analysis is the fast Fourier transform.

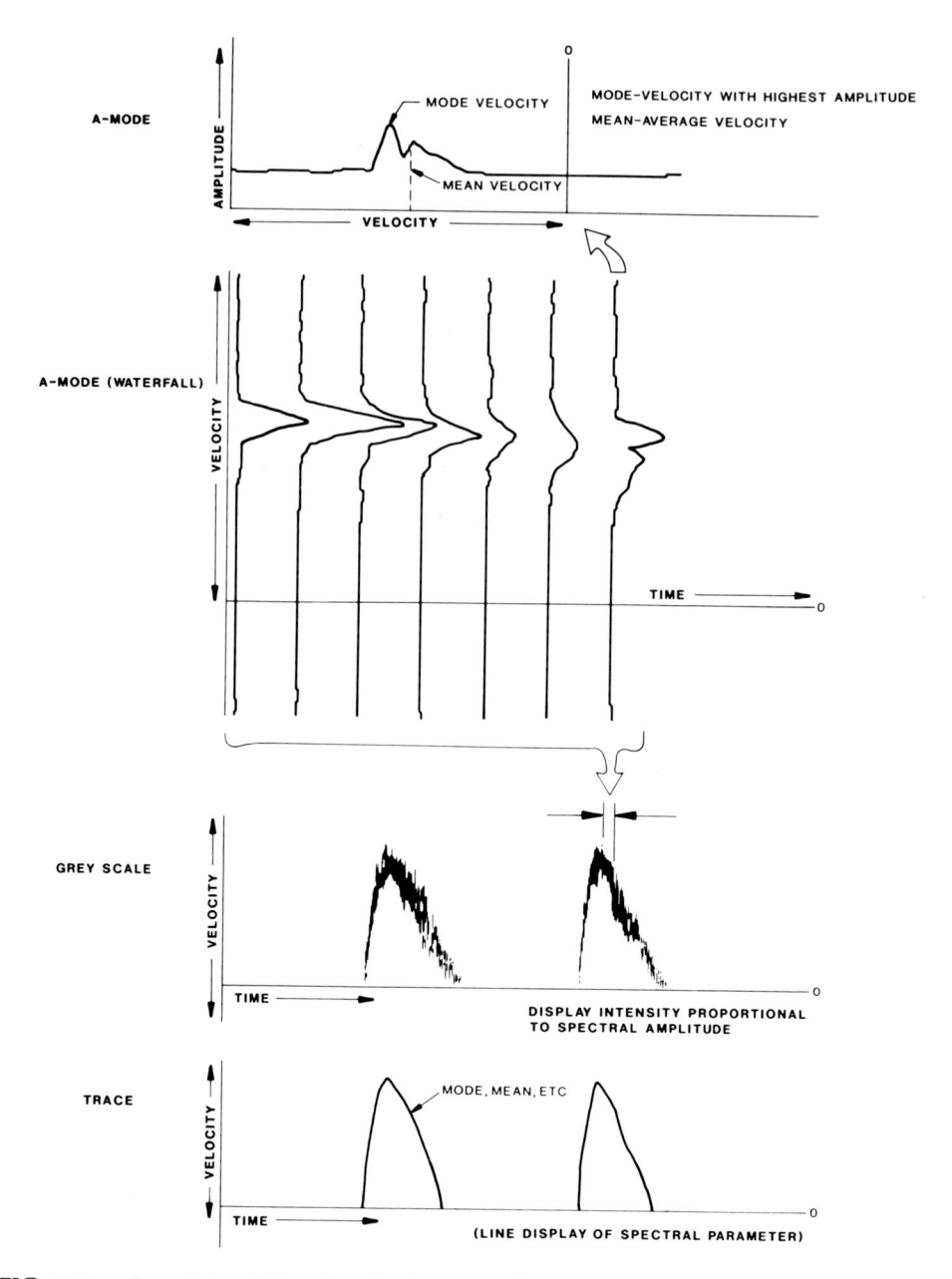

FIG. 12.4. A variety of Doppler displays are illustrated in this figure. At the top an amplitude velocity mode shows the cross section of the spectrum at any one point in time and designates the fact that the most frequently found velocity is the "modal velocity" as opposed to the arithmetic mean velocity. The A-mode waterfall display shows individual amplitude versus velocity cross sections of the spectrum at a variety of instants in time. The third display shown is the gray scale spectrum, with the A-mode waterfall shown above, having been selected from it. Derived arithmetical estimates of the gray scale spectral velocity versus time display, as illustrated at the bottom, are the mode, mean, etc. which may be calculated and shown in addition to the spectral display.

LAMINAR FLOW

DISTURBED FLOW

FIG. 12.5. Laminar flow with organized distribution of velocities across the lumen and relatively uniform direction and velocities of scatters is shown in the upper panel, compared to disturbed flow downstream from the jet where laminar flow at high velocity in the jet breaks up into disturbed or disorganized flow.

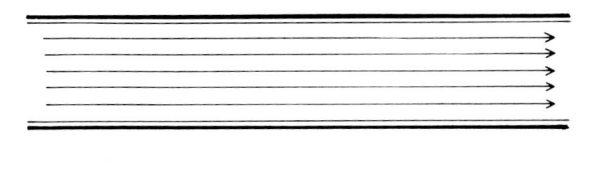

Spectral Width:

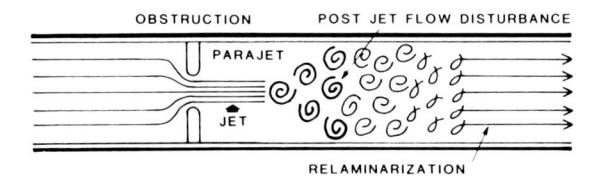

The spectral width can be defined by a variety of statistical terms including: the standard deviation, full width to half maximal amplitude, or 6dB falloff from the modal velocity within the spectrum.

Velocity (Q)-Mode:

A display of Doppler velocities as a function of time (or waveform display), usually with an accompanying EKG.

Velocity Time (Flow Velocity) Integral:

Calculated area under the Doppler curve over a specified period of time.

Section IV

Hydrodynamic Terms

Bernoulli Equation:

Relationship between velocity change across an obstruction and the pressure gradient. Neglecting viscous and early phasic accelerational factors, it is commonly *simplified* to: gradient = 4 × maximal velocity.

Disturbed Flow:

A pattern of flow with a disorganized velocity distribution. It is characterized by marked differences in direction and speed of blood cells within a vessel. The term turbulence can be mathematically defined but has been generally used interchangeably with disturbed flow.

Jet:

A very high (unphysiologic) velocity area downstream from an obstruction where laminar flow proceeds at high velocity.

Laminar Flow:

Flow in which most blood cells are moving with a general uniformity of direction and velocity, and in which there is an organized distribution of velocities across the flow area.

Series Effect:

Extension or propagation of turbulent flow within the circulatory system downstream from an abnormal flow area.

Spatial Velocity Profile:

Plot of velocity distribution across a vessel diameter which may be described as irregular, parabolic or flat, "flat" suggesting that approximately 80–90% of the flow cross-section of the vessel has the same velocity.

Vortex Shed Distance:

The distance distal to a jet orifice after which laminar flow becomes disturbed.

Index

Page numbers followed by *f* represent figures; numbers followed by *t* represent tables.

Acoustic window, beam angle and, 63
Aliasing, 199, 200f
 aortic regurgitation and, 96, 97f
 baseline control and, 57
 blood flow velocity and, 30–34, 31f, 33f
 color flow mapping and, 40–41
 control of, 37t, 38f
 high PRF Doppler and, 39f
 mitral valve regurgitation and, 105f, 106
 Nyquist limit and, 34, 37f
 pulsed wave and, 126
 regurgitant jet and, 93f
American Society of Echocardiography
 Doppler Standards and Nomenclature Committee of
  Doppler signal processing and displays, 204–207
  glossary, 198–204
  hydrodynamic terms, 207–208
  preamble, 197
  section I, 198
  section II, 198–204
  section III, 204–207
  section IV, 207–208
Amplitude, echocardiography and, 19–20
Angiography
 mitral regurgitation and, 111
 valvular regurgitation and, 116
 vs. echocardiography, 93, 95f
Aorta
 ascending, suprasternal window and, 80f, 81
 blood flow in, 8f, 9
  parasternal window and, 84–85
  suprasternal window and, 83
 coarctation of
  continuous wave and, 80f, 82
  in children, 166–167, 168f
 echocardiography of, 17
 insufficiency of
  aliasing and, 32, 33f
  echocardiography of, 42–45, 43f–45f
 mitral regurgitation and, 119–121
 retrograde flow in, 177–178
 stenosis of
  audio output and, 64, 65f
  Bernoulli equation and, 41, 42f
 mitral regurgitation of, 110f, 111
 ultrasound angle and, 21f, 22f, 23
 wall filter and, 55, 56f
 ventricular septal defects and, 162
Aortic root
 cardiac output and, 150–151
 stroke volume and, 150
Aortic valve
 apical window and, 67f, 68–71, 70f
 blood flow and, 123, 124f
 insufficiency, continuous wave and, 73, 75f, 76
 regurgitation of, 91, 92f, 96–103, 97, 100t, 101, 104f
  Bernoulli equation and, 137
  in children, 164
  mitral valve and, 106–107, 107f
  pulsed wave and, 116–117, 117f
  turbulent flow and, 117, 118f, 119
  vs. mitral regurgitation, 107–108, 108t
 stenosis of
  cardiac catheterization and, 133–137, 135f, 136f
  echocardiography and, 128–137, 129, 138f
  in children, 166
  parasternal window and, 85, 86f
  peak gradient and, 133f, 135f
  severity of, 127f
  suprasternal window and, 82f, 83
  valve area calculation and, 167, 170
  vs. mitral insufficiency, 76f, 78
 ventricular echocardiography and, 147, 148
Apex, mitral valve regurgitation and, 104
Apical window
 aortic regurgitation and, 98, 99f, 100f, 103
 aortic stenosis and, 128, 129f, 130f
 cardiac output and, 150
 mitral regurgitation vs. aortic stenosis, 131, 132f
 mitral stenosis and, 138
 regurgitation mapping and, 119
 tricuspid regurgitation and, 111f
 valve disease and, 66f, 67f, 68–81, 69f, 70f, 72f, 73t, 77f
 ventricular echocardiography and, 147, 148

209

Arrhythmia
  fetal, 180–181, 182–183f
  tricuspid regurgitation and, 112, 113f
Astronomy, Doppler effect and, 3–4
Atrioventricular pressure, mitral stenosis and, 140–143, 142f
Atrioventricular valve
  fetal, 174, 175f, 177
  fetal arrhythmia and, 181, 182f
  regurgitation of
    in fetus, 177, 179f
    nonimmune hydrops fetalis and, 178, 180
Atrium
  Bernoulli equation and, 112
  fetal, 177
    isomerism of, 177, 180f
  in children, 162, 163f
  isomerism of, 177, 180f
  pressure of, 112
  septal defects of, 162, 163f
    blood flow measurements in, 164, 165f
    in children, 163f, 182
Audio
  aortic stenosis and, 125
  Doppler display and, 14f, 15–17, 19–20
  ventricular echocardiography and, 148
Audio display, of blood flow, 64, 65f
Auscultation, aortic regurgitation and, 98

Baseline, aliasing control and, 37t, 38f
Baseline control, 55, 57f
Beam
  angle of
    echocardiography and, 20–21, 21f, 22f, 23, 128
    fetal blood flow and, 174
    pulsed, 61f, 62
    tricuspid regurgitation and, 112, 114f
  continuous, 26, 28f
  orientation of, blood flow and, 63, 64f
  pulsed angle of, correction of, 61f, 62
  sample volume and, 30, 31f
  vs. pulsed wave echocardiography, 26, 28f
Bernoulli equation, 41f, 42f, 207
  aortic peak gradient and, 133
  blood flow velocity and, 127f, 136f, 137
  in children, 165
  mitral stenosis and, 138, 140
  regurgitant jet and, 93f
  valvular stenosis and, 165
  ventricle pressure and, 112
  ventricular end-diastolic pressure and, 103, 104f
Blood flow
  abnormalities of, 25
  aortic stenosis and, 127f
  apical window and, 78f, 80
  audio output and, 64, 65f
  beam angle and, 63, 64f
  direction of, 12, 13f, 14f, 15
  echocardiography and, 4–5
  ejection rate of, 151–153, 152f, 154f
  fetal
    arrhythmia and, 181, 183f
    quantitative analysis of, 173–174
  in children, 161–162
    drug management and, 164
    valvular regurgitation and, 165f, 614
  intrauterine growth retardation and, 181, 184f
  left sided, 78f, 80
  mean spectral velocity of, 205
  mitral insufficiency and, 73, 74f, 76
    vs. aortic stenosis, 76f, 78
  mitral stenosis and, 127
  mitral valve and, 79f, 81
  normal values of, 71, 73t
  parasternal window and, 84f, 86f, 87f, 88f
  patterns of, 7–9, 8f
  placental, intrauterine growth retardation and, 181, 184f
  pressure gradient and, 124f, 127f
  pulmonic valve and, 86–88, 87f, 88f
  qualitative analysis of, 174–179, 175–180f
  stenosis and, 123–126, 124–126f
  suprasternal window and, 80f, 81f, 82f
  transducer and, 13f, 14f, 16–17
  tricuspid valve and, 86–88, 87f
  ultrasound angle and, 25
  velocity of
    continuous wave echocardiography and, 26–27, 27f
    determination of, 127f
    echocardiography and, 128, 130–132f, 131
    mitral regurgitation and, 106
    pulsed wave echocardiography and, 30, 32
    ultrasound angle and, 20–21, 21f, 22f, 23
    valvular regurgitation and, 91, 93f
    ventricular echocardiography and, 150
  ventricular hypertrophy and, 67f, 68
  ventricular septal defect and, 85, 86f
Blood pressure, valvular regurgitation and, 91, 93–94f

Cardiac catheterization
  atrioventricular pressure and, 141
  cardiac output and, 151
  ejection rate and, 153
  mitral stenosis and, 140, 141f
  pressure gradient and, 133
    aortic stenosis and, 133–137, 134–136f
  valve area calculation and, 167, 170
  vs. echocardiography, 140, 141f
Cardiac cycle, aortic regurgitation and, 99–100, 101f
Cardiac output
  determination of, 170
  echocardiography and, 150–151
    accuracy of, 151
  ventricular echocardiography and, 149–151, 150f

INDEX

Cardiomyopathy, aortic regurgitation and, 106–107, 107f
Cavitation, ultrasound and, 194
Children
　echocardiography in, 161–162
　flow measurement in, 161–162
　valvular stenosis in, 165–170, 166f, 168–169f
　ventricular septal defects in, 162
Chirp Z transform, 17, 204
Chordae tendinae, mitral valve regurgitation and, 106
Cineangiography, vs. echocardiography, 93, 95f
Coarctation of aorta
　continuous wave and, 80f, 82
　in children, 166–167, 168f
Color flow mapping, 40–41
Congenital heart disease, 159
Continuous wave
　aortic regurgitation and, 98, 99f, 100f
　aortic stenosis and, 125f, 131, 133
　aortic window and, 103
　apical window and, 71, 72f, 73, 74f, 75f
　combined echo-Doppler and, 66, 68
　exposure levels, 189, 190–191f
　mitral regurgitation and, 109f
　mitral stenosis and, 138, 139f, 140f
　parasternal window and, 84–85, 86f, 88f
　pulmonic stenosis and, 125, 126f
　regurgitant jet and, 93, 94f
　regurgitation and, 103
　transducer, 47, 49f
　tricuspid regurgitation and, 111f
　ventricular echocardiography and, 147
　vs. pulsed wave echocardiography, 26–30, 31f, 32t
Continuous wave Doppler, 200
Continuous window, 80f, 81–82
Contrast, display control of, 51–54, 53f, 54f
Coronary artery disease, ejection rate and, 153, 154f
Crosstalk, 51
Cursor position, pulsed wave and, 58, 59f

Diastole
　aortic, vs. mitral regurgitation, 98–99, 100f, 101f
　atrioventricular pressure and, 142f, 143
　fetal, 177, 178f
　intrauterine growth retardation and, 181, 184f
　mitral stenosis and, 138, 139f
　ventricular function and, 155–156
Discrete Fourier transform, 205
Disturbed flow, 207
2D Doppler (Duplex) scanner, 200
Doppler display, illustrations of, 206f
Doppler echocardiography
　general terminology, 199
　in practice, 2
Doppler effect, 199
　description of, 2–4, 3f

　medical applications of, 4–5
　radar and, 11
　sound waves and, 4
Doppler equation, velocity and, 12, 14f, 15
Doppler frequency shift, 199
Doppler gain, 48f, 51, 52f
Doppler gate, pulsed sample depth and, 58–60, 60f
Doppler hypothesis, 2, 3f
Doppler interrogation, modes of, 202f, 203f
Doppler interrogation frequency, 200
Doppler signal, obtaining of, 47–51, 48, 50f
Doppler Standards and Nomenclature Committee
　Doppler signal processing and displays, 204–207
　glossary, 198–204
　hydrodynamic terms, 207–208
　preamble, 197
　section I, 198
　section II, 198–204
　section III, 204–207
　section IV, 207–208
Ductus arteriosus
　in fetus, 176f, 177
　patent, 164

Ebstein's malformation, 177, 179f
Echocardiography
　imaging and, 64–66, 68
　mitral stenosis and, 140, 141f
　two-dimensional, 140, 141f
　ultrasound exposure
　　Doppler levels of, 188–192, 190–191f
　　guidelines for, 187–188
　　safety considerations of, 189, 190f
　vs. angiography, 93, 95f
　vs. cardiac catheterization, 133–137, 134, 136f
Echocardiography examination, 88, 89
Echo-Doppler, combined, 64–66, 68
Ejection rate
　blood flow and, 151–153, 153–154f
　systolic, 153
　timing of, 153
　ventricular echocardiography and, 151–153, 153f, 154f
Electromagnetic wave, Doppler effect and, 2f
Endocarditis, mitral valve regurgitation and, 106f
Erythrocyte
　Doppler effect and, 11f, 12f
　gray scale and, 53f, 54
Extrasystole, fetal, 181, 182–183f

Fast Fourier transform (FFT), 16f, 17, 205
　in spectral analysis, 205
Fetal blood flow
　qualitative analysis of, 174–179, 175–180f
　quantitative analysis of, 173–174

FFT. *See* Fast Fourier transform.
Fick principle, valvular regurgitation and, 116
Flow velocity integral, 207
Foramen ovale, 177
  closure of, 178
Fourier transform, echocardiography and, 16f, 17
Frequency mode, 205
Frequency shift, 10–16

Gorlin equation, valve area calculation and, 167, 170
Gorlin formula, mitral stenosis and, 140–141
Gray scale, 51–54, 53, 54f

Heart
  congenital disease of, 159
  ultrasound and, 189
Heart murmur, 159–161, 160f
Heart rate
  mitral stenosis and, 140
  suprasternal window and, 83f
  ventricular echocardiography and, 149, 150f
High PRF Doppler, 201
Hydrops fetalis, nonimmune, 178, 180

Imaging
  echocardiography and, 25–26, 64–66, 68
  pulsed wave echocardiography and, 29f, 30f
Intermediate window, 88
Intrauterine growth retardation, 181, 184f
Isomerism, atrial, 177, 180f

Jet, 208
Joystick, 58

Laminar flow, 7, 8f, 207f, 208
  blood and, 123, 124f
  fetal echocardiography and, 177
  gray scale and, 53f, 54
  mitral stenosis and, 138, 139f
  sound of, 15
  transducer and, 16f, 17
Leaflet, aortic valve stenosis and, 123

Mapping
  aortic regurgitation and, 117, 118f
  color flow, 40–41
  mitral regurgitation and, 119f
  tricuspid regurgitation and, 119, 120f
  valvular regurgitation and, 116
Maximal velocity, 205
Mean spectral velocity of blood flow, 205
Mean temporal velocity, 205
Mean velocity, time, 205
Mirroring, 51

Mitral valve
  aortic regurgitation and, 98f
  apical window and, 66f, 68, 70f, 71, 72f
  audio output and, 64
  blood flow and, 79f, 81
  closure of, 77f, 78
  insufficiency of
    continuous wave and, 73–76, 74f
    vs. aortic stenosis, 76f, 78
  parasternal window and, 85, 86f
  regurgitation of, 91, 92f, 104, 110f
    mapping of, 119f
    pulsed wave and, 116–117, 117f
    vs. aortic regurgitation, 98–99, 100–101f
    vs. aortic stenosis, 131, 132f
  stenosis of, 20f
    continuous wave and, 73, 75f, 76
    echocardiography and, 138–144, 139, 142f
    severity of, 127
  ventricular diastole and, 155–156
  ventricular septal defects and, 162
M-mode velocity (MQ) display, 205
Modal velocity, 205
Multigate Doppler, 201
Murmur, cardiac, 159–161, 160f

Nyquist frequency, 201
Nyquist limit
  aliasing and, 34–38f, 37t
  blood flow velocity and, 128
  high PRF Doppler and, 39f, 40
  pulsed sample depth and, 58, 60f

Parasternal window
  aortic regurgitation and, 103
  aortic stenosis and, 128
  blood flow and, 84–88, 86f, 87f, 88f
  pulmonic regurgitation and, 113, 115f
  pulmonic stenosis and, 125, 126f
  pulsed wave and, 85–86, 87f
Patent ductus arteriosus, 164
Patient ultrasound exposure
  Doppler exposure levels in, 188–192, 190–192f
  guidelines for, 187–188
  safety considerations in, 193–194
Peak gradient
  aortic stenosis and, 133f, 135
  estimation of, 137
Peak velocity
  atrioventricular pressure and, 142f, 143
  ejection rate and, 152–153
Pitch, frequency and, 10–11
Placental blood flow, intrauterine growth retardation and, 181, 184f
Power output in Doppler mode, 201
Pressure gradient
  aortic coarctation and, 166–167, 168f
  aortic stenosis and, 133f

blood flow and, 124f, 127f
calculation of, 133f
mitral stenosis and, 138, 140f
ventricular septal defects and, 167
PRF. *See* Pulse repetition frequency.
Printout, echocardiography, 42, 44f, 45f
Pulmonary artery, 125, 126f
  atrial isomerism and, 177, 180f
  echocardiography and, 125, 126f
  fetal, 174, 175f
  in children, 165–166, 166f
  pulsed wave and, 87f
  stenosis of, 165–166, 166f
  ventricular septal defects and, 162, 167
Pulmonary valve
  insufficiency of, 88f
  parasternal window and, 86–88, 87f, 88f
  regurgitation of, 113, 115t
  stenosis of, 125, 126f, 167, 170
  valve area calculation and, 167, 170
Pulse
  systolic, 149f
  ventricular echocardiography and, 149f
Pulse repetition frequency (PRF), 201–203
  Nyquist limit and, 34
Pulsed angle, correction of, 61f, 62
Pulsed Doppler, 201
Pulsed sample, depth of, 58–60, 59f, 60f, 62
Pulsed valve, 87
Pulsed wave
  aliasing and, 30–34, 31f, 33f, 126
  aortic regurgitation and, 100, 102f
  apical window and, 71
  exposure levels, 189, 190f
  mitral stenosis and, 138
  parasternal window and, 85–86, 87f
  regurgitant jet and, 93, 94f
  transducer, 48, 49f, 189–190, 191f
  ultrasound exposure and, 189–190, 191f
  valvular regurgitation and, 116–117, 117f
  ventricular echocardiography and, 147
  vs. continuous wave echocardiography, 26–30, 32t

Q wave, ventricular echocardiography and, 149
QP/QS ratio, pediatric echocardiography and, 161

Radar, Doppler effect and, 4, 11
Range gated Doppler, 201
Range gating, 28–29
Records
  freeze-frame image, 198
  standards for, 198
Regurgitant jet
  aortic regurgitation and, 101, 103f
  aortic valve and, 96, 97f
  characteristics of, 91–93, 92, 94f

mitral regurgitation and, 110f, 111
size of, 101, 103f
Regurgitation
  aortic, Bernoulli equation and, 137
  atrioventricular, 177, 179f
  in children, 164, 165f
  in fetus, 177, 179f
  valvular, 164, 165f
Respiratory cycle, aortic regurgitation and, 100, 102

Sample volume, 203
  mitral regurgitation and, 108, 109f
  pulmonic stenosis and, 125, 126f
Sampling angle, 203
Scale factor, 55, 56f
Series effect, 208
Shunting, pediatric, 161
Sonography, quality control of, 88, 89
Sonar, Doppler effect and, 4
Sound, frequency analyzers of, 16
Spatial velocity profile, 208
Spectral analysis, 205
Spectral broadening, 54
Spectral velocity
  baseline control and, 55, 57f
  control of, 37t, 38f, 39
  Nyquist limit and, 36, 37f
  scale factor and, 55, 56f
Spectral width, 207
SPPA intensity, 189
SPTA intensity, 189
Stenosis
  aortic
    audio output and, 64, 65f
    Bernoulli equation and, 41, 42f
    parasternal window and, 85, 86f
    suprasternal window and, 82f, 83
    ultrasound angle and, 21f, 22f, 23
  aortic valve, 166
    cardiac catheterization and, 133–137, 135f, 136f
    echocardiography and, 128–137, 129–138f
    wall filter and, 55, 56f
  blood flow and, 9, 123–126, 124–126f
  mitral valve, 20f
    echocardiography and, 138–144, 139, 142f
  pulmonary artery, 165–166, 166f
  severity of, 127f
  tricuspid valve, 143f, 144
  valvular, 9
Stroke volume, ventricular echocardiography and, 149–150, 150f
Subcostal window, 88
Suprasternal window
  aortic coarctation and, 167
  aortic stenosis and, 128, 129f, 166
  ascending aorta and, 80f, 81
  blood flow and, 81–84, 82f
  cardiac output and, 150

Suprasternal window (*Continued*)
  pulmonary stenosis and, 166
  ventricular echocardiography and, 147, 148f
Systole
  aortic root and, 150–151
  aortic stenosis and, 124f, 137f
  blood flow and, 150
  ejection timing of, 153
  valvular blood flow and, 123, 124f
  ventricular echocardiography and, 149f
Systolic pulse, ventricular echocardiography and, 149f

Tachycardia, fetal, 181, 183f
Teratogenicity, of ultrasound, 193
Terminology
  engineering, 199–204, 200f, 202f, 203f
  general, 199
  hydrodynamic, 207–208
  instrumentation, 199–204, 200f, 202f, 203f
  signal processing and display, 204–207, 206f, 207f
Thump filter, 204
Time-sharing, combined echo-Doppler and, 66
Tissue, speed of sound in, 10
Transcoarctation pressure, 167, 168f
Transducer
  aliasing control and, 37t, 38f, 39
  blood flow and, 12, 13f, 14f
  combined echo-Doppler and, 66
  sample volume and, 81
  suprasternal window and, 81–82, 83
  types of, 189–190, 191f
  ultrasound exposure and, 189–190, 191f
Transducer wave, pulsed, vs. continuous wave, 47–48, 49f
Tricuspid valve, 86–88, 87f
  apical window and, 66f, 68, 69f, 71, 72f
  fetal, 177, 179f
  regurgitation of, 111f, 113f, 114f
    in children, 164
    mapping of, 119, 120f
    vs. mitral regurgitation, 109
  stenosis of, 143f, 144
Turbulent flow, 7–9, 8f
  aortic regurgitation and, 117f
  aortic stenosis and, 124f, 125
  echocardiography of, 124–125, 125f
  gray scale and, 53f, 54
  mitral valve regurgitation and, 105f, 106
  pulmonic stenosis and, 125, 126f
  sound of, 15
  transducer and, 16f, 17
  valvular regurgitation and, 91

Ultrasound
  Doppler vs. standard, 9–12, 12f
  Doppler effect and, 4
  Doppler exposure levels of, 188–192, 190–192f
  Doppler gain and, 51
  exposure guidelines for, 187–188
  safety considerations, 193–194
Umbilical artery, blood flow in, 173–174
Umbilical vein, blood flow in, 173–174

Valve
  evaluation of
    apical window and, 66f, 67f, 68–81, 69f, 70f, 72f, 73t, 74, 79f
    beam angle and, 63
    regurgitant jet and, 91–93, 92, 94f
  regurgitation of
    in children, 164, 165f
    quantitation of, 116–121, 117, 120f
    severity of, 119–120
  stenosis of
    blood flow and, 9
    severity of, 127f
    valve area calculation and, 167, 170
Valve slap, 109f
Velocity
  Doppler equation and, 12, 14f, 15
  spectrum analysis of, 17, 19f
  spectrum analyzers of, 16
  ultrasound angle and, 20–21, 21f, 22f, 23
Velocity (Q) mode, 207
Velocity time integral, 207
Vena cava, fetal, 174, 175f
Ventricle
  blood flow in, 67f, 68, 79f, 80–81
  cardiac output and, 149–151, 150f
  defects of, 85, 86f
  echocardiography of, 147, 148f, 149
  ejection rate, 151–153, 153f, 154f
  filling of, 174, 175f, 177
  functional assessment of, 153, 155f
  hypertrophy of, 67f, 68
  in children, 162, 167
  in fetus, 174, 175f, 177
  left, 79f, 80–81
  parasternal window and, 85, 86f
  pressure of
    aortic regurgitation and, 103, 104f
    tricuspid regurgitation and, 112
  septal defects of, 162, 167
  systole and, 149f
Ventricular echocardiography, 151–153, 153f, 154f
Ventricular end-diastolic pressure, Bernoulli equation and, 103, 104f
Video display, echocardiography and, 42, 43f, 45f
Vortex shed distance, 208

Wall filter, 55, 56f, 204
Wave, pitch, vs. frequency of, 10f

INDEX **215**

Window
  apical
    aortic regurgitation and, 98, 99f, 100f, 103
    aortic stenosis and, 128, 129f, 130f
    aortic valve and, 67f, 68–71, 70f
    cardiac output and, 150
    continuous wave and, 71–73, 72f, 74–75f
    left-sided blood flow and, 78f, 80
    mitral regurgitation and, 131, 132f
    mitral stenosis and, 138
    regurgitation mapping and, 119
    tricuspid regurgitation and, 11f
    valve disease and, 66–67f, 68–81, 69–70f, 73t, 77f
    valve evaluation and, 66–67f, 68–81
    ventricular echocardiography and, 147, 148
  continuous, 80f, 81–82
  parasternal
    aortic blood flow and, 84–85
    aortic regurgitation and, 103
    aortic stenosis and, 128
    blood flow and, 84–88, 86f, 87f, 88f
    pulmonic regurgitation and, 113, 115f
    pulmonic stenosis and, 125, 126f
    pulsed wave and, 85–86, 87f
  suprasternal
    aortic coarctation and, 167
    aortic stenosis and, 82f, 83, 128, 129f, 166
    ascending aorta and, 80f, 81
    blood flow and, 81–84, 82f
    cardiac output and, 150
    heart rate and, 83f
    pulmonary stenosis and, 166
    ventricular echocardiography and, 147, 148f